Pulmonary Hypertension

Editor

RICHARD A. KRASUSKI

CARDIOLOGY CLINICS

www.cardiology.theclinics.com

February 2022 • Volume 40 • Number 1

ELSEVIER

1600 John F. Kennedy Boulevard • Suite 1800 • Philadelphia, Pennsylvania, 19103-2899

http://www.theclinics.com

CARDIOLOGY CLINICS Volume 40, Number 1
February 2022 ISSN 0733-8651, ISBN-13: 978-0-323-84948-7

Editor: Joanna Collett
Developmental Editor: Karen Justine Solomon

Cardiology Clinics (ISSN 0733-8651) is published quarterly by Elsevier Inc., 360 Park Avenue South, New York, NY 10010-1710. Months of issue are February, May, August, and November. Business and Editorial Offices: 1600 John F. Kennedy Blvd., Ste. 1800, Philadelphia, PA 19103-2899. Customer Service Office: 3251 Riverport Lane, Maryland Heights, MO 63043. Periodicals postage paid at New York, NY and additional mailing offices. Subscription prices are $370.00 per year for US individuals, $948.00 per year for US institutions, $100.00 per year for US students and residents, $458.00 per year for Canadian individuals, $967.00 per year for Canadian institutions, $480.00 per year for international individuals, $967.00 per year for international institutions, $100.00 per year for Canadian students/residents and $220.00 per year for international students/residents. To receive student/resident rate, orders must be accompanied by name of affiliated institution, data of term, and the *signature* of program/residency coordinator on institution letterhead. Orders will be billed at individual rate until proof of status is received. Foreign air speed delivery is included in all *Clinics* subscription prices. All prices are subject to change without notice. **POSTMASTER:** Send address changes to *Cardiology Clinics*, Elsevier Health Sciences Division, Subscription Customer Service, 3251 Riverport Lane, Maryland Heights, MO 63043. **Customer Service: 1-800-654-2452 (U.S. and Canada); 314-447-8871 (outside U.S. and Canada). Fax: 314-447-8029. E-mail: journalscustomerservice-usa@elsevier.com (for print support); journalsonlinesupport-usa@elsevier.com (for online support).**

Reprints. For copies of 100 or more, of articles in this publication, please contact the Commercial Reprints Department, Elsevier Inc., 360 Park Avenue South, New York, NY 10010-1710. Tel.: 212-633-3874; Fax: 212-633-3820; E-mail: reprints@elsevier.com.

Cardiology Clinics is also published in Spanish by McGraw-Hill Interamericana Editores S. A., P.O. Box 5-237, 06500, Mexico D. F., Mexico; in Portuguese by Reichmann and Alfonso Editores Rio de Janeiro, Brazil; and in Greek by Dimitrios P. Lagos, 8 Pondon Street, GR115-28 Ilissia, Greece.

Cardiology Clinics is covered in *MEDLINE/PubMed (Index Medicus), Excerpta Medica, The Cumulative Index to Nursing and Allied Health Literature* (CINAHL).

Printed in the United States of America.

Contributors

EDITORIAL BOARD

JAMIL A. ABOULHOSN, MD, FACC, FSCAI
Director, Ahmanson/UCLA Adult Congenital Heart Center, Streisand/American Heart Association Endowed Chair, Divisions of Cardiology and Pediatric Cardiology, David Geffen School of Medicine at UCLA, Los Angeles, California

DAVID M. SHAVELLE, MD, FACC, FSCAI
Associate Professor, Keck School of Medicine of USC, Director, General Cardiovascular Fellowship Program, Director, Cardiac Catheterization Laboratory, LAC + USC Medical Center, Division of Cardiovascular Medicine, University of Southern California, Los Angeles, California

TERRENCE D. WELCH, MD, FACC
Associate Professor of Medicine and Medical Education, Director, Cardiovascular Fellowship Program, Section of Cardiovascular Medicine, Dartmouth-Hitchcock Heart and Vascular Center, Lebanon, New Hampshire; Geisel School of Medicine at Dartmouth, Hanover, New Hampshire

AUDREY H. WU, MD
Associate Professor, Advanced Heart Failure and Transplant Program, Division of Cardiovascular Medicine, Department of Medicine, University of Michigan, Ann Arbor, Michigan

EDITOR

RICHARD A. KRASUSKI, MD
Professor of Medicine and Pediatrics, Director of Adult Congenital Heart Disease Services, Duke University Health System, Durham, North Carolina

AUTHORS

KAREEM AHMAD, MD
Transplant Department, Advanced Lung Disease and Lung Transplant, Inova Fairfax Medical Center, Falls Church, Virginia

AYEDH K. ALAMRI, MBBS
Department of Medicine, University of Utah, University of Utah School of Medicine, Salt Lake City, Utah

RODOLFO M. ALPIZAR-RIVAS, MD
Division of Infectious Diseases, University of Rochester Medical Center, Rochester, New York

MARIE M. BUDEV, DO, MPH, FCCP
Medical Director, Lung and Heart Lung Transplant Program, Professor, Lerner College of Medicine, Macon and Joan Brock Endowed Chair, Cleveland Clinic, Cleveland, Ohio

RICHARD N. CHANNICK, MD
Saul Brandman Endowed Chair in Pulmonary Arterial Hypertension, Co-Director, Pulmonary Vascular Disease Program, Director, Acute and Chronic Thromboembolic Disease Program, Professor of Medicine, Pulmonary and Critical Care Division, Division of Pulmonary, Critical Care, and Sleep Medicine, David Geffen School of Medicine at UCLA, Los Angeles, California

REBECCA EPSTEIN, MD
Pediatric Cardiology, Columbia University Irving Medical Center, NewYork-Presbyterian Hospital, New York, New York

HARRISON W. FARBER, MD
Division of Pulmonary, Critical Care, and Sleep Medicine, Tufts Medical Center, Boston, Massachusetts

SARAH A. GOLDSTEIN, MD
Adult Congenital Heart Disease Fellowship, Division of Cardiology, Duke University Medical Center, Durham, North Carolina

JOHN C. HANEY, MD
Division of Cardiovascular and Thoracic Surgery, Department of Surgery, Duke University Medical Center, Durham, North Carolina

STEPHANIE M. HON, MD
Division of Pulmonary, Critical Care, and Sleep Medicine, Tufts Medical Center, Boston, Massachusetts

VIKRAMJIT KHANGOORA, MD
Transplant Department, Advanced Lung Disease and Lung Transplant, Inova Fairfax Medical Center, Falls Church, Virginia

RICHARD A. KRASUSKI, MD
Professor of Medicine and Pediatrics, Director of Adult Congenital Heart Disease Services, Duke University Health System, Durham, North Carolina

USHA S. KRISHNAN, MD, DM (Card)
Professor of Pediatrics at CUIMC, Pediatric Cardiology, Columbia University Irving Medical Center, NewYork-Presbyterian Hospital, New York, New York

CHRISTY L. MA, PA-C
Division of Cardiovascular Medicine, Department of Medicine, University of Utah, University of Utah School of Medicine, Salt Lake City, Utah

STEPHEN C. MATHAI, MD, MHS
Division of Pulmonary and Critical Care Medicine, Johns Hopkins School of Medicine, Baltimore, Maryland

SHARON L. MCCARTNEY, MD
Division of Cardiothoracic Anesthesia, Department of Anesthesiology, Duke University Medical Center, Durham, North Carolina

STEVEN D. NATHAN, MD
Transplant Department, Advanced Lung Disease and Lung Transplant, Inova Fairfax Medical Center, Falls Church, Virginia

JOSEPH R. NELLIS, MD, MBA
Division of Cardiovascular and Thoracic Surgery, Department of Surgery, Duke University Medical Center, Durham, North Carolina

SUDARSHAN RAJAGOPAL, MD, PhD
Division of Cardiology, Department of Medicine, Duke University Medical Center, Durham, North Carolina

JOHN J. RYAN, MD
Division of Cardiovascular Medicine, Department of Medicine, University of Utah, University of Utah School of Medicine, Salt Lake City, Utah

RAJAN SAGGAR, MD
Director, Pulmonary Hypertension Program, Co-Director, Pulmonary Vascular Disease Program, Lung and Heart-Lung Transplant and Pulmonary Hypertension Programs, Professor of Medicine, Pulmonary and Critical Care Division, Division of Pulmonary, Critical Care, & Sleep Medicine, David Geffen School of Medicine at UCLA, Los Angeles, California

J.D. SERFAS, MD
Section of Adult Congenital Heart Disease, Division of Cardiology, Duke University Medical Center, Durham, North Carolina

ALEXANDER E. SHERMAN, MD
Fellow Physician, Division of Pulmonary, Critical Care, Sleep Medicine, Clinical Immunology and Allergy, David Geffen School of Medicine at UCLA, Los Angeles, California

ANDREW M. VEKSTEIN, MD
Division of Cardiovascular and Thoracic Surgery, Department of Surgery, Duke University Medical Center, Durham, North Carolina

YEN-REI A. YU, MD, PhD
Division of Pulmonary Sciences and Critical Care Medicine, University of Colorado, Aurora, Colorado

JAMES J. YUN, MD, PhD
Assistant Surgical Director, Lung Transplant
Program, Staff Surgeon, Department of
Thoracic and Cardiovascular Surgery,
Cleveland Clinic, Cleveland, Ohio

Contents

The Pathobiology of Pulmonary Arterial Hypertension

1

Sudarshan Rajagopal and Yen-Rei A. Yu

Pulmonary arterial hypertension is characterized by obliteration and obstruction of the pulmonary arterioles that in turn results in high right ventricular afterload and right heart failure. The pathobiology of pulmonary arterial hypertension is complex, with contributions from multiple pathophysiologic processes that are regulated by a variety of molecular mechanisms. This nature likely explains the limited efficacy of our current therapies, which only target a small portion of the pathobiological mechanisms that underlie advanced disease. Here we review the pathobiology of pulmonary arterial hypertension, focusing on the systemic, cellular, and molecular mechanisms that underlie the disease.

Update on Medical Management of Pulmonary Arterial Hypertension

13

Alexander E. Sherman, Rajan Saggar, and Richard N. Channick

Pulmonary arterial hypertension is a rare disease characterized by pulmonary microvasculature remodeling leading to right ventricular failure and death. Medical management of pulmonary hypertension has grown increasingly complex as more therapeutic agents have been developed. Evolving treatment strategies leveraging the endothelin, nitric oxide, and prostacyclin pathways lead to improved exercise capacity and outcomes in patients; however, significant opportunities for advancement remain.

Pulmonary Hypertension Associated with Connective Tissue Disease

29

Stephen C. Mathai

Pulmonary hypertension (PH), a syndrome characterized by elevated pulmonary pressures, commonly complicates connective tissue disease (CTD) and is associated with increased morbidity and mortality. The incidence of PH varies widely between CTDs; patients with systemic sclerosis are most likely to develop PH. Several different types of PH can present in CTD, including PH related to left heart disease and respiratory disease. Importantly, CTD patients are at risk for developing pulmonary arterial hypertension, a rare form of PH that is associated with high morbidity and mortality. Future therapies targeting pulmonary vascular remodeling may improve outcomes for patients with this devastating disease.

Pulmonary Arterial Hypertension in Patients Infected with the Human Immunodeficiency Virus

45

Stephanie M. Hon, Rodolfo M. Alpizar-Rivas, and Harrison W. Farber

It is important to recognize and treat human immunodeficiency virus-associated pulmonary arterial hypertension (HIV-PAH) because of the associated morbidity and mortality. With the introduction of antiretroviral therapies (ART), improved survival has changed the focus of treatment management from immunodeficiency-related opportunistic infections to chronic cardiovascular complications, including HIV-PAH. The 2018 6th World Symposium of Pulmonary Hypertension recommended a revised definition of PAH that might result in a greater number of patients with HIV-PAH; however, the implication of this change is not yet clear. Here, we review the current literature on the diagnosis, management, and outcomes of patients with HIV-PAH.

appropriately selected patients. In this article, the authors review preoperative workup, patient selection, operative technique, postoperative care, and outcomes after PTE.

Chronic thromboembolic pulmonary hypertension is a distinct form of pulmonary hypertension characterized by the nonresolution of thrombotic material in the pulmonary tree; whenever feasible and safe, first-line treatment should be pulmonary thromboendarterectomy. In patients who are not operative candidates, balloon pulmonary angioplasty (BPA) has emerged as an effective treatment modality that results in improvements in functional class, symptoms, hemodynamics, 6-minute walk distance, and right ventricular and pulmonary artery mechanics. Careful attention to procedural technique and rapid identification and treatment of complications are critical for a successful BPA program.

Pediatric pulmonary hypertension (PH) is a rare disease with historically very high morbidity and mortality. In the past 20 years, there has been a growing recognition that pediatric PH, although having similarities to adult PH, is a unique entity with its own particular pathogeneses, presentation, and management. With better understanding and earlier diagnosis of pediatric PH, and as more medications have become available, survival of children with PH has also significantly improved. This article reviews the various forms of PH in childhood, with a focus on both established and investigational therapies that are available for children with PH.

Pulmonary arterial hypertension (PAH) is a progressive fatal disease. Although medical therapies have improved the outlook for these patients, there still exists a cohort of patients with PAH who are refractory to these therapies. Lung transplantation (LT), and in certain cases heart–lung transplantation (HLT), is a therapeutic option for patients with severe PAH who are receiving optimal therapy yet declining. ECMO may serve as a bridge to transplant or recovery in appropriate patients. Although, the mortality within the first 3 months after transplant is higher in PAH recipients than the other indications for LT, and the long-term survival after LT is excellent for this group of individuals. In this review, we discuss the indications for LT in PAH patients, when to refer and list patients for LT, the indications for double lung transplant (DLT) versus HLT for PAH patients, types of advanced circulatory support for severe PAH, and short and long-term outcomes in transplant recipients with PAH.

CARDIOLOGY CLINICS

Preface
Pulmonary Hypertension

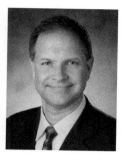

Richard A. Krasuski, MD
Editor

I was a recently minted fellow at Duke University Medical Center in early 1998 when my mentor, Dr Bashore, asked me to come up with a research project utilizing a device he had just purchased for the catheterization laboratory. The INOvent Delivery System (Ohmeda Medical, Laurel, MD, USA) facilitated the controlled delivery of nitric oxide blended with oxygen through a ventilator circuit.[1] I immediately began working on my institutional review board submission with a goal to study patients with what was then known as "primary pulmonary hypertension" and compare them with patients with "secondary pulmonary hypertension."[2] Even then we were careful to exclude patients with elevated pulmonary capillary wedge pressure from our study, as we understood the difference in pathophysiology between precapillary and postcapillary forms of pulmonary hypertension (PH) and that the therapeutic approaches to these conditions greatly differed.

Only a few months later at the 2nd World Symposium on Pulmonary Hypertension (WSPH) in France, the first organized grouping of PH etiologies that shared similar pathologic conditions, clinical features, and therapies was described and became known for many years as the "Evian Classification" and more recently as the "World Health Organization (WHO) Classification."[3] Though several tweaks have been introduced at subsequent WSPH,[4-7] the main structure has persisted and has undoubtedly helped foster a greater understanding of PH for clinicians and researchers alike. In 1998, there were only 2 available therapies that were thought to target the pulmonary vasculature: oral calcium channel blockers and intravenous epoprostenol. Currently there are 14 Food and Drug Administration–approved, advanced medical therapies available to manage pulmonary arterial hypertension (PAH).[8] They fall into 5 major drug classes and are available in oral, inhalational, subcutaneous, and intravenous formulations.

For this issue of *Cardiology Clinics*, I have asked my most esteemed colleagues to share their latest information on the diagnosis and management of PH. A recurring theme in each of these articles is how important it is to make the proper diagnosis. In nearly every article, reference is made to the WHO Classification System, a fundamental building block in understanding pathophysiology and disease progression. Diagnosis should universally include the careful performance of a right heart catheterization, and when necessary, a left heart catheterization to measure the left ventricular end-diastolic pressure. Blindly administering medications can not only lead to unsatisfactory results in these patients but also potentially result in detrimental complications. Referral to a PH Center of Comprehensive Care ensures that the diagnostic evaluation is both comprehensive and appropriate.[9] Involving specialty services, such as rheumatology, infectious disease, hepatology, congenital heart disease, thoracic surgery, and organ transplantation, is often necessary. Furthermore, communication with local providers and subsequent close follow-up are critical components to ensure the best patient outcomes.

Although the proliferation of medications targeting PAH is indeed impressive, current drugs still target only 3 of the pathophysiologic pathways, and Dr Rajagopal and subsequently Dr Channick and colleagues illustrate how we may only be

Cardiol Clin 40 (2022) xi–xii
https://doi.org/10.1016/j.ccl.2021.09.002
0733-8651/22/© 2021 Published by Elsevier Inc.

cardiology.theclinics.com

scratching the surface in terms of potential targets for therapy. We follow with updates on WHO group I diseases, including PH related to connective tissue disorders, HIV infection, and congenital heart disease. We then move into a discussion about group II disease, which continues to be a hot target for clinical trials despite near universal disappointments in this population with advanced medical therapies.[10] The main message remains to focus treatment on the underlying disorder and not the consequent PH. Dr Nathan and colleagues then provide a review of group III disease and share interesting new data regarding the potential role of inhalational therapy for managing PAH in these patients. Group IV disease has the most specifically targeted treatment available (surgery), and chronic thromboembolic pulmonary hypertension (CTEPH) should be assessed for with a ventilation-perfusion scan in any patient presenting with newly diagnosed PH or in patients with prior pulmonary embolism and persisting dyspnea. Pulmonary thromboendarterectomy can be curative in many CTEPH patients, while still others may respond well to transcatheter or medical approaches. Drs Krishnan and Shah then contribute a state-of-the-art discussion regarding diagnosis and management of PH in children. It is exciting to finally see larger trials focusing on this growing patient population.[11] Last, Drs Budev and Yun summarize the approach to organ transplantation when medical options in PAH are unsuccessful.

I have been blessed to participate in the care of so many wonderful patients with this dreaded disease, to take part in clinical research in PAH, and to be involved in educating my colleagues about its diagnosis and management. Every day it seems that new discoveries are made that positively impact clinical care. In fact, the science has moved so quickly that I am becoming more confident that I will see a cure for PH during my lifetime.

Richard A. Krasuski, MD
Adult Congenital Heart Disease Services
Duke University Health System
DUMC 3301
Durham, NC 27710, USA

E-mail address:
richard.krasuski@duke.edu

REFERENCES

1. Kirmse M, Hess D, Fujino Y, et al. Delivery of inhaled nitric oxide using the Ohmeda INOvent Delivery System. Chest 1998;113:1650–7.
2. Krasuski RA, Warner JJ, Wang A, et al. Inhaled nitric oxide selectively dilates pulmonary vasculature in adult patients with pulmonary hypertension, irrespective of etiology. J Am Coll Cardiol 2000;36:2204–11.
3. Fishman AP. Clinical classification of pulmonary hypertension. Clin Chest Med 2001;22:385–91, vii.
4. Simonneau G, Galie N, Rubin LJ, et al. Clinical classification of pulmonary hypertension. J Am Coll Cardiol 2004;43:5S–12S.
5. Simonneau G, Robbins IM, Beghetti M, et al. Updated clinical classification of pulmonary hypertension. J Am Coll Cardiol 2009;54:S43–54.
6. Simonneau G, Gatzoulis MA, Adatia I, et al. Updated clinical classification of pulmonary hypertension. J Am Coll Cardiol 2013;62:D34–41.
7. Simonneau G, Montani D, Celermajer DS, et al. Haemodynamic definitions and updated clinical classification of pulmonary hypertension. Eur Respir J 2019;53(1):1801913.
8. Yaghi S, Novikov A, Trandafirescu T. Clinical update on pulmonary hypertension. J Investig Med 2020;68:821–7.
9. Sahay S, Melendres-Groves L. Pawar L, et al and Pulmonary Vascular Diseases Steering Committee of the American College of Chest P. Pulmonary hypertension care center network: improving care and outcomes in pulmonary hypertension. Chest 2017;151:749–54.
10. Desai A, Desouza SA. Treatment of pulmonary hypertension with left heart disease: a concise review. Vasc Health Risk Manag 2017;13:415–20.
11. Ollivier C, Sun H, Amchin W, et al. New strategies for the conduct of clinical trials in pediatric pulmonary arterial hypertension: outcome of a multistakeholder meeting with patients, academia, industry, and regulators, held at the European Medicines Agency on Monday, June 12, 2017. J Am Heart Assoc 2019;8:e011306.

The Pathobiology of Pulmonary Arterial Hypertension

Sudarshan Rajagopal, MD, PhD[a],*, Yen-Rei A. Yu, MD, PhD[b]

KEYWORDS

- Pulmonary arterial hypertension • Endothelial cell • Smooth muscle cell • Fibroblast • Inflammation

KEY POINTS

- Pulmonary arterial hypertension is a disease of the pulmonary arterioles, characterized by abnormal remodeling and obstruction.
- Pulmonary arterial hypertension leads to increased resistance in the pulmonary vessels and right ventricular afterload, eventually resulting in right heart failure.
- Over the past decades, a number of important pathobiological mechanisms have been found to contribute to pulmonary arterial hypertension.
- These changes are in endothelial function, smooth muscle cell proliferation, fibroblast activation, inflammation, and metabolism.
- A number of molecular mechanisms underlie these pathophysiological changes, including alterations in type II bone morphogenetic protein receptor and transforming growth factor-β signaling, changes in vasoactive mediators, chemokine and cytokine signaling, ion channel activity, transcription factors, and microRNAs and other epigenetic changes.

THE PATHOLOGY OF PULMONARY ARTERIAL HYPERTENSION

Human Pathology

Pulmonary arterial hypertension (PAH) is characterized by lesions in the distal arterioles, ranging from 50 to 500 μm in size.[1,2] Grossly, this results in a decrease in distal perfusion and the classic "pruning" of the distal pulmonary vasculature observed on a chest radiograph or pulmonary angiography.[3] This in turn results in increased right ventricular (RV) afterload and right heart failure. The histopathologic findings of PAH include medial hypertrophy or hyperplasia, intimal and adventitial fibrosis, and plexiform lesions, the pathognomonic lesions for PAH.[1,2] Recent detailed histologic analyses have demonstrated that plexiform lesions are complex lesions that arise from arteriolar obstruction followed by collateralization of the vasa vasorum and bronchial arteries.[4,5] Thus, these lesions represent a compensatory mechanism to maintain distal perfusion through the pulmonary arterial system. In additional to pulmonary arterioles, remodeling of the pulmonary capillaries and venules is also observed in all PH groups.[6] Beyond the pulmonary vasculature, systemic vascular abnormalities in PAH support the emerging paradigm of PAH as a systemic vasculopathy.[7] With their constant exposure to the entire cardiac output, the pulmonary arterioles are most susceptible to vascular remodeling.

Animal Models

Because clinical studies and patient sample studies are limited in offering insights into the pathogenesis of PAH, complementary animal models

[a] Division of Cardiology, Department of Medicine, Duke University Medical Center, Room 128A Hanes House, 330 Trent Drive, Durham, NC 27710, USA; [b] Division of Pulmonary Sciences and Critical Care Medicine, University of Colorado, 12605 E. 16th Avenue, Aurora, CO 80045, USA
* Corresponding author.
E-mail address: sudarshan.rajagopal@duke.edu

Cardiol Clin 40 (2022) 1–12
https://doi.org/10.1016/j.ccl.2021.08.001
0733-8651/22/© 2021 Elsevier Inc. All rights reserved.

are used to better understand the cellular and molecular basis of disease and for testing potential therapies. The earliest and simplest model is chronic, hypoxia-induced PAH. This state was first observed in cattle living at high altitude and was coined "brisket disease."[8] High altitude decreases oxygen tension, causes reactive hypoxic vasoconstriction, and results in abnormal medial hypertrophy of pulmonary arterioles. Although chronic hypoxia-induced PAH was observed initially in large animals, the observations has been extended to small animals (ie, mice and rats). Today, small animals are the most commonly used models for examining PAH.[9,10] Because pathology induced by chronic hypoxia does not recapitulate all the features of human disease, the focus of many studies has been on 2-hit approaches to induce severe pulmonary vascular remodeling. For example, mice are relatively resistant to hypoxic stress and generally develop mild pulmonary remodeling and PH when exposed to chronic hypoxia. However, transgenic technology in mice allows the flexibility to examine the contribution of specific molecules, pathways, and cell types to disease pathogenesis. Genetic modifications in combination with hypoxia can lead to severe PH in mice, for example, exposing mice with lung-specific overexpression of IL-6 to hypoxia.[11] Other 2-hit approaches, including combining SU5416 injections, a vascular endothelial growth factor receptor 2 antagonist that can cause endothelial injury, with hypoxia, pneumonectomy, induction of allergic inflammation, or other genetic modifications,[9] can also enhance the severity of PH.

Similar strategies have also been applied to rat models that, compared with mice, generally develop significantly more extensive vascular remodeling with severe pulmonary hypertension. Although mice are resistant to monocrotaline (MCT) toxicity, MCT administration is commonly used to induce PH in rats, where a single subcutaneous injection of MCT results in progressive, severe pulmonary remodeling, right heart failure, and fatal PH.[10] MCT is thought to act as a toxin to the endothelium, although its effects are complex and not organ-specific. The SU5416-hypoxia model results in severe and sustained PH,[12] which can be fatal depending on the strain of rat used.[13] Together, the use of these models has been invaluable in probing the pathobiology and pathophysiology of PAH.

THE PATHOPHYSIOLOGY OF PULMONARY ARTERIAL HYPERTENSION

The pathophysiology of PAH is complex, with contributions from multiple cell types in the pulmonary vasculature and the right heart. Here we highlight some of the major mechanisms that contribute to pulmonary vascular remodeling (**Fig. 1**) and RV dysfunction in PAH.

Endothelial Dysfunction

PAH is characterized by microvascular rarefaction. Pulmonary artery endothelial cell (PAEC) injury leading to EC dysfunction and apoptosis are triggers for the development of PAH. Both animal models of PH (ie, MCT and SU5416-hypoxia models) and human type II bone morphogenetic protein receptor (BMPR2) mutation-associated PAH are characterized by lung PAEC apoptosis.[14] Chronic PAEC apoptosis results in microvascular destruction and rarefaction. In addition, apoptosis leads to the selection of apoptosis resistance and proliferative PAECs causing occlusive arterial remodeling.[15] Cultured PAECs isolated from human patients with PAH demonstrate increased proliferation compared with nondiseased controls.[16] Idiopathic PAH (IPAH) PAECs also have metabolic abnormalities, with decreased mitochondrial numbers per cell and a higher glycolytic rate.[17] It is unclear as to which of these processes—a primary loss of vessels owing to EC apoptosis versus a secondary loss of vessels owing to obliteration from apoptosis-resistant ECs—is central to PAH pathogenesis.[18] Additionally, these processes may play roles in different phases of the disease.[19] Another aspect by which the EC contributes to PAH is endothelial-to-mesenchymal transition, where ECs can transition to smooth muscle cell (SMC)-like cells that upregulate twist and vimentin.[20]

Smooth Muscle Cell Hypertrophy and Proliferation

Hypertrophy, proliferation, migration, and apoptosis resistance of medial SMCs in the pulmonary arterioles (PASMCs) plays a central role in PAH. PASMCs in normal adult lung are quiescent with a contractile and nonmigratory phenotype. In the setting of tissue injury, SMCs can transition to a proliferative phenotype, resulting in vessel remodeling. Pathologic distal arteriole muscularization results from proliferation of preexisting SMCs and recapitulates many aspects of arterial wall development, including SMC dedifferentiation, distal migration, proliferation, and then redifferentiation.[21] Some of the cues for this process are regulated by nonclassical monocytes and macrophages that sense hypoxia and are predicted to promote pulmonary vascular remodeling and SMC proliferation.[22] For example, macrophage-derived factors such as platelet-derived growth

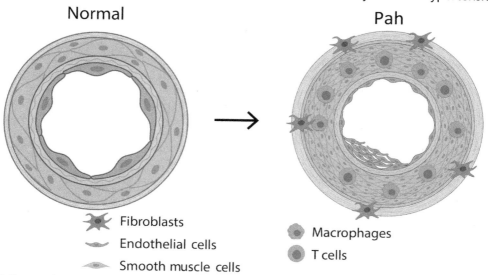

Fig. 1. Cell types that contribute to pulmonary vascular remodeling. Pulmonary vascular remodeling involves all layers of the vascular wall (the intima, primarily composed of ECs; the media, primarily composed of SMCs; and the adventitia, primarily composed of fibroblasts) along with infiltration with immune cells such as macrophages and T cells. This results in the selection of apoptosis-resistant ECs, the proliferation of SMCs, and the activation of fibroblasts. Much of this is driven by signaling from immune cells such as macrophages and T cells. See text for details. Created with BioRender.com.

factor-β are upregulated in PAH and promote SMC proliferation.[23] There are also cell autonomous factors that contribute to SMC proliferation. This process is exemplified by SMC-specific knockout of BMPR1A, which resulted in attenuated SMC proliferation, decreased hypoxia-mediated muscularization of distal vessels, and the preservation of peripheral pulmonary arteries.[24]

Fibroblasts and Fibrosis

Obliterative thickening of vessels in PAH are largely composed of SMCs and myofibroblasts. Frank fibrosis has been noted in PAH pathologic samples, especially in those with PAH associated with connective tissue disease.[2] Adventitial fibroblasts from calves with severe hypoxia-induced PH and humans with IPAH display increased aerobic glycolysis. Treatment of these mice with a pharmacologic agent for an nicotinamide adenine dinucleotide–sensitive transcription corepressor resulted in decreased glycolysis and expression of inflammatory genes, attenuated proliferation, and decreased remodeling of the distal pulmonary vasculature.[25] These fibroblasts also activate macrophages through paracrine signaling via IL-6–activated STAT3 to promote pulmonary vascular remodeling.[26]

Immune Cells and Inflammation

Inflammation is known to be an important mediator of vascular dysfunction in the pathogenesis of PAH. Accumulation of immune cells, including T cells, B cells, monocytes, macrophages, and mast cells, has been observed in all animal models of PH and human disease.[27,28] The predominant cell types are T cells, monocytes, and macrophages. These cells are found mostly in the perivascular regions, but also observed within the plexiform lesions.[29] T cells, monocytes, and macrophages can directly or indirectly, via paracrine signaling, modulate the activation, proliferation, transformation, migration, and survival of vascular mural cells (ie, EC, vascular SMCs, and adventitial fibroblasts), modify extracellular matrix, and regulate remodeling of all parts of the vascular wall. Altering immune cell populations and balance in both adaptive and innate immune compartments modulates vascular remodeling and PH severity. For example, athymic animals develop severe pulmonary remodeling and PH spontaneously owing to the absence of the protective effect of CD4+ T regulatory cells.[30,31] In contrast, Th1 and Th17 cells secrete proinflammatory cytokines such as IL-6, IL-1, IL-21, and tumor necrosis factor-α, and IFN-γ, and promote vascular remodeling.[32,33] Additionally, Th17 cells also promote PH through the secretion of IL-17A.[34] Although Th1 cells and IFN-γ are required for the development of pneumocystis-induced PAH[32]; Th2 cells, through production of IL-4 and IL-13, exacerbate schistosomiasis-induced and other forms of PAH.[35–37] Thus, the balance of Th1 versus Th17 or Th2 versus T regulatory cell populations determine the immune milieu and its effects on vascular remodeling.[33]

Monocytes and macrophages are also involved in multiple aspects of PAH pathogenesis. Recent studies have shown that macrophages are derived from both fetal precursors or circulating monocytes; the function of macrophages depends on their origin, anatomic microenvironment, and specific stimuli.[38–41] Consistent with this paradigm, depletion strategies that differentially affect various populations of monocytes and macrophage can either promote or ameliorate PAH severity.[42–44] Preferential polarization of macrophages to alternative phenotype (M2-like) spectrum, characterized by signaling through STAT3, and promote cellular proliferation and is believed to drive PAH. However, in animal models of PAH, both M1-like and M2-like macrophages have been described.[45] M1-like macrophages are potent producers of interferon, which is a known driver of vascular remodeling and PAH. Moreover, the M1/M2 classification is an oversimplification of macrophage involvement in PAH.[46] Macrophage recruitment and activation are modulated by many factors produced by both vascular mural and other immune cells, including a decrease in BMPR2 signaling, secreted macrophage inhibitory factor by dysfunctional ECs, leukotriene T4, and chemokines (eg, CCL2, CCL1, and CX3CL1).[33,47–50] These molecules and pathways are being explored as potential therapeutic targets for PAH. In addition to T cells and macrophages, mast cells and eosinophils have been implicated in PAH pathogenesis.[51–55] With the complexity of different immune cell populations and responses, immune cell dysregulation generally promotes the abnormal vascular mural cell phenotype in PAH.

Metabolism

As noted elsewhere in this article, many of the cell types in pulmonary vasculature display changes in their metabolic state. Paulin and Michelakis[56] have proposed that many of the pathobiological abnormalities in PAH promote mitochondrial suppression, with an inhibition of glucose oxidation, which in turn results in many of the observed molecular abnormalities noted in PAH. It has been proposed that these metabolic abnormalities are similar to those seen in cancer and explain features of the PAH vascular phenotype, including the enhancement of proliferation and apoptosis resistance. Notably, insulin resistance is also common in PAH and is characterized by alterations in lipid and lipoprotein levels, and elevated levels of circulating medium- and long-chain acylcarnitines.[57,58] These defects in fatty acid oxidation contribute to lipotoxicity in the RV in PAH.[59]

Metabolic profiling has also been used to identify signatures of RV–pulmonary valve dysfunction, consistent with the pulmonary release of tryptophan metabolites.[60] Although it is likely an oversimplification to reduce all of the complex abnormalities in PAH to a single underlying cause of metabolic changes, these studies clearly demonstrate that metabolic abnormalities contribute to PAH pathogenesis and phenotype.

Right Ventricular Dysfunction

The majority of basic pathobiology studies in PAH focus on abnormalities in the pulmonary vasculature, but the RV in PAH also has an abnormal response to increased afterload.[61] The increased afterload from pulmonary vascular remodeling results in right heart failure, characterized by decreased RV function that leads to insufficient cardiac output and/or increased filling pressure at rest or exercise. In response to the increased afterload, the RV displays an adaptive hypertrophic response, but over time this can transition to a maladaptive phenotype.[62] Notably, patients who display preserved RV function in PH have significantly better survival than those who have decreased RV function at follow-up. Adaptive remodeling is characterized by the preservation of a normal cardiac output, RV ejection fraction, filling pressures, and exercise capacity. Adaptive remodeling consists primarily of concentric hypertrophy with minimal dilatation and fibrosis.[62] Maladaptive remodeling is associated with increased filling pressures and a decreased cardiac output and RV ejection fraction; it consists primarily of RV dilatation and fibrosis. With these compensatory mechanisms, RV–pulmonary arterial coupling (typically quantified by the ratio of RV end-systolic elastance and arterial elastance) with efficient energy transfer is maintained initially in adaptive remodeling. However, it is then overwhelmed gradually[61] and transitions from adaptive to maladaptive remodeling. In MCT-induced PH rat models, this transition is associated with a decrease in angiogenesis, a decrease in glucose uptake, and a reversion toward normal metabolism.[63] However, a detailed analysis of human samples with stereology[64] demonstrated that, in advanced PH, there was a significant increase in the RV vasculature in the setting of RV hypertrophy, consistent with compensatory angiogenesis in severe PAH. Similar results were observed in Su5416-hypoxia PH models,[65] where a compensatory angiogenic response was observed, but with a modest decrease in arterial delivery of metabolic substrates owing to an increase in the radius of tissue served per vessel. Metabolomics revealed major metabolic alterations and reprogramming, but without evidence of tissue hypoxia or depletion of key metabolic substrates. This finding suggested that the major driver of RV maladaptation was related to direct changes in cardiomyocytes and not secondary to vascular rarefaction and decreased substrate delivery. Despite these findings supporting the importance of RV function on outcomes, there are currently no PAH therapies that directly target the RV.

MOLECULAR MECHANISMS OF PULMONARY ARTERIAL HYPERTENSION

Multiple molecular mechanisms contribute to the pathophysiological axes discussed elsewhere in this article. We highlight a number of these mechanisms in **Fig. 2** and elsewhere in this discussion.

Type II Bone Morphogenetic Protein Receptor and Transforming Growth Factor-β Signaling

BMPR2 mutations account for 70% of heritable PAH and are also found in 20% of patients with IPAH.[66] BMPR2 is a member of the transforming growth factor (TGF)-β receptor superfamily. While

TGF-β receptors promote signaling through Smad2/3 transcription factors, BMPR2 promotes signaling through Smad1/5 transcription factors.[67] A large meta-analysis also identified that patients with BMPR2 mutations, whether idiopathic, heritable, or anorexigen-associated, presented at a younger age with more severe disease and were at a higher risk of death compared with those without BMPR2 mutations.[68] Mutations of a number of proteins important in the TGF-β superfamily have been identified as potentially pathogenic in next-generation sequencing studies in PAH.[69] Although some of these genetic links have been known for some time,[70] the complex pharmacology of this system has made it difficult to identify the specific receptor hetereomers and their ligands that were responsible for signaling in the pulmonary vascular endothelium.[71] A breakthrough was made with the discovery that BMP9 is the preferred ligand for preventing apoptosis and enhancing endothelial integrity.[72] Additionally, the administration of BMP9 reversed established PAH in mice carrying a heterozygous knock-in allele of human BMPR2 (R899X) mutation.[72] More recently, an approach of targeting the

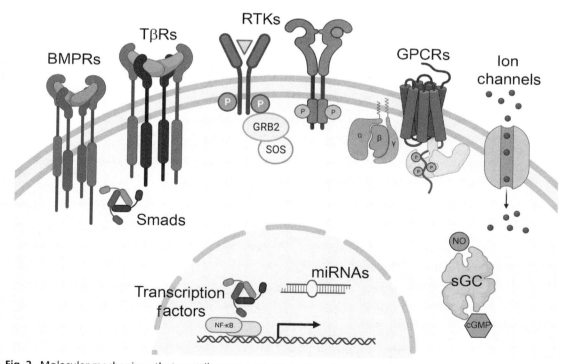

Fig. 2. Molecular mechanisms that contribute to PAH. Multiple molecular mechanisms contribute to the development of PAH, including signaling by BMPRs and TGF-β receptors through Smads, growth factor signaling via receptor tyrosine kinases (RTKs), growth factors and vasoactive mediator signaling via G protein-coupled receptors, the activation of ion channels, nitric oxide signaling via soluble guanylate cyclase (sGC), the activation of transcription factors and epigenetic mechanisms such as microRNAs (miRNAs). See text for details. Created with BioRender.com.

balance of activin/growth differentiation factor and BMP signaling via BMPR2 has demonstrated preclinical efficacy.[73] Although activins and growth differentiation factors promote signaling via Smad2/3, BMPs promote signaling via Smad1/5/9. Treatment with a potent growth differentiation factor 8/11 and activin ligand trap inhibited Smad2/3 signaling, resulting in decreased proliferation and enhancement of apoptosis in the vascular wall, and attenuated PH.[73] These findings suggest that new approaches to target BMPR2 signaling will be useful as a therapeutic strategy in PAH.

Growth Factors

The dysregulation of a range of growth factors, many of which target receptor tyrosine kinases (RTKs), promote abnormal vascular proliferation and play a central role in PAH pathobiology.[74] Markers of angiogenesis, such as vascular endothelial growth factor, have been noted in plexiform lesions.[75] In the setting of vascular destruction and obstruction in PAH, this likely reflects an angiogenic response to form collaterals from bronchial/vasa vasorum to the pulmonary arterial circulation. KDR heterozygosity (the gene encoding vascular endothelial growth factor receptor 2) is strongly associated with PAH that occurs later in life.[76] Levels of fibroblast growth factor 2 (FGF2) are elevated in the remodeled pulmonary vascular endothelium of patients with IPAH; and FGF2 knockdown decreased PASMC growth.[77] In an animal model, the inhibition of FGF receptor 1, a receptor for FGF2, reverses established PH, suggesting this receptor as a potential therapeutic target. Similarly, platelet-derived growth factor (PDGF) promotes PASMC proliferation and migration; and expression of PDGF receptor (PDGFR) is increased in the lung tissue of patients with PAH.[78] The PDGFR antagonist, imatinib, can reverse advanced pulmonary vascular disease in MCT-PH rats and hypoxia mice.[78] Consistent with this finding, imatinib significantly improved exercise capacity and hemodynamics in a clinical trial. Unfortunately, it was also associated with a significant increase in subdural hematomas in patients who were on anticoagulation.[79] In PAH, epidermal growth factor (EGF) activates its receptor (EGFR) to promote cell proliferation and survival. However, the effects of different EGFR antagonists in MCT PH have been noted to be variable, with only some improving RV systolic pressure and hypertrophy.[80] Notably, none of them significantly improved RV systolic pressure or pulmonary vascular remodeling in mice with chronic hypoxic PH. Consistent with this finding, EGFR expression

in lungs was not altered in patients with IPAH. Targeting a range of tyrosine and serine/threonine kinases with sorafenib decreased RV hypertrophy and pulmonary arterial muscularization in MCT-treated rats.[81] An approach using multiple agents to target RTKs (ie, FGFR, EGFR, and PDGFR), was successful in regressing established MCT PH. Treatment decreased the activation of the adapter protein p130(Cas), which works downstream of RTKs to promote cell migration and proliferation.[82] With their central roles in regulating cell migration, proliferation and survival, these growth factors are excellent drug targets in PAH if their potential systemic effects can be limited.

Vasoactive Mediators: Prostacyclins, Endothelins, and Nitric Oxide

Vasoactive mediators have long been known to contribute to PAH pathophysiology, with low levels of vasodilators such as prostacyclin[83] and high levels of vasoconstrictors such as endothelin-1[84] noted in patients with PAH. Only a small percentage of patients with PAH are vasodilator responsive,[85] displaying an acute decrease in pulmonary pressures after treatment with a pulmonary vasodilator such as inhaled nitric oxide, adenosine or epoprostenol.[86] Vasodilator responders display an excellent long-term therapeutic response to calcium channel blockers.[87] Regardless of their acute response to vasodilators, patients with PAH demonstrated a positive response to treatments, such as prostacyclin infusion, in early studies.[88] These initial discoveries translated to the first therapy for PAH, intravenous epoprostenol.[89,90] Although long-term treatment with therapies such as prostacyclins have been shown to be beneficial, they do not seem to reverse PAH pathology fully. As noted in an autopsy study of a PAH patient maintained on longterm therapy who died of a different cause, vascular abnormalities are still evident.[91] All 3 pathways currently targeted by PAH-specific therapies—the prostacyclin pathway (targeted by prostacyclin receptor agonists), the nitric oxide/cyclic guanosine monophosphate axis (targeted by phosphodiesterase 5 inhibitors and soluble guanylate cyclase stimulators), and the endothelin pathway (targeted by endothelin receptor antagonists)—have direct vasoactive effects. It is possible that other vasoactive pathways, such as angiotensin[92,93] and other mediators,[94] would also have beneficial effects in PAH, but they have not been tested in large clinical trials in the PAH population. Notably, although these drugs are thought to primarily act through vasodilation, with prolonged exposure, they likely also act as antiproliferative agents, because vasoconstriction is closely linked to other complex changes in the vasculature.[95]

Chemokines

Chemokines, also known as chemotactic cytokines, are a group of more than 40 small proteins that regulate cell migration and function. Chemokines bind to more than 20 chemokine receptors, which are G protein-coupled receptors. Chemokine receptors are categorized into 5 families based on their activating chemokine ligand (CXCR, CCR, CX3CR, or XCRs), with an additional group of atypical chemokine receptors that bind chemokines of different families, but primarily act as scavenger or decoy receptors. Chemokines bind to negatively charged glycosaminoglycans on the EC surface or extracellular matrix, resulting in a chemokine concentration gradient that promotes immune and inflammatory cell recruitment.[96,97] Chemokine levels have been correlated with disease severity, pulmonary hemodynamics, and RV function in multiple studies. For example, CCL2 and CXCL10 levels are associated with disease severity.[98–101] CCL2, CXCL8, CXCL10, CXCL12, and CXCL13 levels are correlated with hemodynamics such as pulmonary vascular resistance,[100,102–104] right atrial pressure,[98,102] cardiac output,[102] and cardiac index.[98,100,102] With respect to harder outcomes, CCL2, CCL21, and CXCL12 levels have been associated with adverse outcomes and mortality.[105–108] Some of these chemokines may increase as part of an adaptive mechanism; for example, elevated levels of CXCL10 are associated with improved survival in patients with PAH.[109] In addition, some chemokines could serve as biomarkers for monitoring disease progression or treatment effect. For example, the beneficial effects of epoprostenol treatment on functional and hemodynamic status in patients with PAH were associated with increased levels of CCL2.[104] Despite these strong associations with disease severity, chemokines have been challenging to target owing to their complex pharmacology, but novel approaches may make these targets more druggable.[110]

Ion Channels

Ion channels play a central role in the membrane potential and regulate vascular tone of the pulmonary circulation. Voltage-gated potassium channels play a central role in hypoxic vasoconstriction.[111] Mice with mutation of Kv1.5 display impaired hypoxic vasoconstriction.[112] Fawn-hooded rats have a chromosomal abnormality that disrupts a mitochondria–reactive oxygen species–hypoxia inducible factor–Kv pathway, resulting in a loss of voltage-gated potassium channel activity. These rats develop pulmonary hypertension spontaneously.[113] A familial form of PAH is due to heterozygous loss-of-function mutations in KCNK3,[114] which encodes the TASK-1 potassium channel. Consistent with this finding, MCT-treated rats have decreased expression of KCNK3, and the pharmacologic activation of KCNK3 improved PH.[115] Such findings suggest that ion channels may serve as drug targets in PAH treatment.

Transcription Factors and Nuclear Receptors

Transcription factors are the downstream targets of a wide range of signals, such as hypoxia, growth factors, cytokines, and chemokines, that result in the reprogramming of cells to a PAH-promoting phenotype. Hypoxia inducible factor-1α mediates much of the transcriptional response to hypoxia, and its activity in macrophages results in the activation of pro-proliferative signals to PASMCs. For example, FoxO1 is responsible for signaling downstream of many growth factors and inflammatory mediators, and inactivation of specific isoforms results in the pro-proliferative and antiapoptotic phenotype of PASMCs in PAH.[116] Similarly, the related transcription factor FoxM1 promotes PASMC proliferation in PAH.[117] PPAR-γ and β-catenin have been shown to promote BMPR2 signaling via apelin, resulting in improved PAEC survival. In mice, this effect was recapitulated with apelin treatment leading to PAH reversal.[118]

MicroRNAs and Long Noncoding RNAs

A number of epigenetic changes have been noted in PAH. Noncoding RNAs, such as microRNAs (miRNAs) and long noncoding RNAs (lncRNAs), have been identified as being dysregulated in PAH. The miRNAs are small noncoding RNAs that inhibit gene expression and are critical in gene regulation.[119] Recently, a number of groups have identified changes in miRNA expression in PAH that seem to contribute to PAH pathobiology. Of these miRNAs, miR-29, -124, -140, and -204 have been reported as dysregulated in PAH, where they seem to play distinct roles.[120] miR-124, -140, and -240 inhibit cellular proliferation, and miR-29 promotes proliferation but inhibits vasoconstriction. However, it has been challenging to interpret some of these studies, because the effects are not always consistent between patients and different disease models.[120] More recently, lncRNAs have been implicated in PAH pathogenesis. The lncRNA H19 was described recently as a new biomarker for right heart failure in PAH. The lncRNA H19 is upregulated in the decompensated RV of patients with PAH and also in rat disease models.[121] Silencing H19 improved RV fibrosis and capillary rarefaction, suggesting that targeting these lncRNAs could be a potential therapeutic strategy. The lncRNA TYKRIL has been shown to be upregulated in pericytes and PASMCs in cells exposed to hypoxia and patients with IPAH.[122] Expression of PDGFRβ strongly correlated with TYKRIL expression and TYKRIL knockdown decreased PDGFRβ expression, suggesting another approach for targeting pathogenic signaling in PAH.

SUMMARY

The pathobiology of PAH is complex, with contributions from multiple pathophysiologic processes that are regulated by a variety of molecular mechanisms. This finding likely explains the limited efficacy of our current therapies, which only target a small portion of the pathobiological mechanisms that underlie advanced disease. It is likely that different therapies that target these multiple axes will need to be used in combination, as is being used with our currently available therapies,[86] to improve outcomes in this devastating disease.

CLINICS CARE POINTS

- Multiple cellular and molecular mechanisms contribute to vascular remodeling in the development of PAH.
- Current PAH therapies focus on targeting vasoactive mechanisms, including prostacyclin receptor agonists, endothelin receptor antagonists, phosphodiesterase 5 inhibitors, and soluble guanylate cyclase stimulators.
- Novel PAH therapies that are being developed target other signaling pathways including the type II bone morphogenetic protein receptor and growth factor receptors.
- All of these pathways regulate endothelial function, smooth muscle cell proliferation, fibroblast activation, inflammation, and metabolism that underlie PAH pathogenesis.

DISCLOSURE

The authors have no commercial or financial conflicts of interest.

REFERENCES

1. Heath D, Edwards JE. The pathology of hypertensive pulmonary vascular disease; a description of six grades of structural changes in the pulmonary arteries with special reference to congenital cardiac septal defects. Circulation 1958;18:533–47.
2. Stacher E, Graham BB, Hunt JM, et al. Modern age pathology of pulmonary arterial hypertension. Am J Respir Crit Care Med 2012;186:261–72.
3. Gray HH, Morgan JM, Kerr IH, et al. Clinical correlates of angiographically diagnosed idiopathic pulmonary hypertension. Thorax 1990;45:442–6.
4. Galambos C, Sims-Lucas S, Abman SH, et al. Intrapulmonary bronchopulmonary anastomoses and plexiform lesions in idiopathic pulmonary arterial hypertension. Am J Respir Crit Care Med 2016; 193:574–6.
5. Norvik C, Westoo CK, Peruzzi N, et al. Synchrotron-based phase-contrast micro-CT as a tool for understanding pulmonary vascular pathobiology and the 3-D microanatomy of alveolar capillary dysplasia. Am J Physiol Lung Cell Mol Physiol 2020;318: L65–75.
6. Pietra GG, Capron F, Stewart S, et al. Pathologic assessment of vasculopathies in pulmonary hypertension. J Am Coll Cardiol 2004;43:25S–32S.
7. Nickel NP, Yuan K, Dorfmuller P, et al. Beyond the lungs: systemic manifestations of pulmonary arterial hypertension. Am J Respir Crit Care Med 2020;201:148–57.
8. Rhodes J. Comparative physiology of hypoxic pulmonary hypertension: historical clues from brisket disease. J Appl Physiol (1985) 2005;98:1092–100.
9. Gomez-Arroyo J, Saleem SJ, Mizuno S, et al. A brief overview of mouse models of pulmonary arterial hypertension: problems and prospects. Am J Physiol Lung Cell Mol Physiol 2012;302: L977–91.
10. Gomez-Arroyo JG, Farkas L, Alhussaini AA, et al. The monocrotaline model of pulmonary hypertension in perspective. Am J Physiol Lung Cell Mol Physiol 2012;302:L363–9.
11. Steiner MK, Syrkina OL, Kolliputi N, et al. Interleukin-6 overexpression induces pulmonary hypertension. Circ Res 2009;104:236–44, 28p following 244.
12. Abe K, Toba M, Alzoubi A, et al. Formation of plexiform lesions in experimental severe pulmonary arterial hypertension. Circulation 2010;121: 2747–54.
13. Jiang B, Deng Y, Suen C, et al. Marked strain-specific differences in the SU5416 rat model of severe pulmonary arterial hypertension. Am J Respir Cell Mol Biol 2016;54:461–8.
14. Teichert-Kuliszewska K, Kutryk MJ, Kuliszewski MA, et al. Bone morphogenetic

protein receptor-2 signaling promotes pulmonary arterial endothelial cell survival: implications for loss-of-function mutations in the pathogenesis of pulmonary hypertension. Circ Res 2006;98: 209–17.

15. Sakao S, Taraseviciene-Stewart L, Lee JD, et al. Initial apoptosis is followed by increased proliferation of apoptosis-resistant endothelial cells. FASEB J 2005;19:1178–80.

16. Xu W, Erzurum SC. Endothelial cell energy metabolism, proliferation, and apoptosis in pulmonary hypertension. Compr Physiol 2011;1:357–72.

17. Xu W, Koeck T, Lara AR, et al. Alterations of cellular bioenergetics in pulmonary artery endothelial cells. Proc Natl Acad Sci U S A 2007;104:1342–7.

18. Kuebler WM, Nicolls MR, Olschewski A, et al. A pro-con debate: current controversies in PAH pathogenesis at the American Thoracic Society International Conference in 2017. Am J Physiol Lung Cell Mol Physiol 2018;315:L502–16.

19. Michelakis ED. Spatio-temporal diversity of apoptosis within the vascular wall in pulmonary arterial hypertension: heterogeneous BMP signaling may have therapeutic implications. Circ Res 2006;98:172–5.

20. Ranchoux B, Antigny F, Rucker-Martin C, et al. Endothelial-to-mesenchymal transition in pulmonary hypertension. Circulation 2015;131: 1006–18.

21. Sheikh AQ, Lighthouse JK, Greif DM. Recapitulation of developing artery muscularization in pulmonary hypertension. Cell Rep 2014;6:809–17.

22. Yu YA, Malakhau Y, Yu CA, et al. Nonclassical monocytes sense hypoxia, regulate pulmonary vascular remodeling, and promote pulmonary hypertension. J Immunol 2020;204:1474–85.

23. Ntokou A, Dave JM, Kauffman AC, et al. Macrophage-derived PDGF-B induces muscularization in murine and human pulmonary hypertension. JCI Insight 2021;6(6):e139067.

24. El-Bizri N, Wang L, Merklinger SL, et al. Smooth muscle protein 22alpha-mediated patchy deletion of Bmpr1a impairs cardiac contractility but protects against pulmonary vascular remodeling. Circ Res 2008;102:380–8.

25. Li M, Riddle S, Zhang H, et al. Metabolic reprogramming regulates the proliferative and inflammatory phenotype of adventitial fibroblasts in pulmonary hypertension through the transcriptional corepressor C-terminal binding protein-1. Circulation 2016;134:1105–21.

26. El Kasmi KC, Pugliese SC, Riddle SR, et al. Adventitial fibroblasts induce a distinct proinflammatory/profibrotic macrophage phenotype in pulmonary hypertension. J Immunol 2014;193:597–609.

27. Tuder RM, Voelkel NF. Pulmonary hypertension and inflammation. J Lab Clin Med 1998;132:16–24.

28. Dorfmuller P, Perros F, Balabanian K, et al. Inflammation in pulmonary arterial hypertension. Eur Respir J 2003;22:358–63.

29. Tuder RM, Groves B, Badesch DB, et al. Exuberant endothelial cell growth and elements of inflammation are present in plexiform lesions of pulmonary hypertension. Am J Pathol 1994;144:275–85.

30. Taraseviciene-Stewart L, Nicolls MR, Kraskauskas D, et al. Absence of T cells confers increased pulmonary arterial hypertension and vascular remodeling. Am J Respir Crit Care Med 2007;175:1280–9.

31. Chu Y, Xiangli X, Xiao W. Regulatory T cells protect against hypoxia-induced pulmonary arterial hypertension in mice. Mol Med Rep 2015;11:3181–7.

32. Swain SD, Siemsen DW, Pullen RR, et al. CD4+ T cells and IFN-gamma are required for the development of Pneumocystis-associated pulmonary hypertension. Am J Pathol 2014;184:483–93.

33. Rabinovitch M, Guignabert C, Humbert M, et al. Inflammation and immunity in the pathogenesis of pulmonary arterial hypertension. Circ Res 2014; 115:165–75.

34. Schuler R, Efentakis P, Wild J, et al. T cell-derived IL-17a induces vascular dysfunction via perivascular fibrosis formation and dysregulation of (.)NO/cGMP signaling. Oxid Med Cell Longev 2019; 2019:6721531.

35. Kumar R, Mickael C, Kassa B, et al. Th2 CD4(+) T cells are necessary and sufficient for schistosoma-pulmonary hypertension. J Am Heart Assoc 2019; 8:e013111.

36. Chen G, Zuo S, Tang J, et al. Inhibition of CRTH2-mediated Th2 activation attenuates pulmonary hypertension in mice. J Exp Med 2018;215:2175–95.

37. Daley E, Emson C, Guignabert C, et al. Pulmonary arterial remodeling induced by a Th2 immune response. J Exp Med 2008;205:361–72.

38. Tan SY, Krasnow MA. Developmental origin of lung macrophage diversity. Development 2016;143: 1318–27.

39. Mould KJ, Barthel L, Mohning MP, et al. Cell origin dictates programming of resident versus recruited macrophages during acute lung injury. Am J Respir Cell Mol Biol 2017;57:294–306.

40. Gosselin D, Link VM, Romanoski CE, et al. Environment drives selection and function of enhancers controlling tissue-specific macrophage identities. Cell 2014;159:1327–40.

41. Lavin Y, Winter D, Blecher-Gonen R, et al. Tissue-resident macrophage enhancer landscapes are shaped by the local microenvironment. Cell 2014; 159:1312–26.

42. Zawia A, Arnold ND, West L, et al. Altered macrophage polarization induces experimental pulmonary hypertension and is observed in patients with pulmonary arterial hypertension. Arterioscler Thromb Vasc Biol 2021;41:430–45.

43. Frid MG, Brunetti JA, Burke DL, et al. Hypoxia-induced pulmonary vascular remodeling requires recruitment of circulating mesenchymal precursors of a monocyte/macrophage lineage. Am J Pathol 2006;168:659–69.

44. Zaloudikova M, Vytasek R, Vajnerova O, et al. Depletion of alveolar macrophages attenuates hypoxic pulmonary hypertension but not hypoxia-induced increase in serum concentration of MCP-1. Physiol Res 2016;65:763–8.

45. Schweitzer F, Tarantelli R, Rayens E, et al. Monocyte and alveolar macrophage skewing is associated with the development of pulmonary arterial hypertension in a primate model of HIV infection. AIDS Res Hum Retroviruses 2019;35:63–74.

46. Pugliese SC, Kumar S, Janssen WJ, et al. A time- and compartment-specific activation of lung macrophages in hypoxic pulmonary hypertension. J Immunol 2017;198:4802–12.

47. Sawada H, Saito T, Nickel NP, et al. Reduced BMPR2 expression induces GM-CSF translation and macrophage recruitment in humans and mice to exacerbate pulmonary hypertension. J Exp Med 2014;211:263–80.

48. Jalce G, Guignabert C. Multiple roles of macrophage migration inhibitory factor in pulmonary hypertension. Am J Physiol Lung Cell Mol Physiol 2020;318:L1–9.

49. Le Hiress M, Tu L, Ricard N, et al. Proinflammatory signature of the dysfunctional endothelium in pulmonary hypertension. Role of the macrophage migration inhibitory factor/CD74 complex. Am J Respir Crit Care Med 2015;192:983–97.

50. Groth A, Vrugt B, Brock M, et al. Inflammatory cytokines in pulmonary hypertension. Respir Res 2014; 15:47.

51. Farha S, Sharp J, Asosingh K, et al. Mast cell number, phenotype, and function in human pulmonary arterial hypertension. Pulm Circ 2012;2:220–8.

52. Hoffmann J, Yin J, Kukucka M, et al. Mast cells promote lung vascular remodelling in pulmonary hypertension. Eur Respir J 2011;37:1400–10.

53. Bartelds B, van Loon RLE, Mohaupt S, et al. Mast cell inhibition improves pulmonary vascular remodeling in pulmonary hypertension. Chest 2012;141:651–60.

54. Weng M, Baron DM, Bloch KD, et al. Eosinophils are necessary for pulmonary arterial remodeling in a mouse model of eosinophilic inflammation-induced pulmonary hypertension. Am J Physiol Lung Cell Mol Physiol 2011;301:L927–36.

55. Medoff BD, Okamoto Y, Leyton P, et al. Adiponectin deficiency increases allergic airway inflammation and pulmonary vascular remodeling. Am J Respir Cell Mol Biol 2009;41:397–406.

56. Paulin R, Michelakis ED. The metabolic theory of pulmonary arterial hypertension. Circ Res 2014; 115:148–64.

57. Hemnes AR, Luther JM, Rhodes CJ, et al. Human PAH is characterized by a pattern of lipid-related insulin resistance. JCI Insight 2019;4:e123611.

58. Luo N, Craig D, Ilkayeva O, et al. Plasma acylcarnitines are associated with pulmonary hypertension. Pulm Circ 2017;7:211–8.

59. Brittain EL, Talati M, Fessel JP, et al. Fatty acid metabolic defects and right ventricular lipotoxicity in human pulmonary arterial hypertension. Circulation 2016;133:1936–44.

60. Lewis GD, Ngo D, Hemnes AR, et al. Metabolic profiling of right ventricular-pulmonary vascular function reveals circulating biomarkers of pulmonary hypertension. J Am Coll Cardiol 2016;67:174–89.

61. Vonk Noordegraaf A, Chin KM, Haddad F, et al. Pathophysiology of the right ventricle and of the pulmonary circulation in pulmonary hypertension: an update. Eur Respir J 2019;53:1801900.

62. Ryan JJ, Archer SL. The right ventricle in pulmonary arterial hypertension: disorders of metabolism, angiogenesis and adrenergic signaling in right ventricular failure. Circ Res 2014;115:176–88.

63. Sutendra G, Dromparis P, Paulin R, et al. A metabolic remodeling in right ventricular hypertrophy is associated with decreased angiogenesis and a transition from a compensated to a decompensated state in pulmonary hypertension. J Mol Med 2013;91:1315–27.

64. Graham BB, Koyanagi D, Kandasamy B, et al. Right ventricle vasculature in human pulmonary hypertension assessed by stereology. Am J Respir Crit Care Med 2017;196:1075–7.

65. Graham BB, Kumar R, Mickael C, et al. Vascular adaptation of the right ventricle in experimental pulmonary hypertension. Am J Respir Cell Mol Biol 2018;59:479–89.

66. Morrell NW, Aldred MA, Chung WK, et al. Genetics and genomics of pulmonary arterial hypertension. Eur Respir J 2019;53:1801899.

67. Wharton K, Derynck R. TGFbeta family signaling: novel insights in development and disease. Development 2009;136:3691–7.

68. Evans JD, Girerd B, Montani D, et al. BMPR2 mutations and survival in pulmonary arterial hypertension: an individual participant data meta-analysis. Lancet Respir Med 2016;4:129–37.

69. Graf S, Haimel M, Bleda M, et al. Identification of rare sequence variation underlying heritable pulmonary arterial hypertension. Nat Commun 2018; 9:1416.

70. International PPHC, Lane KB, Machado RD, et al. Heterozygous germline mutations in BMPR2, encoding a TGF-beta receptor, cause familial primary pulmonary hypertension. Nat Genet 2000;26:81–4.

71. Upton PD, Morrell NW. TGF-beta and BMPR-II pharmacology–implications for pulmonary vascular diseases. Curr Opin Pharmacol 2009;9:274–80.

72. Long L, Ormiston ML, Yang X, et al. Selective enhancement of endothelial BMPR-II with BMP9 reverses pulmonary arterial hypertension. Nat Med 2015;21:777–85.

73. Yung LM, Yang P, Joshi S, et al. ACTRIIA-Fc rebalances activin/GDF versus BMP signaling in pulmonary hypertension. Sci Transl Med 2020;12:eaaz5660.

74. Hassoun PM, Mouthon L, Barbera JA, et al. Inflammation, growth factors, and pulmonary vascular remodeling. J Am Coll Cardiol 2009;54:S10–9.

75. Tuder RM, Chacon M, Alger L, et al. Expression of angiogenesis-related molecules in plexiform lesions in severe pulmonary hypertension: evidence for a process of disordered angiogenesis. J Pathol 2001;195:367–74.

76. Swietlik EM, Greene D, Zhu N, et al. Bayesian inference associates rare KDR Variants with specific phenotypes in pulmonary arterial hypertension. Circ Genom Precis Med 2020;14(1):e003155.

77. Izikki M, Guignabert C, Fadel E, et al. Endothelial-derived FGF2 contributes to the progression of pulmonary hypertension in humans and rodents. J Clin Invest 2009;119:512–23.

78. Schermuly RT, Dony E, Ghofrani HA, et al. Reversal of experimental pulmonary hypertension by PDGF inhibition. J Clin Invest 2005;115:2811–21.

79. Hoeper MM, Barst RJ, Bourge RC, et al. Imatinib mesylate as add-on therapy for pulmonary arterial hypertension: results of the randomized IMPRES study. Circulation 2013;127:1128–38.

80. Dahal BK, Cornitescu T, Tretyn A, et al. Role of epidermal growth factor inhibition in experimental pulmonary hypertension. Am J Respir Crit Care Med 2010;181:158–67.

81. Klein M, Schermuly RT, Ellinghaus P, et al. Combined tyrosine and serine/threonine kinase inhibition by sorafenib prevents progression of experimental pulmonary hypertension and myocardial remodeling. Circulation 2008;118:2081–90.

82. Tu L, De Man FS, Girerd B, et al. A critical role for p130Cas in the progression of pulmonary hypertension in humans and rodents. Am J Respir Crit Care Med 2012;186:666–76.

83. Christman BW, McPherson CD, Newman JH, et al. An imbalance between the excretion of thromboxane and prostacyclin metabolites in pulmonary hypertension. N Engl J Med 1992;327:70–5.

84. Stewart DJ, Levy RD, Cernacek P, et al. Increased plasma endothelin-1 in pulmonary hypertension: marker or mediator of disease? Ann Intern Med 1991;114:464–9.

85. Brittain EL, Hemnes AR. Vasodilator-responsive idiopathic pulmonary arterial hypertension: evidence for a new disease? Ann Intern Med 2015;162:148–9.

86. Galie N, Humbert M, Vachiery JL, et al. 2015 ESC/ERS guidelines for the diagnosis and treatment of pulmonary hypertension: the Joint Task Force for the Diagnosis and Treatment of Pulmonary Hypertension of the European Society of Cardiology (ESC) and the European Respiratory Society (ERS): endorsed by: Association for European Paediatric and Congenital Cardiology (AEPC), International Society for Heart and Lung Transplantation (ISHLT). Eur Heart J 2016;37:67–119.

87. Rich S, Brundage BH. High-dose calcium channel-blocking therapy for primary pulmonary hypertension: evidence for long-term reduction in pulmonary arterial pressure and regression of right ventricular hypertrophy. Circulation 1987;76:135–41.

88. Rubin LJ, Groves BM, Reeves JT, et al. Prostacyclin-induced acute pulmonary vasodilation in primary pulmonary hypertension. Circulation 1982;66:334–8.

89. Rubin LJ, Mendoza J, Hood M, et al. Treatment of primary pulmonary hypertension with continuous intravenous prostacyclin (epoprostenol). Results of a randomized trial. Ann Intern Med 1990;112:485–91.

90. Barst RJ, Rubin LJ, Long WA, et al. A comparison of continuous intravenous epoprostenol (prostacyclin) with conventional therapy for primary pulmonary hypertension. N Engl J Med 1996;334:296–301.

91. Pogoriler JE, Rich S, Archer SL, et al. Persistence of complex vascular lesions despite prolonged prostacyclin therapy of pulmonary arterial hypertension. Histopathology 2012;61:597–609.

92. Morrell NW, Morris KG, Stenmark KR. Role of angiotensin-converting enzyme and angiotensin II in development of hypoxic pulmonary hypertension. Am J Physiol 1995;269:H1186–94.

93. de Man FS, Tu L, Handoko ML, et al. Dysregulated renin-angiotensin-aldosterone system contributes to pulmonary arterial hypertension. Am J Respir Crit Care Med 2012;186:780–9.

94. Iyinikkel J, Murray F. GPCRs in pulmonary arterial hypertension: tipping the balance. Br J Pharmacol 2018;175:3063–79.

95. Humbert M, Guignabert C, Bonnet S, et al. Pathology and pathobiology of pulmonary hypertension: state of the art and research perspectives. Eur Respir J 2019;53:1801887.

96. Rot A. Endothelial cell binding of NAP-1/IL-8: role in neutrophil emigration. Immunol Today 1992;13:291–4.

97. Tanaka Y, Adams DH, Shaw S. Proteoglycans on endothelial cells present adhesion-inducing cytokines to leukocytes. Immunol Today 1993;14:111–5.

98. Yang T, Li ZN, Chen G, et al. Increased levels of plasma CXC-Chemokine Ligand 10, 12 and 16 are associated with right ventricular function in patients with idiopathic pulmonary arterial hypertension. Heart Lung 2014;43:322–7.

99. Hashimoto K, Nakamura K, Fujio H, et al. Epoprostenol therapy decreases elevated circulating levels of monocyte chemoattractant protein-1 in patients with primary pulmonary hypertension. Circ J 2004;68:227–31.

100. George PM, Oliver E, Dorfmuller P, et al. Evidence for the involvement of type I interferon in pulmonary arterial hypertension: novelty and significance. Circ Res 2014;114:677–88.

101. Zabini D, Heinemann A, Foris V, et al. Comprehensive analysis of inflammatory markers in chronic thromboembolic pulmonary hypertension patients. Eur Respir J 2014;44:951–62.

102. Olsson KM, Olle S, Fuge J, et al. CXCL13 in idiopathic pulmonary arterial hypertension and chronic thromboembolic pulmonary hypertension. Respir Res 2016;17:21.

103. Kimura H, Okada O, Tanabe N, et al. Plasma monocyte chemoattractant protein-1 and pulmonary vascular resistance in chronic thromboembolic pulmonary hypertension. Am J Respir Crit Care Med 2001;164:319–24.

104. Damas JK, Otterdal K, Yndestad A, et al. Soluble CD40 ligand in pulmonary arterial hypertension: possible pathogenic role of the interaction between platelets and endothelial cells. Circulation 2004; 110:999–1005.

105. Duncan M, Wagner BD, Murray K, et al. Circulating cytokines and growth factors in pediatric pulmonary hypertension. Mediators Inflamm 2012;2012: 143428.

106. McCullagh BN, Costello CM, Li L, et al. Elevated plasma CXCL12α is associated with a poorer prognosis in pulmonary arterial hypertension. PLoS One 2015;10:e0123709.

107. Kazimierczyk R, Blaszczak P, Jasiewicz M, et al. Increased platelet content of SDF-1alpha is associated with worse prognosis in patients with pulmonary arterial hypertension. Platelets 2018;30(4): 445–51.

108. Hoffmann-Vold AM, Hesselstrand R, Fretheim H, et al. CCL 21 as a potential serum biomarker for pulmonary arterial hypertension in Systemic Sclerosis. Arthritis Rheumatol 2018;70(10):1644–53.

109. Heresi GA, Aytekin M, Newman J, et al. CXC-chemokine ligand 10 in idiopathic pulmonary arterial hypertension: marker of improved survival. Lung 2010;188:191–7.

110. Mamazhakypov A, Viswanathan G, Lawrie A, et al. The role of chemokines and chemokine receptors in pulmonary arterial hypertension. Br J Pharmacol 2021;178(1):72–89.

111. Post JM, Hume JR, Archer SL, et al. Direct role for potassium channel inhibition in hypoxic pulmonary vasoconstriction. Am J Physiol 1992;262:C882–90.

112. Archer SL, London B, Hampl V, et al. Impairment of hypoxic pulmonary vasoconstriction in mice lacking the voltage-gated potassium channel Kv1.5. FASEB J 2001;15:1801–3.

113. Bonnet S, Michelakis ED, Porter CJ, et al. An abnormal mitochondrial-hypoxia inducible factor-1alpha-Kv channel pathway disrupts oxygen sensing and triggers pulmonary arterial hypertension in fawn hooded rats: similarities to human pulmonary arterial hypertension. Circulation 2006;113: 2630–41.

114. Ma L, Roman-Campos D, Austin ED, et al. A novel channelopathy in pulmonary arterial hypertension. N Engl J Med 2013;369:351–61.

115. Antigny F, Hautefort A, Meloche J, et al. potassium channel subfamily K member 3 (KCNK3) contributes to the development of pulmonary arterial hypertension. Circulation 2016;133:1371–85.

116. Savai R, Al-Tamari HM, Sedding D, et al. Pro-proliferative and inflammatory signaling converge on FoxO1 transcription factor in pulmonary hypertension. Nat Med 2014;20:1289–300.

117. Bourgeois A, Lambert C, Habbout K, et al. FOXM1 promotes pulmonary artery smooth muscle cell expansion in pulmonary arterial hypertension. J Mol Med 2018;96:223–35.

118. Alastalo TP, Li M, Perez Vde J, et al. Disruption of PPARgamma/beta-catenin-mediated regulation of apelin impairs BMP-induced mouse and human pulmonary arterial EC survival. J Clin Invest 2011; 121:3735–46.

119. Chun HJ, Bonnet S, Chan SY. Translational advances in the field of pulmonary hypertension. Translating MicroRNA biology in pulmonary hypertension. It will take more than "miR" words. Am J Respir Crit Care Med 2017;195:167–78.

120. Santos-Ferreira CA, Abreu MT, Marques CI, et al. Micro-RNA analysis in pulmonary arterial hypertension: current knowledge and challenges. JACC Basic Transl Sci 2020;5:1149–62.

121. Omura J, Habbout K, Shimauchi T, et al. Identification of long noncoding RNA H19 as a new biomarker and therapeutic target in right ventricular failure in pulmonary arterial hypertension. Circulation 2020;142:1464–84.

122. Zehendner CM, Valasarajan C, Werner A, et al. Long noncoding RNA TYKRIL plays a role in pulmonary hypertension via the p53-mediated regulation of PDGFRbeta. Am J Respir Crit Care Med 2020;202:1445–57.

Update on Medical Management of Pulmonary Arterial Hypertension

Alexander E. Sherman, MD[a], Rajan Saggar, MD[b],
Richard N. Channick, MD[b],*

KEYWORDS

- Pulmonary arterial hypertension • Pulmonary hypertension • Medical management • Therapy
- Treatment

KEY POINTS

- Translational research over the past 25 years has led to targeted therapies for pulmonary arterial hypertension
- Upfront combination therapy targeting the endothelin, nitric oxide, and prostacyclin pathways have demonstrated significant clinical benefit
- Aggressive, goal-directed therapy improves patient outcomes and medical therapy has changed pulmonary arterial hypertension from an untreatable fatal disease to a highly manageable condition.

INTRODUCTION

Pulmonary arterial hypertension (PAH) is characterized by pulmonary microvascular remodeling, leading to a progressive increase in pulmonary vascular resistance (PVR); untreated, it results in right ventricular failure and death. In 2019, the World Symposium on Pulmonary Hypertension updated the hemodynamic definitions and clinical classifications of pulmonary hypertension to include a mean pulmonary arterial pressure of 20 mm Hg or greater with pulmonary artery occlusion pressure of 15 mm Hg or less and PVR of more than 3 Wood units.[1] Risk stratification using clinical and hemodynamic parameters drives management decisions, and the progressive nature of PAH has led to recommendations involving aggressive combination therapy earlier in the disease course.

The pathogenesis of PAH (group 1 of the clinical classification of pulmonary hypertension) is complex and the implicated pathways remain central to modern medical therapy. Vasculature remodeling causes smooth muscle cell proliferation, intimal hyperplasia, and inflammation. Currently approved medical therapies target 3 mechanistic pathways: excess endothelin (ET) activity, abnormal nitric oxide (NO) activity, and prostacyclin (PGI$_2$) deficiency.

DISCUSSION

Endothelin Receptor Antagonists

ETs are an important class of regulatory molecules involved in vascular smooth muscle tone. Since the discovery of ET-1 in 1988,[2,3] 2 additional peptides, ET-2 and ET-3, have been identified.[4] The 2 receptors for these molecules are ET receptor A (ET$_A$) and ET receptor B, which are both expressed on pulmonary vascular smooth muscle and endothelial cells. Targeting these receptors with ET

[a] Division of Pulmonary, Critical Care, Sleep Medicine, Clinical Immunology and Allergy, David Geffen School of Medicine at UCLA, 650 Charles E. Young Drive South 43-229 CHS, Los Angeles, CA 90095-1690, USA;
[b] Pulmonary Vascular Disease Program, Acute and Chronic Thromboembolic Disease Program, Pulmonary and Critical Care Division, Division of Pulmonary, Critical Care, & Sleep Medicine, David Geffen School of Medicine at UCLA, 650 Charles E. Young Drive South 43-229 CHS, Los Angeles, CA 90095-1690, USA
* Corresponding author.
E-mail address: rchannick@mednet.ucla.edu

Cardiol Clin 40 (2022) 13–27
https://doi.org/10.1016/j.ccl.2021.08.002

receptor antagonists (ERAs) remains a fundamental component of PAH treatment.[5]

ET-1 production is regulated by vascular endothelial cells to control vascular tone, and its interaction with ET_A in pulmonary vascular smooth muscle cells results in the release of intracellular calcium and vasoconstriction that persists beyond the ET-1–ET_A receptor interaction.[6] Under normal physiologic circumstances, ET-1 activates ET receptor B receptors on endothelial cells resulting in vasodilation mediated by PGI_2 and NO pathways, negative feedback and downregulation of ET-1 production, and ET-1 clearance. In pulmonary hypertension, ET-1 serum concentrations are elevated and ET-1 is found in higher amounts in pulmonary arterial smooth muscle cells.[7–9]

All 3 currently approved ERAs carry a risk of embryo–fetal toxicity and are likely to cause major birth defects based on animal studies. Pregnancy must be excluded before the initiation of treatment in women and prevented with 2 reliable forms of birth control during and up to at least 1 month after stopping therapy. A decrease in sperm counts have been observed in patients on ERA therapy. Peripheral edema is common in the progression of pulmonary hypertension, has been observed after initiation of ERA therapy, and may necessitate drug discontinuation if refractory to medical management.

Bosentan (Tracleer) is an ERA with slight affinity for ET_A over ET receptor B and was the first oral medication approved for the management of PAH. In BREATHE-1, bosentan demonstrated improved PVR, patient exercise capacity by the 6-minute walk test (6MWT), and time to clinical worsening.[10,11] Unlike other currently approved ERAs, bosentan is available for twice daily dosing in both tablet form (62.5 mg and 125.0 mg) and oral suspension (32 mg), allowing for nasogastric administration; however, it carries a risk of hepatotoxicity[12] and requires monthly monitoring of liver function tests. Owing to its significant induction of CYP3A and CYP2C9, bosentan is contraindicated with cyclosporin A and glyburide.

Ambrisentan (Letairis) predominantly affects ET_A and was approved in 2007 at 5 or 10 mg once daily dosing after the ARIES-1 and ARIES-2 randomized placebo-controlled trials demonstrated improvement in 6MWT and time to clinical worsening.[13] Ambrisentan is contraindicated in patients with idiopathic pulmonary fibrosis after it demonstrated an increased risk of disease progression or death in patients with idiopathic pulmonary fibrosis, regardless of pulmonary hypertension in the ARTEMIS-IPF study.[14]

Macitentan (Opsumit) is a dual ERA approved at 10 mg once daily dosing in 2013 after the SERAPHIN trial demonstrated a decrease in morbidity and mortality in patients with PAH.[15] The composite primary outcomes of events related to PAH or any-cause death was reduced by 45% in patients on 10 mg macitentan compared with placebo (**Fig. 1**). A PAH-related event was worsening PAH, need for intravenous or subcutaneous PGI_2 medication, lung transplantation, or atrial septostomy. Worsening PAH was defined as a decrease of 15% in the 6MWT from baseline, worsening symptoms of PAH, and the need for additional PAH treatment. Secondary end points included demonstrated improvement in World Health Organization (WHO) functional class and 6MWT.

Nitric Oxide Pathway Agents

NO production is chronically impaired in PAH. NO, produced in endothelial cells, is a vasoactive mediator that increases cyclic guanosine monophosphate (cGMP) production by activating soluble guanylate cyclase. Release of cGMP results in vasodilation and inhibits smooth muscle cell proliferation.[16,17] An increase in cGMP is accomplished either by the phosphodiesterase type-5 inhibitors (PDE5i) sildenafil and tadalafil, which block cGMP breakdown, or directly by the soluble guanylate cyclase stimulator, riociguat.

Sildenafil (Revatio) is a PDE5i approved for PAH at 20 mg based on improvement of exercise capacity by 6MWT in the SUPER trial.[18] The 20-mg 3 times daily regimen improved 6MWT equivalently to higher doses, despite a dose-dependent improvement in the mean pulmonary artery pressure, cardiac index, and PVR up to 80 mg 3 times

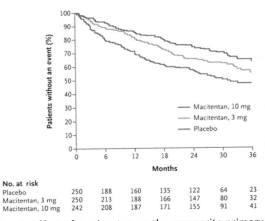

Fig. 1. Effect of macitentan on the composite primary end point of a first event related to PAH or death from any cause. (*From* Pulido T, Adzerikho I, Channick RN, et al. Macitentan and Morbidity and Mortality in Pulmonary Arterial Hypertension. N Engl J Med. 2013;369(9):809-818; with permission.)

daily. Some clinicians do use higher doses in practice. Sildenafil is available as a tablet, oral suspension, or for intravenous use.

Tadalafil (Adcirca, Alyq) is a longer acting PDE5i approved for PAH in 2009. The PHIRST trial demonstrated that 40 mg once daily of tadalafil increased 6MWT after 16 weeks of therapy, even in patients already on background therapy with bosentan.[13] Time to clinical worsening (defined as death, lung or heart–lung transplantation, atrial septostomy, hospitalization owing to worsening PAH, initiation of new PAH therapy, or worsening WHO functional class) was improved in the tadalafil 40 mg group compared with placebo, with incidence of clinical worsening demonstrating a relative risk reduction of 68% ($P = .038$). Similar to sildenafil, tadalafil is contraindicated with the use of nitrates, and both medications carry similar adverse effect profiles. These include headache, flushing, myalgia, and dyspepsia, which typically improve or resolve over time and rarely result in the need for drug discontinuation. Transitions between sildenafil and tadalafil are generally well-tolerated.[19]

Riociguat (Adempas) is an soluble guanylate cyclase stimulator and directly increases cGMP, acting downstream of endogenous NO.[20] To date, it is the only agent approved for inoperable or postoperative chronic thromboembolic pulmonary hypertension. The PATENT-1[21] and CHEST-1[22] trials showed improvement in 6MWT in patients with PAH and patients with chronic thromboembolic pulmonary hypertension with 2.5 mg 3 times daily therapy, respectively. This effect was shown in both treatment-naïve patients and those on background ERA or PGI₂ analogue therapy in PATENT-1. A decrease in PVR and N-terminal pro brain natriuretic peptide and improvement in WHO functional class were also observed in both trials. The adverse effects of riociguat include headache, dyspepsia, dizziness, and hypotension. The average decrease in mean arterial pressure in both trials was 9 mm Hg, thus requiring a slow uptitration to the target dose of 2.5 mg 3 times daily. Riociguat is typically started at 1 mg 3 times daily and increased every 2 weeks by 0.5 mg 3 times daily if systolic blood pressure remains greater than 95 mm Hg. When studied in combination with sildenafil, there was no evidence of a positive benefit–risk ratio and more pronounced hypotension.[23] As such, riociguat is contraindicated with nitrates and PDE5i. Unlike PDE5i medications, riociguat is contraindicated in pregnancy.

Given its known deficiency in PAH and the role of drugs indirectly increasing NO, inhaled NO (iNO) is a logical therapeutic agent; iNO was approved in 1999 for the treatment of neonates with pulmonary hypertension.[24,25] Despite a lack of clinical trial data, iNO is recommended for use in acute vasoreactivity testing to identify patients with PAH who may have a long-term clinical and hemodynamic effect from calcium channel blockers[26] and is also used postoperatively after cardiothoracic surgery and for acute right ventricular failure.[27,28] The inhaled route offers theoretic advantages over systemic administration of medication. By directly delivering medication to the target organ, a greater local concentration may be attained with lower systemic levels, decreasing systemic toxicity. Portable iNO has demonstrated hemodynamic effects,[29] and strategies to leverage this factor for long-term ambulatory use are still under investigation.[30]

Prostacyclin Pathway Agents

PGI₂ is a potent vasodilator and inhibitor of platelet aggregation, with an important role in maintaining vascular homeostasis. Its actions are mediated by the IP receptor, causing cyclic adenosine monophosphate production, leading to marked vasodilation and inhibition of smooth muscle cell proliferation.[31,32] There are currently 3 FDA-approved PGI₂ analogues: epoprostenol, iloprost, and treprostinil, as well as an IP receptor agonist, selexipag.

Epoprostenol (Veletri, Flolan), a synthetic form of PGI₂, was the first approved PAH-specific drug in 1996. It requires a pH of 10 for stability in solution and its half-life is 3 to 6 minutes at physiologic conditions, requiring a continuous infusion by intravenous pump.[33] Epoprostenol is a highly effective therapy and is the only PAH therapy shown to improve survival in a randomized controlled trial. The primary end point of this 12-week prospective trial in 81 patients with severe PAH was the 6MWT, where it showed a 31-m improvement compared with placebo, and no patients on epoprostenol died compared with 8 patients in the conventional therapy group.[34] Given its proven efficacy in severe PAH, epoprostenol is recommended as the first-line therapy for patients with WHO functional class IV symptoms and a high risk profile with evidence of right heart failure.[35] PGI₂ side effects are common, may be dose limiting, and include headache, jaw pain, flushing, diarrhea, nausea, and vomiting.[36] Infusions are typically initiated at 1 to 2 ng/kg/min and may be increased in small increments until dose-limiting effects are elicited. Pretreatment or aggressive treatment of transient side effects may improve tolerability during dose escalation. This treatment efficacy must be balanced against significant challenges associated with treatment, including the need for a chronic indwelling venous catheter, daily preparation of the medication, and experience operating a pump with fleeting windows for troubleshooting owing to the short medication half-life.

Treprostinil (Remodulin [IV/SQ], Tyvaso [IH], Orenitram [PO]) is a more stable PGI_2 analogue with a half-life of 4 to 6 hours. It is approved as a continuous intravenous or subcutaneous infusion and also as an intermittent inhaled or oral formulation. Subcutaneous delivery was shown to improve 6MWT by 16 m versus placebo and avoids the need for an indwelling intravenous catheter, but may cause significant infusion site reactions and pain in some patients.[37] As with epoprostenol, a gradual dose escalation to ensure tolerance is required to achieve maximal efficacy. Transitions between epoprostenol and treprostinil infusions have been shown to be safe and effective.[38,39]

Inhaled treprostinil is administered 4 times daily with a goal dose of 9 inhalations (54 μg) at each dose by handheld nebulizer. Primarily studied as an add-on therapy to oral agents, inhaled treprostinil gained FDA approval in 2011 after showing an improved 6MWT in patients with PAH.[40] More recent data in patients with pulmonary hypertension owing to interstitial lung disease not on background therapy found the 6MWT to be increased at 12 weeks compared with placebo.[41] Inhaled treprostinil is dosed in 4 equally spaced treatment sessions during waking hours, with initial therapy typically starting with 3 breaths per treatment session. If tolerated, regular dose increases until the target dose of 9 breaths per treatment is recommended. If adverse events prevent reaching 9 breaths 4 times per day, the maximum tolerated dose should be continued.

Iloprost (Ventavis) is a shorter acting inhaled PGI_2 that requires 6 to 9 inhalations of 2.5 to 5.0 μg each day, which may limit its widespread use despite also being shown to improve exercise capacity.[42] Inhaled therapy has theoretic advantages, including direct delivery to the site of action, ideally with fewer systemic side effects, although transient cough and throat irritation have been noted.

There are currently 2 FDA-approved oral agents acting on the PGI_2 pathway that are particularly appealing given the challenges associated with parenteral and inhaled therapy. Initially approved by the FDA in 2002, oral treprostinil (Orenitram) monotherapy demonstrated improved 6MWT in treatment-naïve patients with PAH with WHO functional class II or III symptoms in the FREEDOM-M trial.[43] The FREEDOM-C trial examined oral treprostinil as add-on therapy to background ERA and/or PDE5i therapy, but failed to meet its primary exercise tolerance end point. Although this outcome was attributed to the dosing strategy and high rates of adverse events

limiting tolerability, the follow-up FREEDOM C2 trial also did not show significant improvement in 6MWT or time to clinical worsening despite having smaller doses available for slower uptitration.[44,45] The more recent FREEDOM-EV trial demonstrated lower rates of clinical worsening (26% vs 36% for placebo; $P = .039$) in patients with PAH on background nonprostanoid monotherapy. A post hoc analysis restratified the group into a higher versus lower risk group (defined by at least 2 of 3: WHO functional class I–II, 6MWT >440 m, and N-terminal pro brain natriuretic peptide of <300) showing a more pronounced effect of oral treprostinil therapy in the higher risk group with hazard ratio 0.64 (95% confidence interval, 0.46–0.88; $P = .006$)[46] The recommended starting dose for oral treprostinil is 0.250 mg 2 times a day or 0.125 mg 3 times daily and is usually increased by either 0.25 to 0.50 mg 2 times a day or 0.125 mg 3 times daily every 3 to 4 days as tolerated. The maximum dose is determined by tolerability. Assuming a 70-kg patient, 1 mg 2 times a day of oral treprostinil is approximately equivalent to 10 ng/kg/min of infused treprostinil. Similar to other PGI_2 agents, the most common adverse events are headache, diarrhea, flushing, nausea, and vomiting.

Selexipag (Uptravi) is a selective PGI_2 receptor (IP receptor) agonist approved in 2015 based on the GRIPHON trial. The GRIPHON trial demonstrated a composite end point of mortality or morbidity, including disease progression or worsening of PAH resulting in hospitalization, initiation of parenteral prostanoid therapy or long-term oxygen therapy, or need for either lung transplantation or atrial septostomy (**Fig. 2**).[47] The starting dose is 200 μg twice daily, increased by 200 μg at weekly intervals to a maximum of 1600 μg twice daily as tolerated. The maintenance dose is determined by tolerability of side effects, the most common of which are headache, diarrhea, jaw pain, nausea, myalgias, vomiting, extremity pain, and flushing. If side effects cannot be tolerated, then a dose decrease should occur. Ingestion with food increases the time to maximum plasma levels and may improve tolerability. CYP2C8 inhibitors increase exposure of selexipag and its active metabolites, and the drug is dosed only once daily in patients with moderate (Childs–Pugh class B) hepatic impairment, and it should be avoided in patients with severe hepatic impairment.

TREATMENT STRATEGIES
Risk Stratification

After making a diagnosis of PAH, the use of risk stratification in determining the optimal treatment strategy for patients is paramount, and in line

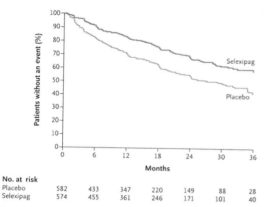

Fig. 2. Effect of selexipag on composite end point of death from any cause or a complication related to PAH (disease progression or worsening of PAH that resulted in hospitalization, initiation of parenteral prostanoid therapy or long-term oxygen therapy, or the need for lung transplantation or balloon atrial septostomy). (*From* Sitbon O, Channick R, Chin KM, et al. Selexipag for the Treatment of Pulmonary Arterial Hypertension. N Engl J Med. 2015;373(26):2522-2533; with permission.)

with recommendations from the World Symposium on Pulmonary Hypertension.[35] There are several registries used for risk stratification including the REVEAL, COMPERA, and French Pulmonary Hypertension Network. Low-risk profiles are associated with improved outcomes and achieving these parameters may serve as a guide for medical therapy.

The REVEAL 2.0 calculator defines low risk patients as 12-month mortality of 2.6% or less and uses a multimodality approach, including clinicodemographic data, vital signs, history of all-cause hospitalizations, 6MWT, brain natriuretic peptide, presence of pericardial effusion on echocardiogram, diffusion capacity for carbon monoxide, and hemodynamic parameters.[48] The COMPERA registry was used to distinguish low-, medium-, and high-risk patients with PAH based on WHO functional class, 6MWT, brain natriuretic peptide or *N*-terminal pro brain natriuretic peptide, right atrial pressure, cardiac index, and mixed venous oxygen saturation.[49] The European Society of Cardiology/European Respiratory Society guidelines use the French registry with 4 criteria defining low risk: WHO functional class I or II, 6MWT of greater than 440 m, right atrial pressure of less than 8 mm Hg, and cardiac index of 2.5 L/min/m² or greater. Assessed at baseline and at the first follow-up visit within 1 year, patients who achieved all 4 low-risk criteria had transplant-free survival rate of 91% at 5 years. Patients with 3 or 4 low-risk criteria at first follow-up

had a 1-year mortality risk of 0% to 1% compared with those who met zero or 1 low-risk feature with a 1-year mortality of between 13% and 30%.[50]

Combination Therapy Strategies

The majority of patients with PAH will require combination therapy using agents targeting the ERA, PDE5i, and PGI₂ pathways, and there have been several studies examining the tolerability and outcomes associated with combination therapy. In all of the recent large trials, including SERAPHIN[15] and GRIPHON,[47] the majority of the patients were on background PAH therapy. Although these studies examined sequential combination therapy, the landmark AMBITION trial compared upfront combination oral therapy with monotherapy with favorable results, serving as key evidence for the recommendation for upfront dual oral therapy for most patients (**Fig. 3**).[35]

The AMBITION trial examined combination tadalafil and ambrisentan therapy with a combined primary end point of any-cause mortality, hospitalization for worsening PAH, disease progression (worsening WHO functional class and 6MWT), or unsatisfactory long-term clinical response. This study showed that combination therapy had a hazard ratio of 0.5 (95% confidence interval, 0.35–0.72) versus pooled monotherapy, with 18% of combination therapy patients reaching the primary end point versus 34% on ambrisentan monotherapy and 28% on tadalafil monotherapy.[51] **Table 1** summaries the currently available medications for PAH.[52]

Use of Pulmonary Arterial Hypertension Therapy in Non–Group 1 Pulmonary Hypertension

The accurate identification of the underlying etiology is a crucial step in the diagnosis and treatment of PAH. This review discussed the currently approved drugs for the medical management of PAH (ie, group 1 pulmonary hypertension) and how they are used in modern treatment strategies; however, it is essential that targeted therapies are used in patients with appropriate types of pulmonary hypertension. For instance, the most common cause of pulmonary hypertension in developed countries is group 2, owing to left heart disease; however, the FIRST trial was halted early owing to increased mortality in these patients when treated with epoprostenol.[53] Agents targeting the ET and NO pathways have shown mixed results when used in group 2 pulmonary hypertension and targeted PAH therapy is not recommended.[54] As discussed elsewhere in this article, IH treprostinil was recently found to improve 6MWT in patients with

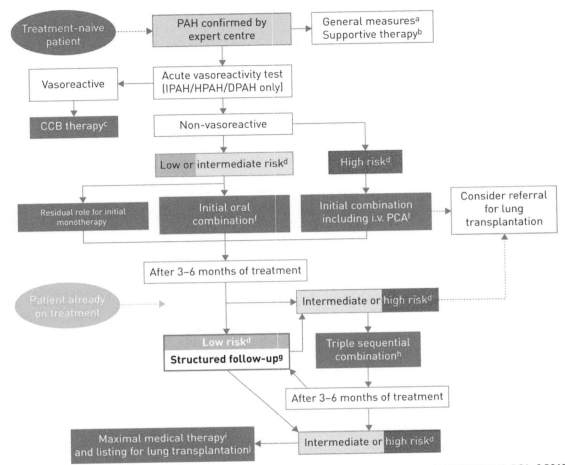

Fig. 3. Treatment algorithm for PAH from the sixth World Symposium on PH. CCB, IPAH/HPAH/DPAH, PCA. [a] 2015 ESC/ERS PH guidelines Table 16; [b] 2015 ESC/ERS PH guidelines Table 17; [c] 2015 ESC/ERS PH guidelines Table 18; [d] 2015 ESC/ERS PH guidelines Table 13; [e] 2015 ESC/ERS PH guidelines Table 19; [f] 2015 ESC/ERS PH guidelines Table 20; [g] 2015 ESC/ERS PH guidelines Table 14; [h] 2015 ESC/ERS PH guidelines Table 21; [i] maximal medical therapy is considered triple combination therapy including a s.c. or an i.v. PCA (i.v. preferred in high-risk status); [j] 2015 ESC/ERS PH guidelines Table 22. (*From* Galiè N, Channick RN, Frantz RP, et al. Risk stratification and medical therapy of pulmonary arterial hypertension. Eur Respir J. 2019;53(1). Reproduced with permission of the © ERS 2021; DOI: 10.1183/13993003.01889-2018 Published 24 January 2019.)

underlying interstitial lung disease. Treatment with sildenafil is not recommended for patients with group 5 pulmonary hypertension associated with sickle cell disease after sildenafil was associated with increased rates of hospitalization for pain episodes in the Walk-PHaSST trial.[55]

EMERGING THERAPIES AND FUTURE DIRECTIONS

As discussed elsewhere in this article, currently approved medications for PAH target 3 pathways: ET, NO, and PGI$_2$. Still, the pathogenesis of PAH and its downstream effects leading to pulmonary vascular remodeling and ultimately right

ventricular failure are complex and involve inflammation, oxidative stress, growth factor activation, imbalance of proliferative and anti-proliferative signaling, and altered hormonal signaling. New pathways and drugs are under investigation for PAH treatment.[56]

Mutations affecting the bone morphogenetic protein receptor type II are the most common genetic causes of PAH with poorer outcomes compared with other causes of PAH.[57] Bone morphogenetic protein receptor type II mutations lead to transforming growth factor-β receptor overexpression, making it a viable therapeutic target. Sotatercept—a fusion protein that sequesters transforming growth factor-β ligands, thereby

Table 1
Clinical trials of PAH-specific therapies

Clinical Trials	No.	Duration (Weeks)	Background PAH-Specific Therapy	Comparator Group(s)	Primary End Point	Results (S or NS)	PMID
Oral PAH-specific therapies							
Sildenafil							
SUPER 2005	277	12	No	Placebo	Δ 6MWD	6MWD improved (S), TTCW not improved (NS)	16291984
SERAPH 2005	26	16	No	Bosentan	Δ RV mass	Significant reduction in RV mass (S), 6MWD improved (S)	15750042
Singh et al. 2006	20	6	No	Placebo	Δ 6MWD	6MWD improved (S)	16569546
Badesch et al. 2007	84	12	No	Placebo	Δ 6MWD	6MWD improved (S)	17985403
PACES 2008	267	16	Epoprostenol	Placebo	Δ 6MWD	6MWD improved (S), TTCW improved (S)	18935500
Vizza et al. 2017	103	12	Bosentan	Placebo	Δ 6MWD	6MWD not improved (NS)	28874133
Tadalafil							
PHIRST 2009	405	16	No, or bosentan (54%)	Placebo	Δ 6MWD	6MWD improved (S), TTCW improved (S)	19470885
AMBITION 2015	500	78	No (but 1 of the 3 study arms was upfront combination therapy with tadalafil and ambrisentan)	Ambrisentan monotherapy or tadalafil monotherapy	TTCF (including death)	TTCF improved (S), 6MWD improved (S)	26308684
Ambrisentan							
ARIES-1 2008	202	12	No	Placebo	Δ 6MWD	6MWD improved (S), TTCW not improved (NS)	18506008

(continued on next page)

Table 1
(continued)

Clinical Trials	No.	Duration (Weeks)	Background PAH-Specific Therapy	Comparator Group(s)	Primary End Point	Results (S or NS)	PMID
ARIES-2 2008	192	12	No	Placebo	Δ 6MWD	6MWD improved (S), TTCW improved (S)	18506008
AMBITION 2015	500	78	No (but 1 of the 3 study arms was upfront combination therapy with tadalafil and ambrisentan)	Ambrisentan monotherapy or tadalafil monotherapy	TTCF (including death)	TTCF improved (S), 6MWD improved (S)	26308684
Bosentan							
Channick et al.[11] 2001	32	12	No	Placebo	Δ 6MWD	6MWD improved (S), TTCW improved (S)	11597664
BREATHE-1 2002	213	16	No	Placebo	Δ 6MWD	6MWD improved (S), TTCW improved (S)	11907289
BREATHE-2 2004	33	16	Epoprostenol	Placebo	Δ PVR	PVR not improved (NS), 6MWD not improved (NS)	15358690
BREATHE-5 2006	54	16	No	Placebo	SaO_2, PVR	SaO_2 not reduced, PVR improved (S), 6MWD improved (S)	16801459
EARLY 2008	185	24	No, or sildenafil (16%)	Placebo	Δ PVR and Δ 6MWD	PVR improved (S), 6MWD not improved (NS)	18572079
COMPASS-2 2015	334	16	Sildenafil	Placebo	TTCW (including death)	TTCW not improved (NS), 6MWD improved (S)	26113687
Macitentan							
SERAPHIN 2013	742	115	No, or PDESi (61%), or oral (5%) or inhaled prostanoid	Placebo	TTCW (including death)	TTCW improved (S)	23984728

Study	N	Duration (weeks)	Background therapy	Comparator	Primary endpoint	Results	Reference
MERIT-1 2017	80	16	No, or PDE5i only (46%), or PDE5i + oral or inhaled prostanoid (13%), or oral or inhaled prostanoid alone (3%)	Placebo	Δ PVR	PVR improved (S), 6MWD improved (S)	28919201
Riociguat							
PATENT-1 2013	443	12	No, or ERA (44% - mostly bosentan), or prostanoid (6% - mostly inhaled iloprost)	Placebo	Δ 6MWD	6MWD improved (S), TTCW improved (S), PVR improved (S)	23383378
CHEST-1 2013	261	16	No	Placebo	Δ 6MWD	6MWD improved (S), PVR improved (S)	23383377
PATENT PLUS 2015	18	12	Sildenafil	Placebo	Δ Supine SBP	Terminated owing to excess SAE in the treatment group and no clear benefit	25657022
RESPITE 2017	61	24	ERA	None	Δ 6MWD, Δ NT-proBNP, Δ WHO-FC, Δ hemodynamics	6MWD improved (S), NT-proBNP WHO-FC improved (S), hemody	28889107
REPLACE 2020	226	24	ERA	PDE5i	Clinical improvement	Clinical improvement (S)	33773120
Selexipag							
GRIPHON 2015	1156	71	No, or ERA (15%), PDE5i (32%), or both (33%)	Placebo	TTCW (including death)	TTCW improved (S)	26699168
TRITON 2020	247	26	Macitentan and tadalafil	Placebo	Δ PVR	PVR not improved (NS), 6MWD not improved (NS), TTCW not improved (NS)	NCT02558231

(continued on next page)

Table 1
(continued)

Clinical Trials	No.	Duration (Weeks)	Background PAH-Specific Therapy	Comparator Group(s)	Primary End Point	Results (S or NS)	PMID
Oral treprostinil							
FREEDOM-C 2012	350	16	ERA and/or PDE-5i	Placebo	Δ 6MWD	6MWD not improved (NS), TTCW not improved (NS)	22628490
FREEDOM-C2 2013	310	16	ERA and/or PDE-5i	Placebo	Δ 6MWD	6MWD not improved (NS), TTCW not improved (NS)	23669822
FREEDOM-M 2013	349	12	No	Placebo	Δ 6MWD	6MWD improved (S), TTCW not improved (NS)	23307827
FREEDOM-EV 2020	690	22	ERA alone (28%), or PDE5i or soluble guanylate cyclase stimulator alone (72%)	Placebo	TTCW	TTCW improved (S), 6MWD not improved (NS)	31765604
Parenteral and inhaled PAH-specific therapies							
Epoprostenol							
Rubin et al.[20] 1990	23	8	No	Conventional therapy[a]	Δ 6MWD and Δ pulmonary hemodynamics	6MWD improved (NS), pulmonary hemodynamics improved (NS)	2107780
Barst et al.[34] 1996	81	12	No	Conventional therapy[a]	Δ 6MWD	6MWD improved (S), PVR and mPAP improved (S), survival improved (S)	8532025
Badesch et al. 2000	111	12	No	Conventional therapy[a]	Δ 6MWD	6MWD improved (S), PVR and mPAP improved (S)	10733441

Treprostinil

Study	N	Duration	Background therapy	Comparator	Primary endpoint	Results	PMID
Simonneau et al. 2002	470	12	No	Placebo	Δ 6MWD	6MWD improved (S), PVR and mPAP improved (S)	11897647
TRUST 2010	44	12	No	Placebo	Δ 6MWD	6MWD improved (S), TTCW improved in a post hoc analysis (S)	20022264
TRIUMPH I 2010	235	12	Bosentan (70%) or sildenafil (30%)	Placebo	Δ 6MWD	6MWD improved (S), TTCW not improved (NS)	20430262

Iloprost

Study	N	Duration	Background therapy	Comparator	Primary endpoint	Results	PMID
AIR 2002	203	12	No	Placebo	Δ 6MWD and WHO-FC	6MWD & WHO-FC improved (S), PVR improved (S), TTCW not improved (NS)	12151469
STEP 2006	67	12	Bosentan	Placebo	Δ 6MWD	6MWD improved (S), TTCW improved (S)	16946127
COMBI 2006	40	12	Bosentan	Bosentan monotherapy	Δ 6MWD	Terminated for futility, 6MWD not improved (NS)	17012628

Abbreviations: 6MWD, 6-min walk distance; CCB, calcium channel blocker; IPAH, idiopathic PAH; mPAP, mean pulmonary artery pressure; N/A, not applicable; NS, not statistically significant; NT-pro BNP, N-terminal pro brain natriuretic peptide; S, statistically significant; SAE, serious adverse effect; SaO$_2$, systemic arterial blood oxygen saturation; TTCF, time to clinical failure; TTCW, time to clinical worsening.

[a] Could include CCB, warfarin, supplemental oxygen, digoxin, and/or diuretics, as deemed appropriate.

Adapted from Mayeux JD, Pan IZ, Dechand J, Jacobs JA, Jones TL, McKellar SH, Beck E, Hatton ND, Ryan JJ. Management of Pulmonary Arterial Hypertension. Curr Cardiovasc Risk Rep. 2021;15(1):2; adapted with permission.

decreasing transforming growth factor-β signaling—is being investigated as a novel therapy for PAH. The PULSAR phase II clinical trial (https://clinicaltrials.gov/ct2/show/NCT03496207) enrolled 106 patients with PAH on standard therapy, and preliminary results indicated improvements after 6 weeks in right heart strain, exercise capacity, and a decrease in PVR compared with placebo.[58] SPECTRA (https://clinicaltrials.gov/ct2/show/NCT03738150), a related trial, is examining the effects of sotatercept in adults with PAH and WHO functional class III symptoms.

The role of inflammation in vascular remodeling and progression of PAH is being further recognized, leading to clinical trials targeting signaling factors involved in implicated pathways (eg, IL-1, IL-6, C-reactive protein, tumor necrosis factor-α, monocyte chemoattractant protein-1).[59–61] Anti–IL-1 and anti–IL-6 therapies such as anakinra and tocilizumab have been examined for their use in PAH.[62,63]

Plasmablasts in idiopathic PAH have shown clonality similar to that seen in autoimmune diseases, leading to investigation of rituximab, a B-cell–depleting medication for the treatment of PAH associated with systemic sclerosis. Initial studies have demonstrated safety and biomarkers may identify patients more likely to respond to treatment.[64]

Imatinib, a medication approved for some forms of cancer, has potential benefits on pulmonary blood flow and exercise tolerance, but has only been prescribed for compassionate use owing to safety and tolerability concerns.[65] It remains under investigation, including alternate routes of delivery (ie, inhaled).[66]

SUMMARY

Over the past 25 years, PAH has evolved from an untreatable fatal disease to a highly manageable condition. Translational research has led to breakthroughs in targeted therapies directed toward the ET, NO, and PGI$_2$ pathways. These treatments produce clinically important benefits, especially when used in combination in a goal-directed approach.

CLINICS CARE POINTS

- Multimodality risk stratification should guide initial therapy for patients with PAH with a goal to achieve low-risk status.
- Combination therapy leveraging the ET, NO, and/or PGI$_2$ pathways is appropriate for the majority of patients with PAH.

- Individual medications for PAH have varying adverse effect profiles and degrees of patient burden, which should be considered to maximize treatment tolerability.
- Calcium channel blocker therapy provides a sustained hemodynamic benefit in less than 10% of patients, and vasoreactivity testing to identify this uncommon group is recommended in idiopathic PAH, heritable PAH, or drug-induced PAH.
- Intravenous epoprostenol is the recommended therapy for patients with severe PAH and evidence of right ventricular failure given its proven efficacy and mortality benefit.
- Uptitration of PAH therapy, especially for agents acting on the PGI$_2$ pathway, requires careful attention to adverse side effects.

DISCLOSURE

A.E. Sherman has no relevant financial disclosures. R. Saggar is a consultant for Altavant, Third Pole, Acceleron, Janssen. Consultant and Speaker for United Therapeutics. R.N. Channick is a consultant for several companies producing PAH medications, including Janssen, Bayer, Gossamer, United Therapeutics, and Third Pole. He is a speaker on pulmonary arterial hypertension for Janssen and Bayer.

REFERENCES

1. Simonneau G, Montani D, Celermajer DS, et al. Haemodynamic definitions and updated clinical classification of pulmonary hypertension. Eur Respir J 2019;53(1):1801913.
2. Yanagisawa M, Inoue A, Takuwa Y, et al. The human preproendothelin-1 gene: possible regulation by endothelial phosphoinositide turnover signaling. J Cardiovasc Pharmacol 1989;13(Suppl 5):S13–7 [discussion S18].
3. Clarke JG, Benjamin N, Larkin SW, et al. Endothelin is a potent long-lasting vasoconstrictor in men. Am J Physiol 1989;257(6 Pt 2):H2033–5.
4. Firth JD, Ratcliffe PJ. Organ distribution of the three rat endothelin messenger RNAs and the effects of ischemia on renal gene expression. J Clin Invest 1992;90(3):1023–31.
5. Dupuis J, Hoeper MM. Endothelin receptor antagonists in pulmonary arterial hypertension. Eur Respir J 2008;31(2):407–15.
6. Channick RN, Sitbon O, Barst RJ, et al. Endothelin receptor antagonists in pulmonary arterial hypertension. J Am Coll Cardiol 2004;43(12 Suppl S):62S–7S.

7. Stewart DJ, Levy RD, Cernacek P, et al. Increased plasma endothelin-1 in pulmonary hypertension: marker or mediator of disease? Ann Intern Med 1991;114(6):464–9.

8. Giaid A, Yanagisawa M, Langleben D, et al. Expression of endothelin-1 in the lungs of patients with pulmonary hypertension. N Engl J Med 1993;328(24): 1732–9.

9. Davie N, Haleen SJ, Upton PD, et al. ETA and ETB receptors modulate the proliferation of human pulmonary artery smooth muscle cells. Am J Respir Crit Care Med 2002;165(3):398–405.

10. Rubin LJ, Badesch DB, Barst RJ, et al. Bosentan therapy for pulmonary arterial hypertension. N Engl J Med 2002;346(12):896–903.

11. Channick RN, Simonneau G, Sitbon O, et al. Effects of the dual endothelin-receptor antagonist bosentan in patients with pulmonary hypertension: a randomised placebo-controlled study. Lancet 2001; 358(9288):1119–23.

12. Humbert M, Segal ES, Kiely DG, et al. Results of European post-marketing surveillance of bosentan in pulmonary hypertension. Eur Respir J 2007;30(2): 338–44.

13. Nazzareno G, Horst O, Oudiz Ronald J, et al. Ambrisentan for the treatment of pulmonary arterial hypertension. Circulation 2008;117(23):3010–9.

14. Raghu G, Behr J, Brown KK, et al. Treatment of idiopathic pulmonary fibrosis with ambrisentan: a parallel, randomized trial. Ann Intern Med 2013;158(9): 641–9.

15. Pulido T, Adzerikho I, Channick RN, et al. Macitentan and morbidity and mortality in pulmonary arterial hypertension. N Engl J Med 2013;369(9):809–18.

16. Humbert M, Morrell NW, Archer SL, et al. Cellular and molecular pathobiology of pulmonary arterial hypertension. J Am Coll Cardiol 2004;43(12 Supplement):S13–24.

17. Sitbon O, Morrell N. Pathways in pulmonary arterial hypertension: the future is here. Eur Respir Rev 2012;21(126):321–7.

18. Galiè N, Ghofrani HA, Torbicki A, et al. Sildenafil citrate therapy for pulmonary arterial hypertension. N Engl J Med 2005;353(20):2148–57.

19. Frantz RP, Durst L, Burger CD, et al. Conversion from sildenafil to tadalafil: results from the sildenafil to tadalafil in pulmonary arterial hypertension (SITAR) study. J Cardiovasc Pharmacol Ther 2014; 19(6):550–7.

20. Ghofrani H-A, Humbert M, Langleben D, et al. Riociguat: mode of action and clinical development in pulmonary hypertension. Chest 2017;151(2):468–80.

21. Ghofrani H-A, Galiè N, Grimminger F, et al. Riociguat for the treatment of pulmonary arterial hypertension. N Engl J Med 2013;369(4):330–40.

22. Ghofrani H-A, D'Armini AM, Grimminger F, et al. Riociguat for the treatment of chronic thromboembolic pulmonary hypertension. N Engl J Med 2013; 369(4):319–29.

23. Galiè N, Müller K, Scalise A-V, et al. Patent plus: a blinded, randomised and extension study of riociguat plus sildenafil in pulmonary arterial hypertension. Eur Respir J 2015;45(5):1314–22.

24. Clark RH, Kueser TJ, Walker MW, et al. Low-dose nitric oxide therapy for persistent pulmonary hypertension of the newborn. N Engl J Med 2000;342(7): 469–74.

25. Inhaled nitric oxide in full-term and nearly full-term infants with hypoxic respiratory failure. N Engl J Med 1997;336(9):597–604.

26. Olivier S, Marc H, Xavier J, et al. Long-term response to calcium channel blockers in idiopathic pulmonary arterial hypertension. Circulation 2005; 111(23):3105–11.

27. Winterhalter M, Simon A, Fischer S, et al. Comparison of inhaled iloprost and nitric oxide in patients with pulmonary hypertension during weaning from cardiopulmonary bypass in cardiac surgery: a prospective randomized trial. J Cardiothorac Vasc Anesth 2008;22(3):406–13.

28. Bhorade S, Christenson J, O'connor M, et al. Response to inhaled nitric oxide in patients with acute right heart syndrome. Am J Respir Crit Care Med 1999;159(2):571–9.

29. Channick RN, Newhart JW, Johnson FW, et al. Pulsed delivery of inhaled nitric oxide to patients with primary pulmonary hypertension: an ambulatory delivery system and initial clinical tests. Chest 1996;109(6):1545–9.

30. Yu B, Ferrari M, Schleifer G, et al. Development of a portable mini-generator to safely produce nitric oxide for the treatment of infants with pulmonary hypertension. Nitric Oxide 2018;75:70–6.

31. Mitchell JA, Ahmetaj-Shala B, Kirkby NS, et al. Role of prostacyclin in pulmonary hypertension. Glob Cardiol Sci Pract 2014;2014(4):382–93.

32. Lang IM, Gaine SP. Recent advances in targeting the prostacyclin pathway in pulmonary arterial hypertension. Eur Respir Rev 2015;24(138):630–41.

33. Barst R. How has epoprostenol changed the outcome for patients with pulmonary arterial hypertension? Int J Clin Pract 2010;64(s168):23–32.

34. Barst RJ, Rubin LJ, Long WA, et al. A comparison of continuous intravenous epoprostenol (prostacyclin) with conventional therapy for primary pulmonary hypertension. N Engl J Med 1996;334(5): 296–301.

35. Galiè N, Channick RN, Frantz RP, et al. Risk stratification and medical therapy of pulmonary arterial hypertension. Eur Respir J 2019;53(1):1801889.

36. Kingman M, Archer-Chicko C, Bartlett M, et al. Management of prostacyclin side effects in adult patients with pulmonary arterial hypertension. Pulm Circ 2017;7(3):598–608.

37. Simonneau G, Barst RJ, Galie N, et al. Continuous sub-cutaneous infusion of treprostinil, a prostacyclin analogue, in patients with pulmonary arterial hypertension. Am J Respir Crit Care Med 2002;165(6):800–4.

38. Gomberg-Maitland M, Tapson VF, Benza RL, et al. Transition from intravenous epoprostenol to intravenous treprostinil in pulmonary hypertension. Am J Respir Crit Care Med 2005;172(12):1586–9.

39. Mouratoglou SA, Patsiala A, Feloukidis C, et al. Transition protocol from subcutaneous treprostinil to intravenous epoprostenol in deteriorating patients with pulmonary arterial hypertension. Int J Cardiol 2020;306:187–9.

40. McLaughlin VV, Benza RL, Rubin LJ, et al. Addition of inhaled treprostinil to oral therapy for pulmonary arterial hypertension: a randomized controlled clinical trial. J Am Coll Cardiol 2010;55(18):1915–22.

41. Waxman A, Restrepo-Jaramillo R, Thenappan T, et al. Inhaled treprostinil in pulmonary hypertension due to interstitial lung disease. N Engl J Med 2021; 384(4):325–34.

42. Olschewski H, Simonneau G, Galiè N, et al. Inhaled iloprost for severe pulmonary hypertension. N Engl J Med 2002;47(5):322–9.

43. Zhi-Cheng J, Parikh K, Tomas P, et al. Efficacy and safety of oral treprostinil monotherapy for the treatment of pulmonary arterial hypertension. Circulation 2013;127(5):624–33.

44. Tapson VF, Torres F, Kermeen F, et al. Oral treprostinil for the treatment of pulmonary arterial hypertension in patients on background endothelin receptor antagonist and/or phosphodiesterase type 5 inhibitor therapy (the FREEDOM-C study): a randomized controlled trial. Chest 2012;142(6): 1383–90.

45. Tapson VF, Jing Z-C, Xu K-F, et al. Oral treprostinil for the treatment of pulmonary arterial hypertension in patients receiving background endothelin receptor antagonist and phosphodiesterase type 5 inhibitor therapy (the FREEDOM-C2 study): a randomized controlled trial. Chest 2013;144(3):952–8.

46. White RJ, Jerjes-Sanchez C, Bohns Meyer GM, et al. Combination therapy with oral treprostinil for pulmonary arterial hypertension. A double-blind placebo-controlled clinical trial. Am J Respir Crit Care Med 2020;201(6):707–17.

47. Sitbon O, Channick R, Chin KM, et al. Selexipag for the treatment of pulmonary arterial hypertension. N Engl J Med 2015;373(26):2522–33.

48. Benza RL, Gomberg-Maitland M, Elliott CG, et al. Predicting survival in patients with pulmonary arterial hypertension: the REVEAL risk score calculator 2.0 and comparison with ESC/ERS-based risk assessment strategies. Chest 2019;156(2):323–37.

49. Hoeper MM, Kramer T, Pan Z, et al. Mortality in pulmonary arterial hypertension: prediction by the 2015 European pulmonary hypertension guidelines risk stratification model. Eur Respir J 2017;50(2): 1700740.

50. Boucly A, Weatherald J, Savale L, et al. Risk assessment, prognosis and guideline implementation in pulmonary arterial hypertension. Eur Respir J 2017;50(2):1700889.

51. Galiè N, Barberà JA, Frost AE, et al. Initial Use of ambrisentan plus tadalafil in pulmonary arterial hypertension. N Engl J Med 2015;373(9):834–44.

52. Mayeux JD, Pan IZ, Dechand J, et al. Management of pulmonary arterial hypertension. Curr Cardiovasc Risk Rep 2021;15(1):2.

53. Califf RM, Adams KF, McKenna WJ, et al. A randomized controlled trial of epoprostenol therapy for severe congestive heart failure: the Flolan International Randomized Survival Trial (FIRST). Am Heart J 1997;134(1):44–54.

54. Desai A, Desouza SA. Treatment of pulmonary hypertension with left heart disease: a concise review. Vasc Health Risk Manag 2017;13:415–20.

55. Machado RF, Barst RJ, Yovetich NA, et al. Hospitalization for pain in patients with sickle cell disease treated with sildenafil for elevated TRV and low exercise capacity. Blood 2011;118(4):855–64.

56. George MP, Gladwin MT, Graham BB. Exploring new therapeutic pathways in pulmonary hypertension. Metabolism, proliferation, and personalized medicine. Am J Respir Cell Mol Biol 2020;63(3): 279–92.

57. Evans JDW, Girerd B, Montani D, et al. BMPR2 mutations and survival in pulmonary arterial hypertension: an individual participant data meta-analysis. Lancet Respir Med 2016;4(2):129–37.

58. Humbert M, McLaughlin V, Gibbs JSR, et al. Sotatercept for the treatment of pulmonary arterial hypertension. N Engl J Med 2021;384(13):1204–15.

59. Huertas A, Tu L, Humbert M, et al. Chronic inflammation within the vascular wall in pulmonary arterial hypertension: more than a spectator. Cardiovasc Res 2020;116(5):885–93.

60. Tamura Y, Phan C, Tu L, et al. Ectopic upregulation of membrane-bound IL6R drives vascular remodeling in pulmonary arterial hypertension. J Clin Invest 2018;128(5):1956–70.

61. Le Hiress M, Tu L, Ricard N, et al. Proinflammatory signature of the dysfunctional Endothelium in pulmonary hypertension. Role of the macrophage migration inhibitory factor/CD74 complex. Am J Respir Crit Care Med 2015;192(8):983–97.

62. Trankle CR, Canada JM, Kadariya D, et al. IL-1 blockade reduces inflammation in pulmonary arterial hypertension and right ventricular failure: a single-arm, open-label, phase IB/II pilot study. Am J Respir Crit Care Med 2018;199(3):381–4.

63. Hernández-Sánchez J, Harlow L, Church C, et al. Clinical trial protocol for TRANSFORM-UK: a therapeutic open-label study of tocilizumab in the

treatment of pulmonary arterial hypertension. Pulm Circ 2018;8(1). 2045893217735820.

64. Zamanian RT, Badesch D, Chung L, et al. Safety and efficacy of B-cell depletion with rituximab for the treatment of systemic sclerosis associated pulmonary arterial hypertension: a multi-center, double-blind, randomized, placebo-controlled trial. Am J Respir Crit Care Med 2021. https://doi.org/10.1164/rccm.202009-3481OC.

65. Hoeper Marius M, Barst Robyn J, Bourge Robert C, et al. Imatinib mesylate as add-on therapy for pulmonary arterial hypertension. Circulation 2013; 127(10):1128–38.

66. Pitsiou G, Zarogoulidis P, Petridis D, et al. Inhaled tyrosine kinase inhibitors for pulmonary hypertension: a possible future treatment. Drug Des Devel Ther 2014;8:1753–63.

Pulmonary Hypertension Associated with Connective Tissue Disease

Stephen C. Mathai, MD, MHS

KEYWORDS

- Pulmonary hypertension • Connective tissue disease • Epidemiology • Diagnosis • Outcomes

KEY POINTS

- Pulmonary hypertension commonly complicates connective tissue disease.
- Connective tissue disease predisposes patients to development of all five groups of the World Health Organization clinical classification.
- Pulmonary hypertension of any type portends a poor prognosis in connective tissue disease.
- Advances in therapies for certain forms of pulmonary hypertension have improved outcomes in connective tissue disease patients.

INTRODUCTION

Pulmonary hypertension (PH) is a syndrome characterized by elevated pulmonary pressures leading to increased pulmonary vascular resistance (PVR) that ultimately causes right ventricular (RV) dysfunction, failure, and death.[1] PH can develop in association with many different diseases and can result from processes that primarily affect systems distinct from the pulmonary vasculature, such as the heart, lung parenchyma, liver, and kidneys, in addition to processes that affect the pulmonary vasculature directly, such as thromboembolism.[2] Patients with connective tissue disease (CTD) are at particularly high risk for the development of PH and in certain forms of CTD, such as systemic sclerosis or scleroderma (SSc), pulmonary arterial hypertension (PAH), the most rare form of PH.[3] The presence of PH in any form is associated with increased morbidity and mortality. Unfortunately, patients with CTD-associated PH tend to have poorer survival compared with patients with PH without CTD. The reasons for the increased risk of development of PH, attenuated response to therapy, and poorer outcomes are poorly understood.

DEFINITION AND CLASSIFICATION OF PULMONARY HYPERTENSION

According to the most recent consensus guidelines, PH is defined hemodynamically as a mean pulmonary artery pressure (mPAP) greater than 20 mm Hg.[4] This threshold for elevated pulmonary pressures was lowered from 25 mm Hg based on studies demonstrating the normal range of pulmonary pressures in healthy subjects and poor outcomes for patients with mean pulmonary pressures greater than 20 mm Hg.[5–7]

Furthermore, the risk of progression from mild to more severe hemodynamic impairment appears to be high in CTD, with 2 cohort studies suggesting up to one-third of patients with mPAP between 21 and 24 mm Hg progressing to mPAP greater than 25 mm Hg over 3 years.[8,9] Right heart catheterization (RHC) is required to diagnose PH, as mPAP cannot be directly measured by echocardiography. In hemodynamic terms, PH is often divided in to precapillary, postcapillary, and combined precapillary and postcapillary disease based on the pulmonary capillary wedge pressure (PCWP) and PVR.[4] Current guidelines further refine this classification and incorporate hemodynamic criteria with clinical and associated characteristics (**Table 1**).

Division of Pulmonary and Critical Care Medicine, Johns Hopkins University School of Medicine, 1830 E. Monument Street, Room 540, Baltimore, MD 21205, USA
E-mail address: smathai4@jhmi.edu

Cardiol Clin 40 (2022) 29–43
https://doi.org/10.1016/j.ccl.2021.08.003
0733-8651/22/
© 2021 Elsevier Inc. All rights reserved.

Table 1
Hemodynamic classification of pulmonary hypertension

Definition	Mean PAP (mm Hg)	PCWP (mm Hg)	PVR (Wu)	WHO Group
Normal hemodynamics	14.0 ± 3.3	8.0 ± 2.9	0.93 ± 0.38	N/A
Precapillary PH	>20	≤15	≥3	1, 3, 4, 5
Isolated postcapillary PH	>20	>15	<3	2 and 5
Combined precapillary and postcapillary PH	>20	>15	≥3	2 and 5

Because CTD in general can affect multiple organ systems, PH related to CTD can be associated with any of the 5 World Health Organization (WHO) groups (**Fig. 1**).[3,10–17] The most common CTDs associated with PH are listed in **Fig. 1** and include mixed connective tissue disease (MCTD), polymyositis/dermatomyositis (PM/DM), rheumatoid arthritis (RA), Sjogren syndrome (SS), systemic lupus erythematosus (SLE), and SSc. The risk of development of PH of any form varies by underlying CTD; the risk of PAH in particular seems to be higher in certain CTDs, such as SSc. Thus, recommendations for screening for PH in CTD vary by type of CTD. Importantly, it does not appear that the change in mPAP threshold defining PH has had a significant impact on the prevalence of PAH in SSc, as 2 recent cohort studies demonstrated that less than 2% of patients with SSc were reclassified as PAH based on the new definition.[10,18] In general, the presence of PH of any severity complicating any CTD is associated with a poorer prognosis.[11–14]

PATHOPHYSIOLOGY AND PATHOBIOLOGY

The pathophysiology and pathobiology of PH remain poorly understood. PAH develops as a consequence of progressive remodeling of the small- to medium-sized pulmonary vasculature. Plexiform lesions, medial hypertrophy with muscularization of the arterioles, concentric intimal proliferation, and in situ thrombosis are the pathologic hallmarks of the disease.[15] Although the exact

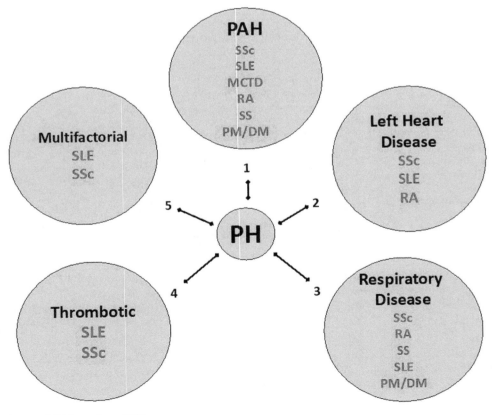

Fig. 1. Types of PH in various CTDs.

mechanisms of this remodeling remain unclear, multiple factors are thought to be involved.[16] Genetic factors demonstrated to predispose to the development of PAH or to the progression of disease and disease severity have not been routinely shown to be present in PAH-CTD.[17] Inflammation and autoimmunity are thought to play a central role in the development of PAH, both in the idiopathic pulmonary arterial hypertension (IPAH) and in PAH-CTD.[19,20] Autoimmunity and subsequent immune dysregulation may lead to activation of pathogenic autoreactive B cells and T cells and thus may be involved in the pathobiology of PAH, and in particular, PAH-CTD.

The pathobiology of other forms of PH outside of PAH is less well characterized. Patients with group 2 PH can have either passive PH (due solely to increased pressure downstream of the pulmonary arteries) or reactive/mixed PH (due to a combination of increased downstream pressure and structural and/or functional abnormalities of the pulmonary vasculature).[4] Pathologically, pulmonary veins are enlarged, dilated, and thickened with pulmonary capillary dilatation, interstitial edema, alveolar hemorrhage, and enlarged lymphatics. Distal pulmonary arteries can show evidence of medial hypertrophy, smooth muscle cell proliferation, and eccentric intimal lesions, but do not have classic plexiform lesions. Patients with CTD may be particularly prone to developing group 2 PH because of high prevalence of diastolic dysfunction of the left ventricle; additionally, valvular disorders, particularly those affecting the mitral valve, may also be present in certain CTDs and lead to increased pulmonary venous pressures.[3]

Group 3 PH can result from several entities, including obstructive lung disease, restrictive lung disease, neuromuscular disease, or obstructive sleep apnea. Within this category, PH related to interstitial lung disease (ILD) is most commonly encountered clinically in patients with CTD. Vascular obliteration related to parenchymal destruction and hypoxia contributes to the development of PH related to ILD. There exist commonalities in pathobiology between PH and ILD, and in particular, SSc-related ILD (SSc-ILD), that may explain the frequent copresentation of these 2 entities.[21] The same factors that lead to fibrosis in the vasculature may be influencing fibrosis in the interstitium, mediated by several pathways, including the transforming growth factor-β superfamily, and factors such as the CXC chemokines, platelet-derived growth factor, and angiotensin II, among others. Whether endothelial injury in SSc predisposes these patients to a higher risk of development of PH-ILD compared with other forms of ILD remains to be determined.[22]

CHARACTERISTICS OF PULMONARY HYPERTENSION BY CONNECTIVE TISSUE DISEASE TYPE
Scleroderma

SSc is a heterogeneous disorder characterized by endothelial dysfunction, fibroblast dysregulation, and immune system abnormalities that lead to progressive fibrosis of the skin and internal organs.[23] SSc is classified as limited or diffuse based on the extent of skin involvement. In either form, SSc can involve multiple organ systems, including the heart, lungs, gastrointestinal tract, and kidneys.[24] Although the incidence and prevalence of SSc are lower than other CTDs, such as RA and SLE, PH more commonly complicates SSc compared with other CTDs.[25] Whether this is related to specific differences in the pathobiology of SSc remains to be determined.[19,20] PH in SSc can be classified in any of the 5 WHO group classifications. PAH occurs in about 8% to 14% of patients with SSc when the diagnosis is based on RHC.[11] Higher estimates of PAH (up to 45% in certain series) have overestimated the prevalence because the diagnosis relied on echocardiography and not RHC. Although echocardiography can be useful to suggest the presence of PH and to identify potential causes of PH (eg, valvular disease, left ventricular dysfunction, congenital heart disease), echocardiography cannot establish the diagnosis of PH because of the inaccuracy of the Doppler signal in assessing true RV systolic pressure and the frequent inability to obtain an adequate Doppler signal, particularly in patients with CTD.[26] However, despite the potential for overdiagnosis of PAH based on the limitations of echocardiography, PAH in SSc is still likely to be underrecognized and underdiagnosed as suggested by its lower than expected prevalence in PH registries.

In addition, patients with SSc can develop pulmonary veno-occlusive disease (PVOD, World Symposium on Pulmonary Hypertension [WSPH] group 1.6), a rare form of PAH.[27] PVOD is a severe form of PAH characterized by both pulmonary arterial and pulmonary venule remodeling. In general, PVOD is a rare phenomenon, occurring in an estimated 0.1 to 0.2 persons per million.[28] Although genetic factors contribute to the development of PVOD in some cases, the genetic mutations have yet to be described in CTD patients with PVOD. PVOD can occur in various forms of CTD, including RA, SLE, SS, MCTD, but is most commonly seen in SSc, reported in up to 75% of autopsies in patients with SSc with PAH.[27]

Clinically, PVOD is characterized by a low diffusion capacity for carbon monoxide, and classical chest computed tomographic (CT) evidence of mediastinal lymphadenopathy, septal thickening, and centrilobular ground-glass opacities. Patients with PVOD may have a more rapid disease progression and thus require close evaluation and consideration of advanced therapy.

Screening and early detection

Because patients with SSc are at high risk of developing PAH, routine screening for this disease has been recommended.[29] Many support the use of the DETECT algorithm, a 2-step algorithm incorporating pulmonary function testing parameters, serum biomarkers, clinical characteristics (presence of telangiectasias), and electrocardiogram findings to generate a risk score to determine the need for echocardiography (**Fig. 2**).[29] Subsequent findings on echocardiography (right atrial enlargement, TR jet $\geq$2.5 m/s) in combination with step 1 score determine the need for RHC. Using this algorithm, the false negative rate for PAH was 4% compared with a nearly 30% false negative rate when using the European Society of Cardiology/European Respiratory Society (ESC/ERS) guidelines for screening in this population. Still, this algorithm has limitations: (1) it was developed in a high-risk subset of patients with SSc (those with a diffusing capacity for carbon monoxide [DLCO] < 60% predicted and >3 years duration of SSc) and (2) it was designed to detect PH defined as a mean PAP $\geq$ 25 mm Hg rather than the current definition of PH (mean PAP > 20 mm Hg). Therefore, this approach may not apply to all patients with SSc, nor have the same test characteristics (sensitivity and specificity) for the new definition of PH.

Outcomes

Outcomes in patients with SSc with PAH are poor, particularly in comparison to other forms of PAH. Modern era cohort studies have reported 3-year survival ranging from 50% to 75%.[30–33] The improved survival in the PHAROS registry may reflect inclusion of patients with less severe disease, as more than half of the subjects were in WHO functional class 1 or 2 at enrollment. Prior studies have also demonstrated that survival remains worse in SSc with PAH than in patients with the idiopathic form of PAH, despite seemingly less severe hemodynamic perturbations at diagnosis. This may reflect differences in the RV adaptation to increased afterload. In 1 cohort study, N-terminal pro b-type natriuretic peptide (NT-proBNP) levels were significantly higher in PAH because of SSc compared with IPAH despite less severe hemodynamic impairment; this

difference persisted when controlling for potential confounders, such as age and renal function.[34] Because NT-proBNP is released from the ventricles in response to increased wall stress, the observation suggested that responses to increased afterload on the RV may differ between PAH in SSc and IPAH. In line with this, physiologic studies have shown depressed RV function for a similar afterload in compared with IPAH.[35,36] Using pressure-volume measurements in the RV, Tedford and colleagues[36] demonstrated significantly lower contractility in PAH from SSc compared with patients with IPAH, despite similar pulmonary vascular resistive and pulsatile loading characteristics as assessed by resistance-compliance relationships and arterial elastance measures. This may reflect intrinsic differences in RV contractility. Furthermore, Hsu and colleagues[37] demonstrated a "dose-response" relationship in RV contractility assessed using isolated myocyte preparations from RV biopsies between patients with SSc without PAH, patients with SSc with PAH, and patients with IPAH. These findings suggest intrinsic RV dysfunction may contribute to the clinical differences in presentation and outcomes. **Box 1** shows predictors of outcomes in patients with SSc and PAH.

Pulmonary hypertension related to interstitial lung disease and other comorbidities in systemic sclerosis

Patients with SSc can also develop PH related to ILD, but there are limited data describing its prevalence. The presence of PH in SSc-ILD portends a poor prognosis.[11,19] In a cohort of 59 patients with SSc with PH, 20 of whom had significant ILD (defined as a total lung capacity [TLC] < 60% predicted or TLC between 60% and 70% predicted combined with moderate to severe fibrosis on high-resolution CT of the chest), survival was significantly worse in the SSc-ILD cohort with 1-, 2-, and 3-year survival rates of 82%, 49%, and 39% compared with 87%, 79%, and 64% in the PH alone group, respectively (P<.01)[11] and presence of ILD portended a 5-fold increased risk of death compared with PAH. Occult left heart disease may also be common in patients with SSc with PH and impacts outcomes. Fox and colleagues[20] demonstrated that nearly 40% of patients with SSc who were diagnosed with PAH based on PCWP $\leq$ 15 mm Hg actually had postcapillary PH after fluid challenge during RHC. Furthermore, patients with evidence of diastolic dysfunction and precapillary PH had a 2-fold increased risk of death compared with patients with PAH-SSc after adjusting for hemodynamic severity of PH.[38]

Other Connective Tissue Diseases

Although PH can complicate other CTDs, these have been less well characterized, largely because of the lower overall prevalence of PH in patients with other CTDs or the lower overall prevalence of these CTDs in the general population.

Mixed Connective Tissue Disease

Patients with MCTD have clinical features of several CTDs, including SSc, SLE, RA, and PM/DM. The characteristic laboratory feature is the presence of antibodies to uridine-rich (U1) RNP polypeptides, which is required to establish the diagnosis.[39] Lung disease in MCTD is common and can manifest as parenchymal disease, pulmonary vascular disease, or both.[14,40] Cohort studies have provided estimates of the prevalence of PAH in MCTD ranging from 1% to as high as 50% and of ILD in up to 50%.[14,41] Thromboembolism may be more common in MCTD; in 1 study, 19.9% of patients with MCTD had venous clots.[41] Whether these patients

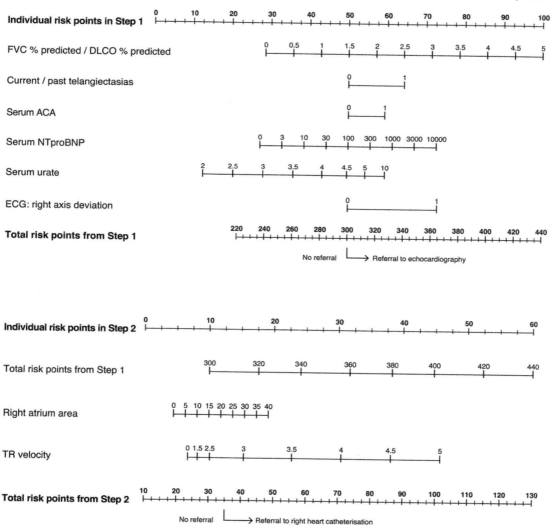

Fig. 2. The DETECT algorithm. Nomograms for the DETECT algorithm. Two-step algorithm for determining referral for RHC or suspected PAH in systemic sclerosis. At step 1 (*top*), risk points for each of the 6 nonechocardiographic variables are calculated and summed. If the total risk points from step 1 are greater than 300, the patient is referred for echocardiography. Similarly, at step 2, risk points for the carried forward and the 2 echocardiographic variables are calculated. If the total risk points from step 2 is greater than 35, the patient is referred to RHC. If a single step 1 variable is missing, it should be assigned 50 risk points, with the exception of current/past telangiectasias, which should be assigned 65 points. If a single step 2 variable is missing, it should be assigned 10 points. The nomograms cannot be reliably used if more than 1 variable out of the 8 total variables is missing. ACA, anticentromere antibody; FVC, forced vital capacity; TR, tricuspid regurgitant jet. (*From* Coghlan JG, Denton CP, Grunig E, Bonderman D, Distler O, Khanna D, et al. Evidence-based detection of pulmonary arterial hypertension in systemic sclerosis: the DETECT study. Ann Rheum Dis 2014 Jul;73(7):1340-9.)

with venous thrombosis developed chronic thromboembolic disease and PH is unknown.

Patients with MCTD and PAH tend to be diagnosed late in their disease course, with nearly 70% having WHO FC 3 symptoms at diagnosis.[42] Compared with patients with SSc with PAH, patients with MCTD with PAH are younger and more likely to be black or Hispanic. Biomarkers of disease severity in PAH, such as brain natriuretic peptide, are lower, and DLCO is higher in MCTD compared with SSc, suggesting less severe disease. Hemodynamics do not differ significantly between the 2 groups, except that right atrial pressure tends to be lower in MCTD.[42]

Outcomes

PAH appears to be the most common cause of death in patients with MCTD.[41,43] Two cohort studies have reported outcomes in RHC-proven PAH in MCTD. In a national registry from the United Kingdom, survival in PAH from MCTD was similar to PAH from SSc at 1 year (83% vs 77%) but perhaps better at 3 years (66% vs 47%).[44] In the REVEAL registry, 1-year survival did not differ between PAH related to MCTD or SSc (88% vs 82%).[42] However, when compared with other forms of CTD-related PAH, such as SLE, survival was worse in the MCTD cohorts in both studies. Based on these studies showing the impact of PAH on outcomes, expert consensus recommends screening for PAH in patients with MCTD, particularly those with SSc features.[43]

Systemic Lupus Erythematous

SLE is a multisystem disease that can affect the lungs and lead to several forms of pulmonary vascular disease, including ILD-related PH, PAH, and chronic thromboembolic pulmonary hypertension (CTEPH). In addition, PH can result from SLE-associated cardiomyopathy or from renal failure requiring hemodialysis and placement of arteriovenous fistulas.[45] Thus, PH in SLE can also be classified in any of the 5 PH categories (see **Fig. 1**).

Prevalence estimates of PH in SLE vary widely, from 0.0005% to 14% of patients.[45] Patients who develop the disease tend to be young (average age around 30 at diagnosis) and often have Raynaud phenomenon.[46] Risk factors for the development of PAH related to SLE are not well described, but blacks, those with anti-smooth muscle or anti-cardiolipin antibodies, and history of pericarditis appear more likely to have PH.

Outcomes

As expected, outcomes in patients with SLE with PH are worse than for those without PH. Cohort studies report survival for PAH in patients with SLE that range from 50% to 75% at 3 years; however, there may be geographic differences in outcomes, as deaths attributable to PAH seem to be lower in European and North American cohorts compared with Asian cohorts.[45,46] Risk factors for poor outcomes have been described in a systematic review and include both PH-specific and SLE-specific parameters.[47] Higher mPAP at diagnosis, vascular manifestations of SLE such as Raynaud phenomenon, pulmonary vasculitis, thrombosis, thrombocytopenia, and presence of anticardiolipin antibodies all portend a poorer prognosis. Interestingly, neither lupus disease activity nor nephritis was associated with poorer outcome.

Sjogren Syndrome

SS is a chronic inflammatory disease characterized by lymphocytic infiltration of exocrine glands and extraglandular tissues. It can present as primary disease or in association with other CTDs, such as RA or SSc, and predominantly affects women.[48] Although the sicca syndrome (xerophthalmia and/or keratoconjunctivitis sicca and xerostomia) is most commonly present in patients with SS, extraglandular involvement of the lungs is common, typically manifesting as ILD. Various types of ILD have been described in SS, including lymphocytic interstitial pneumonia, nonspecific interstitial pneumonitis, usual interstitial pneumonitis, and organizing pneumonia.[48]

In contrast to other CTDs, PAH is rare in SS. Relatively large cohort studies have estimated the prevalence of PH at around 20%; however, the diagnosis of PH was based on echocardiography. In the largest case series of patients with

SS-associated PH, Launay and colleagues[49] describe associations between anti-Ro and RNP antibodies and hypergammaglobulinemia in patients with SS with PAH. Survival in this cohort was poor with 1-year and 3-year survival at 73% and 66%, respectively, similar to survival seen in patients with PAH from SSc.

Rheumatoid Arthritis

RA is an autoimmune disease characterized by a symmetric, inflammatory polyarthritis that leads to joint destruction. RA is more prevalent that most other CTDs, occurring in 40 out of 100,000 persons in the United States. Women in the United States have a nearly 4% lifetime risk of developing RA.[50] Extra-articular disease affects multiple organs, and cardiopulmonary involvement is common. There is a high risk of coronary artery disease, myocardial infarction, heart failure, and sudden death compared with age-matched persons without RA. Pulmonary manifestations include ILD, rheumatoid nodules, airways disease with bronchiolitis obliterans and organizing pneumonia, and pleural disease.[50] Lung disease may also result from disease-modifying antirheumatic drugs, with complications such as pneumonitis, fibrosis, obliterative bronchiolitis, infection, and bronchospasm, among others.

PH in RA has been reported in association with left heart disease, ILD, and chronic thromboembolic disease. Isolated PH, that is, PH in the absence of overt left heart disease, ILD, and chronic thromboembolic disease, has been infrequently reported in the literature. In the UK registry, only 12 patients with RA with PAH were identified, whereas in the REVEAL registry, 28 cases of RHC-proven PAH owing to RA were included.[42,44] When compared with patients with SSc-related PAH in the REVEAL cohort, RA patients with PAH tended to be younger (54 ± 15.8 vs 61.8 ± 11.1 years). Raynaud phenomenon was less likely to be present (3.6% vs 32.6% of the cohort); renal insufficiency was less frequent, and b-type natriuretic peptide levels were significantly lower. Functional class at baseline, 6-minute walk distance (6MWD), and hemodynamics were similar. Although spirometry and lung volumes were similar when compared with PAH in SSc, diffusing capacity was higher in the PAH owing to RA cohort. One-year survival in the RA cohort was significantly better than the SSc cohort (96% vs 82%, $P = .01$).

Polymyositis/Dermatomyositis

PM and DM are idiopathic inflammatory myopathies that are characterized by proximal muscle weakness. DM has characteristic skin manifestations, although clinical features of both DM and PM vary among affected individuals. The estimated prevalence of these diseases varies from 5 to 22 per 100,000 persons, with an annual incidence of 2 per 100,000.[51] The most common pulmonary manifestation of PM/DM is ILD, occurring in about 10% of patients, although respiratory symptoms, such as dyspnea and orthopnea, can also arise from muscle weakness affecting the diaphragm.[52]

PH appears to be a rare complication of PM/DM, and if present, may be more related to underlying ILD.[52] In the UK registry, only 7 patients (2% of the entire PAH-CTD cohort) had PAH related to PM/DM, and there were no cases of PAH related to PM/DM seen in the REVEAL registry.[42,44] No clinical demographic or hemodynamic characteristics of these patients were reported in the UK registry; however, the 1- and 3-year survival was 100% for these patients, suggesting better outcomes compared with other PAH-CTD.

DIAGNOSIS

Given the need for precision in the classification of PH phenotype in patients with underlying CTD, a detailed diagnostic algorithm should be followed. Clinical suspicion for PH should be informed by the risk inherent to the underlying CTD. However, in many cases, a thorough evaluation for CTD has not been undertaken before evaluation for PH and thus should be completed. In addition to history and physical examination focusing on identifying features of CTD, serologic evaluation including screening tests for CTD should be completed. Current guidelines recommend anti-nuclear antibody testing using immunofluorescence.[53] If CTD is suggested by results of serologies or if clinical suspicion remains high despite negative screening serologies, additional testing, including anticentromere, antitopoisomerase, anti-RNA polymerase III, double-stranded DNA, anti-Ro, anti-La, and U-1 RNP, antibodies should be sent, and referral to rheumatology should be considered. Furthermore, given the high prevalence of left heart disease, ILD, and thromboembolism in CTD, evaluation for each of these entities should be undertaken before proceeding to RHC given the implications for clinical management. If CTEPH is identified in a CTD patient, further evaluation for thrombophilia should be undertaken.

TREATMENT

Currently, specific pulmonary vasodilator therapy for PH in the setting of CTD is approved by the Food and Drug Administration (FDA) only for patients with PAH, PH due to ILD, and CTEPH. These therapies have been developed by targeting pathways in the putative pathogenesis of PAH and then tested in the PH due to ILD and the CTEPH populations. Randomized clinical trials of novel therapeutics for PAH have included patients with various forms of PAH-CTD, although most patients enrolled likely have SSc. Subgroup analyses in the PAH-CTD cohorts of these studies have not been consistently reported.[54–60] Given the differences in demographic and hemodynamic characteristics between PAH-CTD types, the results from these clinical trials are unlikely to be generalizable to all forms of PAH-CTD and thus should be interpreted with caution in most cases. Still, the PAH therapies discussed later are commonly used in all forms of CTD-PAH, even though the evidence base for diseases other than SSc is minimal.

General Measures

Despite a lack of specific data for PAH of any form, consensus guidelines recommend the use of supplemental oxygen in patients who are hypoxic (peripheral oxygen saturation <90%) at rest or with exercise, largely based on extrapolation of data from chronic obstructive lung disease.[61,62] In addition, diuretics are recommended for the management of right heart failure and volume overload. Digoxin may also be useful for management of refractory right heart failure complicated by atrial arrhythmias. Exercise, and in particular, pulmonary rehabilitation, may also be beneficial as demonstrated in a clinical trial of prescribed exercise in a population of patients with IPAH and PAH-CTD.[63,64]

Anticoagulation

Anticoagulation is recommended in the treatment of IPAH based primarily on retrospective, observational data showing improved survival in patients on warfarin therapy. However, no such data exist for PAH-CTD, and there may be increased risk of harm with anticoagulation.[65] Thus, routine anticoagulation for PAH-CTD in the absence of other comorbidities for which anticoagulation is necessary is not recommended by current expert consensus.[2,66]

Immunosuppression

As discussed previously, inflammatory and immunologic mechanisms are likely involved in the pathogenesis of both CTD and PAH. Given this potential commonality in pathobiology, anti-inflammatory agents have been used in various types of PAH-CTD. However, there are no randomized, clinical trials in patients with PAH-CTD

to support its use in this patient population. Still, several case series have suggested efficacy in certain populations within PAH-CTD. In the report by Jais and colleagues,[67] 23 patients with either SLE- or MCTD-associated PAH were treated with combination therapy including cyclophosphamide and glucocorticoids; nearly half of the patients with SLE and patients with MCTD demonstrated clinical improvement in functional capacity and hemodynamics, although patients with SSc did not. Other investigators have reported improvements in functional capacity, hemodynamics, and survival with immunosuppressant therapy.[68–70] A recently completed randomized controlled double-masked trial in patients with SSc with PAH of rituximab, a monoclonal antibody targeting CD20 on B cells, did not meet its primary endpoint of change in 6MWD (NCT01086540).

Pulmonary Vasodilator Therapy

There are now more than a dozen FDA-approved pulmonary vasodilator therapies for PAH, one for CTEPH, and most recently, one for PH-ILD. According to expert consensus, selection of therapy for patients with PAH should be based on risk stratification at diagnosis and follow-up.[66] There are numerous risk-stratification tools that have been developed and applied in various cohorts. A recent comparison of the predictive value of these tools suggests fair to good discrimination, defined as the ability of the model to separate individuals who develop an event from those who do not, across models.[71] However, the relevance of these predictive models in PAH-CTD is less certain, as some of these models were derived from populations that specifically excluded patients with PAH-CTD or had small proportions of PAH-CTD. Specific analyses of the REVEAL 1.0 model and the ESC/ERS model suggest poor to acceptable predictive utility when applied specifically to PAH-CTD.[72,73] Future studies examining risk in PAH-CTD should be undertaken to better inform prediction model development in this population. Regardless, as shown in **Fig. 3**, current treatment recommendations for patients with PAH, including PAH-CTD, depend on risk assessment.

Historically, response to pulmonary vasodilator therapy in PAH-CTD was thought to be less robust than in other PAH populations. An analysis of patient-level data from registration trials for PAH medications reports a higher rate of adverse events in patients with PAH-CTD and attenuated effect on quality of life compared with IPAH.[74] Subsequently, Rhee and colleagues[75] found the treatment effect, as assessed by change in 6MWD, was similar in magnitude between patients with PAH-CTD and patients with IPAH, but patients with PAH-CTD on therapy had minimal improvement. Interestingly, patients with PAH-CTD treated with placebo had a significant decline in 6MWD in contrast to patients with IPAH. Several factors, specific to patients with PAH-CTD, may influence the observed response to therapy, as shown in **Table 2**. Similarly, interpretation of the clinical relevance of response to therapy for a given outcome measure may differ between PAH-CTD and IPAH. Analysis of change in 6MWD from the registration study for tadalafil in PAH suggests that the minimal clinically important

difference (MCID), the smallest change in an outcome measure that is noticeable to a patient and would lead to a change in therapy, is smaller for PAH-CTD than IPAH.[76] Thus, although not statistically significant in the context of the clinical trial data, smaller changes in 6MWD may be more clinically relevant for PAH-CTD.

Recent data from combination therapy trials suggest that response to therapy may not differ significantly between PAH-CTD and IPAH.[77] This may be particularly true when considering morbidity outcomes, such as time to clinical worsening. In the GRIPHON study of selexipag in combination with other PAH therapy, outcome event rates were similar between PAH-CTD and IPAH

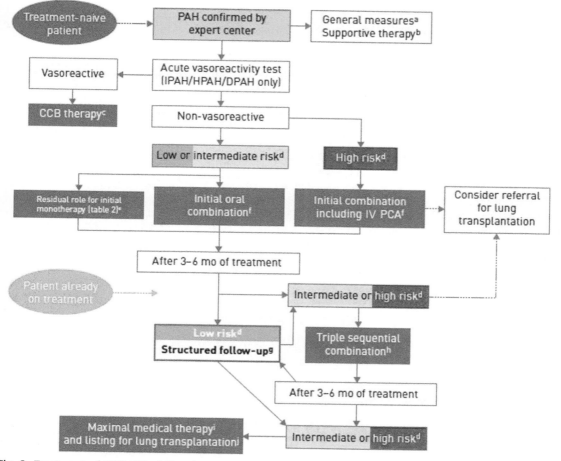

Fig. 3. Treatment of PAH-CTD. CCB, calcium channel blocker; DPAH, drug-induced PAH; HPAH, heritable PAH; PCA, prostacyclin analogue. [a]2015 ESC/ERS PH guidelines Table 16. [b]2015 ESC/ERS PH guidelines Table 17. [c]2015 ESC/ERS PH guidelines Table 18. [d]2015 ESC/ERS PH guidelines Table 13. [e]2015 ESC/ERS PH guidelines Table 19. [f]2015 ESC/ERS PH guidelines Table 20. [g]2015 ESC/ERS PH guidelines Table 14. [h]2015 ESC/ERS PH guidelines Table 21. [i]Maximal medical therapy is considered triple combination therapy, including a subcutaneous or an IV PCA (IV preferred in high-risk status). [j]2015 ESC/ERS PH guidelines Table 22. (*From* Galiè N, Channick RN, Frantz RP, Grünig E, Jing ZC, Moiseeva O, Preston IR, Pulido T, Safdar Z, Tamura Y, McLaughlin VV. Risk stratification and medical therapy of pulmonary arterial hypertension. Eur Respir J. 2019 Jan 24;53(1):1801889. Reproduced with permission of the © ERS 2021.)

Table 2
Disease-specific considerations in connective tissue disease–associated pulmonary hypertension

Domain	Tool	Application to CTD-PAH
Hemodynamics	RHC, Echo	Group II and III disease confound assessment
Exercise testing	6MWD	Musculoskeletal disease/deconditioning
Dyspnea	Borg dyspnea	Non-PAH causes for dyspnea (ILD, anemia, and similar)
Adherence with therapy	Adverse events	Concomitant medications for CTD may interact
Pharmacodynamics	Bioavailability	Different due to gastrointestinal motility, malabsorption
Quality of life	SF-36/CAMPHOR	Extrapulmonary involvement affects quality of life
Global state	Survival	Poorer survival overall compared with IPAH

Adapted from Denton, C.P., Avouac, J., Behrens, F. et al. Systemic sclerosis-associated pulmonary hypertension: why disease-specific composite endpoints are needed. Arthritis Res Ther 13, 114 (2011).

groups.[59] Furthermore, although adverse events were numerically higher in the PAH-CTD group, there were no significant differences in rates between groups. This trial also offered the unique opportunity to examine responses in patients with SLE with PAH. Importantly, no difference in magnitude of response between SLE and other PAH-CTD or IPAH was seen. Robust data from the AMBITION study also support the use of initial combination therapy with phosphodiesterase inhibitors and endothelin receptor antagonists in PAH-CTD to improve time to clinical worsening.[60] In a 36-week open-label study of newly diagnosed patients with PAH owing to SSc, Hassoun and colleagues[78] found significant improvement in symptoms, 6MWD, RV function assessed by echocardiography and cardiac MRI, and hemodynamics with initial combination therapy of tadalafil and ambrisentan. The improvements noted for some of these parameters significantly exceed the reported MCID, for example, RV ejection fraction on cardiac MRI. Taken together, these data suggest with initial combination therapy, patients with CTD-PAH experience significant improvement in symptoms, functional capacity, RV function, hemodynamics, and morbidity that is of similar magnitude to patients with IPAH.

Treatment of Pulmonary Hypertension-Interstitial Lung Disease in Connective Tissue Disease

Recently, the FDA approved inhaled treprostinil for use in patients with PH-ILD, including CTD-ILD. This recommendation was based on the results of the INCREASE study, a 16-week, randomized, double-masked controlled study of inhaled treprostinil versus placebo in patients with PH in the setting of ILD.[79] PH was defined as an mPAP $\geq$ 25 mm Hg with a PCWP $\leq$ 15 mm Hg and a PVR greater than 3 WU. Although patients with other forms of ILD were permitted to enroll if there was evidence of diffuse parenchymal disease on CT of the chest, patients with CTD also had to have a forced vital capacity less than 70% predicted to fulfill inclusion criteria. Of the 326 patients enrolled, 72 (22%) had CTD. At 16 weeks, the change in 6MWD between treatment and placebo was statistically significant (30.1 m, 95% confidence interval [CI] 16.8–45.4 m), and importantly, oxygenation did not significantly change with pulmonary vasodilator therapy. Interestingly, patients with CTD on average demonstrated greater improvement in 6MWD compared with other ILD groups (mean change 43.5 m, 95% CI 9.6–77.4 m). However, there were no improvements in secondary outcome measures such as quality of life.

TREATMENT OF OTHER FORMS OF PULMONARY HYPERTENSION
Pulmonary Hypertension Related to Left Heart Disease in Connective Tissue Disease

Unfortunately, there are no approved therapies for PH in the setting of left heart disease. Identifying the underlying cause of PH will be helpful and allow for directed therapy where appropriate, such as valve-related disease in SLE. Patients with SSc may be prone to more rapid progression of aortic stenosis, which can lead to PH as well.[80] Valve repair or replacement may be of use in select patients. Heart failure with either reduced or preserved ejection fraction (HFrEF vs HFpEF) can lead to PH, but HFpEF is more commonly encountered in CTD. Specific therapy should be directed at the underlying condition, as there are no data to support use of pulmonary vasodilator therapies for this indication.

Chronic Thromboembolic Pulmonary Hypertension in Connective Tissue Disease

Patients with CTEPH in the setting of CTD should be treated according to guideline-based recommendations.[81] When CTEPH is identified, treatment for at least 3 months with anticoagulation should be undertaken before initiating medical or surgical therapy for PH. Evaluation for surgical thromboendarterectomy should be pursued, as this is the definitive treatment for CTEPH. If the patient is not a surgical candidate, interventional therapy with balloon angioplasty or medical therapy with riociguat may be feasible and effective.[82,83] However, neither therapy is definitive, and as such, thromboendarterectomy remains the treatment of choice in appropriate candidates with appropriate anatomy.

Exercise-Induced Pulmonary Hypertension

Although the definition of PH is based on a resting mPAP at least 20 mm Hg, it is estimated that 50% to 70% of the pulmonary vasculature needs to be affected before resting mPAP is elevated. An abnormal pulmonary hemodynamic response to exercise, or exercise-induced pulmonary hypertension (Ex-PH), has therefore been postulated to represent early pulmonary vascular disease. There remains controversy regarding the appropriate definition of Ex-PH based on the hemodynamic criteria and exercise challenge used. Still, an mPAP more than 30 mm Hg and transpulmonary gradient more than 3 WU at maximal exercise have been proposed as the most suitable definition.[84,85] Using this definition applied to a retrospective cohort of patients with SSc, patients with Ex-PH not only had a worse outcome than if Ex-PH was not present but also had survival similar to patients with SSc with PAH.[86] A recent study by Zeder and colleagues[87] demonstrated that exercise hemodynamics, but not resting hemodynamics, predicted outcomes in a cohort of patients with SSc without resting PH (mPAP > 25 mm Hg), suggesting clinical relevance of exercise hemodynamics in patients without significantly elevated pulmonary pressures. However, there are limited data to support treatment of Ex-PH in SSc with pulmonary vasodilators.[88] One recent randomized controlled study examining the role of ambrisentan in a cohort of 38 patients with SSc with mild resting PH (mPAP 21–24 mm Hg) or Ex-PH did not find improvement in the primary outcome of mPAP, but did find improvement in other hemodynamic measures, both at rest and with exercise.[89] However, subgroup analyses by patients with Ex-PH alone were not reported.

Pulmonary Hypertension with Mildly Elevated Pressures (Mean Pulmonary Artery Pressure 21–24 mm Hg)

One of the major limitations to the 6th WSPH recommendations for lowering the mPAP threshold to fulfill the definition of PH is that there are no approved therapies for patients with pulmonary pressure elevations in this range. All currently approved therapies were evaluated in patients with mPAP $\geq$ 25 mm Hg. Furthermore, aside from the study by Pan and colleagues,[89] there are no randomized controlled trial data evaluating the role of pulmonary vasodilator therapy in this population. A small randomized clinical trial of sildenafil in patients with SSc with early pulmonary vascular disease is planned, but is not yet enrolling (NCT04797286).

Pulmonary Veno-Occlusive Disease in Connective Tissue Disease

PVOD is a severe form of PAH characterized by both pulmonary arterial and pulmonary venule remodeling. Patients with PVOD may have a more rapidly progressive decline and may be prone to developing pulmonary edema with pulmonary vasodilator therapy.[27] As such, careful initiation of low-dose monotherapy is generally recommended for patients with PVOD. Given the propensity for rapid progression and risk of pulmonary edema with dose escalation, patients with PVOD should be referred for lung transplantation evaluation if the diagnosis is considered possible based on the clinical scenario.

LUNG TRANSPLANTATION

Current International Society of Heart and Lung Transplantation guidelines recommend lung transplant for patients with CTD if no extrapulmonary contraindications to transplantation exist.[90] Typically, these criteria include uncontrolled gastroesophageal reflux disease or dysphagia, renal dysfunction, or significant LV dysfunction. Largely owing to these concerns, patients with CTD continue to comprise only a minority of transplant recipients. However, when recent short- and long-term outcomes are considered, outcomes for patients with CTD are comparable to other transplant recipients with similar indications for transplantation (ie, ILD and PAH).[91,92] Therefore, patients with PH in the setting of CTD should be referred for lung transplant evaluation.

SUMMARY

PH remains a common complication of CTD and can present in various forms, most commonly in the setting of left heart disease, lung disease, or PAH. The presence of PH in any form portends a poor outcome. Advances in screening for PAH in high-risk cohorts, such as SSc, along with increased awareness of treatment options for non-PAH forms of PH may help support efforts to identify pulmonary vascular disease earlier in this at-risk population and allow for intervention. Initial combination therapy is now recommended as standard of care for treatment-naive, intermediate-risk patients with PAH-CTD, and pulmonary vasodilator therapy is approved for both patients with CTEPH and patients with PH-ILD with CTD. Furthermore, lung transplant remains an option in the appropriate patient. Still, despite these advances, there remains an ongoing need to improve outcomes for patients with CTD with PH.

CLINICS CARE POINTS

- Routine, yearly screening for development of pulmonary hypertension in certain forms of connective tissue disease, such as scleroderma, is recommended.
- Thorough evaluation for pulmonary hypertension should be undertaken to ensure proper classification according to the World Health Organization Classification as treatment strategies vary between pulmonary hypertension types.
- New therapies for pulmonary hypertension in the setting of interstitial lung disease have been approved by the Federal Drug Agency recently and should be considered in the management of these patients.

DISCLOSURE

Consultancies: Actelion, Acceleron, Bayer, United Therapeutics. Funding to institution: Actelion, United Therapeutics. NHLBI: U01HL125175 (Co-PI); R01HL134905 (Co-I); R01HL11490 (Co-I). DOD: PR191839 (PI). The clinical trial (NCT04797286) referenced in the article is supported by DOD grant PR191839 (PI-Mathai).

REFERENCES

1. Chin KM, Kim NH, Rubin LJ. The right ventricle in pulmonary hypertension. Coron Artery Dis 2005; 16(1):13–8.

2. Galiè N, Humbert M, Vachiery JL, et al, ESC Scientific Document Group. 2015 ESC/ERS guidelines for the diagnosis and treatment of pulmonary hypertension: the Joint Task Force for the Diagnosis and Treatment of Pulmonary Hypertension of the European Society of Cardiology (ESC) and the European Respiratory Society (ERS): endorsed by: Association for European Paediatric and Congenital Cardiology (AEPC), International Society for Heart and Lung Transplantation (ISHLT). Eur Heart J 2016; 37(1):67–119.

3. Mathai SC, Hassoun PM. Pulmonary arterial hypertension in connective tissue diseases. Heart Fail Clin 2012;8(3):413–25.

4. Simonneau G, Montani D, Celermajer DS, et al. Haemodynamic definitions and updated clinical classification of pulmonary hypertension. Eur Respir J 2019;53(1):1801913.

5. Kovacs G, Berghold A, Scheidl S, et al. Pulmonary arterial pressure during rest and exercise in healthy subjects: a systematic review. Eur Respir J 2009;34: 888–94.

6. Maron BA, Hess E, Maddox TM, et al. Association of borderline pulmonary hypertension with mortality and hospitalization in a large patient cohort: insights from the Veterans Affairs Clinical Assessment, Reporting and Tracking program. Circulation 2016; 133:1240–8.

7. Assad TR, Maron BA, Robbins IM, et al. Prognostic effect and longitudinal hemodynamic assessment of borderline pulmonary hypertension. JAMA Cardiol 2017. https://doi.org/10.1001/jamacardio. 2017.3882.

8. Valerio CJ, Schreiber BE, Handler CE, et al. Borderline mean pulmonary artery pressure in patients with systemic sclerosis: transpulmonary gradient predicts risk of developing pulmonary hypertension. Arthritis Rheum 2013;65(4):1074–84.

9. Coghlan JG, Wolf M, Distler O, et al. Incidence of pulmonary hypertension and determining factors in patients with systemic sclerosis. Eur Respir J 2018; 51(4):1701197.

10. Xanthouli P, Jordan S, Milde N, et al. Haemodynamic phenotypes and survival in patients with systemic sclerosis: the impact of the new definition of pulmonary arterial hypertension. Ann Rheum Dis 2020; 79(3):370–8.

11. Mathai SC, Hummers LK, Champion HC, et al. Survival in pulmonary hypertension associated with the scleroderma spectrum of diseases: impact of interstitial lung disease. Arthritis Rheum 2009; 60(2):569–77.

12. Chung SM, Lee CK, Lee EY, et al. Clinical aspects of pulmonary hypertension in patients with systemic lupus erythematosus and in patients with idiopathic pulmonary arterial hypertension. Clin Rheumatol 2006;25(6):866–72.

13. Hatron PY, Tillie-Leblond I, Launay D, et al. Pulmonary manifestations of Sjogren's syndrome. Presse Med 2011;40(1 Pt 2):e49–64.

14. Szodoray P, Hajas A, Kardos L, et al. Distinct phenotypes in mixed connective tissue disease: subgroups and survival. Lupus 2012;21(13):1412–22.

15. Stewart S, Rassl D. Advances in the understanding and classification of pulmonary hypertension. Histopathology 2009;54(1):104–16.

16. Voelkel NF, Gomez-Arroyo J, Abbate A, et al. Pathobiology of pulmonary arterial hypertension and right ventricular failure. Eur Respir J 2012;40(6):1555–65.

17. Morrell NW, Aldred MA, Chung WK, et al. Genetics and genomics of pulmonary arterial hypertension. Eur Respir J 2019;53(1):1801899.

18. Jaafar S, Visovatti S, Young A, et al. Impact of the revised haemodynamic definition on the diagnosis of pulmonary hypertension in patients with systemic sclerosis. Eur Respir J 2019;54(2):1900586.

19. Launay D, Montani D, Hassoun PM, et al. Clinical phenotypes and survival of pre-capillary pulmonary hypertension in systemic sclerosis. PLoS One 2018;13(5):e0197112.

20. Fox BD, Shimony A, Langleben D, et al. High prevalence of occult left heart disease in scleroderma-pulmonary hypertension. Eur Respir J 2013;42: 1083–91.

21. Farkas L, Gauldie J, Voelkel NF, et al. Pulmonary hypertension and idiopathic pulmonary fibrosis: a tale of angiogenesis, apoptosis, and growth factors. Am J Respir Cell Mol Biol 2011;45(1):1–15.

22. Lewandowska K, Ciurzynski M, Gorska E, et al. Antiendothelial cells antibodies in patients with systemic sclerosis in relation to pulmonary hypertension and lung fibrosis. Adv Exp Med Biol 2013;756:147–53.

23. Gabrielli A, Avvedimento EV, Krieg T. Scleroderma. N Engl J Med 2009;360(19):1989–2003.

24. van den Hoogen F, Khanna D, Fransen J, et al. 2013 classification criteria for systemic sclerosis: an American College of Rheumatology/European League Against Rheumatism Collaborative Initiative. Ann Rheum Dis 2013;72:1747–55.

25. Ranque B, Mouthon L. Geoepidemiology of systemic sclerosis. Autoimmun Rev 2010;9(5):A311–8.

26. Mathai SC, Sibley CT, Forfia PR, et al. Tricuspid annular plane systolic excursion is a robust outcome measure in systemic sclerosis-associated pulmonary arterial hypertension. J Rheumatol 2011; 38(11):2410–8.

27. Dorfmuller P, Humbert M, Perros F, et al. Fibrous remodeling of the pulmonary venous system in pulmonary arterial hypertension associated with connective tissue diseases. Hum Pathol 2007;38(6):893–902.

28. Montani D, Lau EM, Dorfmuller P, et al. Pulmonary veno-occlusive disease. Eur Respir J 2016;47: 1518–34.

29. Coghlan JG, Denton CP, Grunig E, et al. Evidence-based detection of pulmonary arterial hypertension in systemic sclerosis: the DETECT study. Ann Rheum Dis 2014;73(7):1340–9.

30. Hachulla E, Carpentier P, Gressin V, et al. Risk factors for death and the 3-year survival of patients with systemic sclerosis: the French ItinerAIR-Sclerodermie study. Rheumatology (Oxford) 2009;48(3):304–8.

31. Campo A, Mathai SC, Le PJ, et al. Hemodynamic predictors of survival in scleroderma-related pulmonary arterial hypertension. Am J Respir Crit Care Med 2010;182(2):252–60.

32. Rubenfire M, Huffman MD, Krishnan S, et al. Survival in systemic sclerosis with pulmonary arterial hypertension has not improved in the modern era. Chest 2013;144(4):1282–90.

33. Chung L, Domsic RT, Lingala B, et al. Survival and predictors of mortality in systemic sclerosis associated pulmonary arterial hypertension: outcomes from the PHAROS registry. Arthritis Care Res (Hoboken) 2013;65(3):454–63.

34. Mathai SC, Bueso M, Hummers LK, et al. Disproportionate elevation of N-terminal pro-brain natriuretic peptide in scleroderma-related pulmonary hypertension. Eur Respir J 2010;35(1):95–104.

35. Overbeek MJ, Lankhaar JW, Westerhof N, et al. Right ventricular contractility in systemic sclerosis-associated and idiopathic pulmonary arterial hypertension. Eur Respir J 2008;31(6):1160–6.

36. Tedford RJ, Mudd JO, Girgis RE, et al. Right ventricular dysfunction in systemic sclerosis associated pulmonary arterial hypertension. Circ Heart Fail 2013;6(5):953–63.

37. Hsu S, Kokkenen-Simon KM, Kirk JA, et al. Right ventricular myofilament functional differences in humans with systemic sclerosis-associated versus idiopathic pulmonary arterial hypertension. Circulation 2018;137:2360–70.

38. Bourji KI, Kelemen BW, Mathai SC, et al. Poor survival in patients with scleroderma and pulmonary hypertension due to heart failure with preserved ejection fraction. Pulm Circ 2017;7(2):409–20.

39. Sharp GC, Irvin WS, Tan EM, et al. Mixed connective tissue disease—an apparently distinct rheumatic disease syndrome associated with a specific antibody to an extractable nuclear antigen (ENA). Am J Med 1972;52(2):148–59.

40. Gunnarsson R, Andreassen AK, Molberg O, et al. Prevalence of pulmonary hypertension in an unselected, mixed connective tissue disease cohort: results of a nationwide, Norwegian cross-sectional multicentre study and review of current literature. Rheumatology (Oxford) 2013;52(7):1208–13.

41. Gunnarsson R, Aalokken TM, Molberg O, et al. Prevalence and severity of interstitial lung disease in mixed connective tissue disease: a nationwide, cross-sectional study. Ann Rheum Dis 2012;71(12):1966–72.

42. Chung L, Liu J, Parsons L, et al. Characterization of connective tissue disease-associated pulmonary arterial hypertension from REVEAL: identifying systemic sclerosis as a unique phenotype. Chest 2010;138(6):1383–94.

43. Khanna D, Gladue H, Channick R, et al. Recommendations for screening and detection of connective-tissue disease associated pulmonary arterial hypertension. Arthritis Rheum 2013;65(12):3194–201.

44. Condliffe R, Kiely DG, Peacock AJ, et al. Connective tissue disease-associated pulmonary arterial hypertension in the modern treatment era. Am J Respir Crit Care Med 2009;179(2):151–7.

45. Hannah JR, D'Cruz DP. Pulmonary complications of systemic lupus erythematosus. Semin Respir Crit Care Med 2019;40(2):227–34.

46. Hachulla E, Jais X, Cinquetti G, et al, French Collaborators Recruiting Members(*). Pulmonary arterial hypertension associated with systemic lupus erythematosus: results from the French Pulmonary Hypertension Registry. Chest 2018;153(01):143–51.

47. Johnson SR, Gladman DD, Urowitz MB, et al. Pulmonary hypertension in systemic lupus. Lupus 2004; 13(7):506–9.

48. Flament T, Bigot A, Chaigne B, et al. Pulmonary manifestations of Sjögren's syndrome. Eur Respir Rev 2016;25(140):110–23.

49. Launay D, Hachulla E, Hatron PY, et al. Pulmonary arterial hypertension: a rare complication of primary Sjogren syndrome: report of 9 new cases and review of the literature. Medicine (Baltimore) 2007;86(5): 299–315.

50. Crowson CS, Matteson EL, Myasoedova E, et al. The lifetime risk of adult-onset rheumatoid arthritis and other inflammatory autoimmune rheumatic diseases. Arthritis Rheum 2011;63(3):633–9.

51. Bernatsky S, Joseph L, Pineau CA, et al. Estimating the prevalence of polymyositis and dermatomyositis from administrative data: age, sex and regional differences. Ann Rheum Dis 2009;68(7):1192–6.

52. Mathai SC, Danoff SK. Management of interstitial lung disease associated with connective tissue disease. BMJ 2016;352:h6819.

53. Frost A, Badesch D, Gibbs JSR, et al. Diagnosis of pulmonary hypertension. Eur Respir J 2019;53(1): 1801904.

54. Girgis RE, Frost AE, Hill NS, et al. Selective endothelin A receptor antagonism with sitaxsentan for pulmonary arterial hypertension associated with connective tissue disease. Ann Rheum Dis 2007;66(11):1467–72.

55. Oudiz RJ, Schilz RJ, Barst RJ, et al. Treprostinil, a prostacyclin analogue, in pulmonary arterial hypertension associated with connective tissue disease. Chest 2004;126(2):420–7.

56. Denton CP, Humbert M, Rubin L, et al. Bosentan treatment for pulmonary arterial hypertension related to connective tissue disease: a subgroup analysis of the pivotal clinical trials and their open-label extensions. Ann Rheum Dis 2006;65(10):1336–40.

57. Denton CP, Pope JE, Peter HH, et al. Long-term effects of bosentan on quality of life, survival, safety and tolerability in pulmonary arterial hypertension related to connective tissue diseases. Ann Rheum Dis 2008;67(9):1222–8.

58. Badesch DB, Hill NS, Burgess G, et al. Sildenafil for pulmonary arterial hypertension associated with connective tissue disease. J Rheumatol 2007; 34(12):2417–22.

59. Coghlan JG, Channick R, Chin K, et al. Targeting the prostacyclin pathway with selexipag in patients with pulmonary arterial hypertension receiving double combination therapy: insights from the randomized controlled GRIPHON study. Am J Cardiovasc Drugs 2018;18(1):37–47.

60. Coghlan JG, Galiè N, Barberà JA, et al, AMBITION Investigators. Initial combination therapy with ambrisentan and tadalafil in connective tissue disease-associated pulmonary arterial hypertension (CTD-PAH): subgroup analysis from the AMBITION trial. Ann Rheum Dis 2017;76(7):1219–27.

61. Continuous or nocturnal oxygen therapy in hypoxemic chronic obstructive lung disease: a clinical trial. Nocturnal Oxygen Therapy Trial Group. Ann Intern Med 1980;93(3):391–8.

62. Long term domiciliary oxygen therapy in chronic hypoxic cor pulmonale complicating chronic bronchitis and emphysema. Report of the Medical Research Council Working Party. Lancet 1981; 1(8222):681–6.

63. Mereles D, Ehlken N, Kreuscher S, et al. Exercise and respiratory training improve exercise capacity and quality of life in patients with severe chronic pulmonary hypertension. Circulation 2006;114(14):1482–9.

64. Grunig E, Maier F, Ehlken N, et al. Exercise training in pulmonary arterial hypertension associated with connective tissue diseases. Arthritis Res Ther 2012;14(3):R148.

65. Khan MS, Usman MS, Siddiqi TJ, et al. Is anticoagulation beneficial in pulmonary arterial hypertension? Circ Cardiovasc Qual Outcomes 2018;11(9):e004757.

66. Galiè N, Channick RN, Frantz RP, et al. Risk stratification and medical therapy of pulmonary arterial hypertension. Eur Respir J 2019;53(1):1801889.

67. Jais X, Launay D, Yaici A, et al. Immunosuppressive therapy in lupus- and mixed connective tissue disease-associated pulmonary arterial hypertension: a retrospective analysis of twenty-three cases. Arthritis Rheum 2008;58(2):521–31.

68. Sanchez O, Sitbon O, Jais X, et al. Immunosuppressive therapy in connective tissue diseases-associated pulmonary arterial hypertension. Chest 2006;130(1):182–9.

69. Kato M, Kataoka H, Odani T, et al. The short-term role of corticosteroid therapy for pulmonary arterial

hypertension associated with connective tissue diseases: report of five cases and a literature review. Lupus 2011;20(10):1047–56.

70. Miyamichi-Yamamoto S, Fukumoto Y, Sugimura K, et al. Intensive immunosuppressive therapy improves pulmonary hemodynamics and long-term prognosis in patients with pulmonary arterial hypertension associated with connective tissue disease. Circ J 2011;75(11):2668–74.

71. Benza RL, Gomberg-Maitland M, Elliott CG, et al. Predicting survival in patients with pulmonary arterial hypertension: the REVEAL risk score calculator 2.0 and comparison with ESC/ERS-based risk assessment strategies. Chest 2019;156(2):323–37.

72. Mercurio V, Diab N, Peloquin G, et al. Risk assessment in scleroderma patients with newly diagnosed pulmonary arterial hypertension: application of the ESC/ERS risk prediction model. Eur Respir J 2018; 52(4):1800497.

73. Mullin CJ, Khair RM, Damico RL, et al, PHAROS Investigators. Validation of the REVEAL prognostic equation and risk score calculator in incident systemic sclerosis-associated pulmonary arterial hypertension. Arthritis Rheumatol 2019;71(10):1691–700.

74. Rhee RL, Gabler NB, Praestgaard A, et al. Adverse events in connective tissue disease-associated pulmonary arterial hypertension. Arthritis Rheum 2015; 67(09):2457–65.

75. Rhee RL, Gabler NB, Sangani S, et al. Comparison of treatment response in idiopathic and connective tissue disease-associated pulmonary arterial hypertension. Am J Respir Crit Care Med 2015;192(09):1111–7.

76. Mathai SC, Puhan MA, Lam D, et al. The minimal important difference in the 6-minute walk test for patients with pulmonary arterial hypertension. Am J Respir Crit Care Med 2012;186(5):428–33.

77. McLaughlin V, Zhao C, Coghlan JG, et al. Outcomes associated with modern treatment paradigms in connective tissue disease (CTD)-associated pulmonary arterial hypertension (PAH): a meta-analysis of randomized controlled trials (RCTs). Eur Heart J 2020;41(2). ehaa946.2282.

78. Hassoun PM, Zamanian RT, Damico R, et al. Ambrisentan and tadalafil up-front combination therapy in scleroderma-associated pulmonary arterial hypertension. Am J Respir Crit Care Med 2015;192(9):1102–10.

79. Waxman AB, Restrepo-Jarmillo R, Thenappan T, et al. Inhaled treprostinil in pulmonary hypertension due to interstitial lung disease. N Eng J Med 2021; 384:325–34.

80. e Groote P, Gressin V, Hachulla E, et al, ItinerAIR-Scleroderma Investigators.. Evaluation of cardiac abnormalities by Doppler echocardiography in a large nationwide multicentric cohort of patients with systemic sclerosis. Ann Rheum Dis 2008;67(1):31–6.

81. Kim NH, Delcroix M, Jais X, et al. Chronic thromboembolic pulmonary hypertension. Eur Respir J 2019; 53(1):1801915.

82. Ghofrani HA, D'Armini AM, Grimminger F, et al, CHEST-1 Study Group. Riociguat for the treatment of chronic thromboembolic pulmonary hypertension. N Engl J Med 2013;369(04):319–29.

83. Lang I, Meyer BC, Ogo T, et al. Balloon pulmonary angioplasty in chronic thromboembolic pulmonary hypertension. Eur Respir Rev 2017;26(143):160119.

84. Herve P, Lau EM, Sitbon O, et al. Criteria for diagnosis of exercise pulmonary hypertension. Eur Respir J 2015;46:728–37.

85. Kovacs G, Avian A, Olschewski H. Proposed new definition of exercise pulmonary hypertension decreases false-positive cases. Eur Respir J 2016;47: 1270–3.

86. Stamm A, Saxer S, Lichtblau M, et al. Exercise pulmonary haemodynamics predict outcome in patients with systemic sclerosis. Eur Respir J 2016; 48:1658–67.

87. Zeder K, Avian A, Bachmaier G, et al. Exercise pulmonary resistances predict long-term survival in systemic sclerosis. Chest 2021;159(2):781–90.

88. Ulrich S, Mathai SC. Performance under pressure: the relevance of pulmonary vascular response to exercise in scleroderma. Chest 2021;159:481–3.

89. Pan Z, Marra AM, Benjamin N, et al. Early treatment with ambrisentan of mildly elevated mean pulmonary arterial pressure associated with systemic sclerosis: a randomized, controlled, double-blind, parallel group study (EDITA study). Arthritis Res Ther 2019;21:217.

90. Yusen RD, Edwards LB, Dipchand AI, et al, International Society for Heart and Lung Transplantation. The Registry of the International Society for Heart and Lung Transplantation: thirty-third adult lung and heart-lung transplant report-2016; focus theme: primary diagnostic indications for transplant. J Heart Lung Transpl 2016;35:1170–84.

91. Bernstein EJ, Peterson ER, Sell JL, et al. Survival of adults with systemic sclerosis following lung transplantation: a nationwide cohort study. Arthritis Rheumatol 2015;67:1314–22.

92. Eberlein M, Mathai SC. Lung transplantation in scleroderma. Time for the pendulum to swing? Ann Am Thorac Soc 2016;13(6):767–9.

Pulmonary Arterial Hypertension in Patients Infected with the Human Immunodeficiency Virus

Stephanie M. Hon, MD[a],*, Rodolfo M. Alpizar-Rivas, MD[b], Harrison W. Farber, MD[a]

KEYWORDS

- Pulmonary arterial hypertension • HIV • Management • Outcomes

KEY POINTS

- It is important to recognize and treat human immunodeficiency virus-associated pulmonary arterial hypertension (HIV-PAH) because of the associated morbidity and mortality.
- With the introduction of antiretroviral therapies (ART), improved survival has changed the focus of treatment management from immunodeficiency-related opportunistic infections to chronic cardiovascular complications, including HIV-PAH.
- The 2018 6th World Symposium of Pulmonary Hypertension recommended a revised definition of PAH that might result in a greater number of patients with HIV-PAH; however, the implication of this change is not yet clear.

INTRODUCTION

Pulmonary arterial hypertension (PAH) was first suspected in 1891 when Dr E. Romberg reported a case of a patient with pulmonary artery thickening without other heart or lung disease findings on autopsy. Later in 1951, Dr D.T. Dresdale described an additional series of 3 patients and named the condition primary pulmonary hypertension.[1] Since then, the understanding and characterization of PAH have evolved with multiple etiologies identified and categorized into 5 groups by the 2018 6th World Symposium of Pulmonary Hypertension (**Table 1**). Group 1 PAH includes idiopathic, heritable, drug/toxin-induced, and PAH associated with certain conditions such as connective tissue disease, congenital heart disease, portal hypertension, schistosomiasis, and human immunodeficiency virus (HIV) infection.[2] The diagnosis of PAH requires the appropriate hemodynamic criteria, most currently defined in 2018 by consensus at the World Symposium of Pulmonary Hypertension: mean pulmonary artery (mPA) pressure greater than 20 mm Hg with a pulmonary capillary wedge pressure (PCWP) <15 mm Hg and a pulmonary vascular resistance (PVR) $\geq$3 Woods Units (WU), measured by right heart catheterization (RHC).[2]

HIV is a member of the Retroviridae family with a genome composed of 2 identical copies of single-stranded RNA. There are 2 types of HIV: HIV-1 that is most commonly found worldwide and HIV-2 that is mainly prevalent in western and central Africa.[3] First reports of acquired immune deficiency syndrome (AIDS) from HIV infection appeared in 1981 when a case series of 19 previously healthy men who had sex with men presented with Kaposi sarcoma and/or pneumocystis pneumonia in California.[4] In 1987, the AZT trial demonstrated that antiretroviral therapy (ART) could alter mortality

[a] Division of Pulmonary, Critical Care, and Sleep Medicine, Tufts Medical Center, 800 Washington Street, Box 257, Boston, MA 02111, USA; [b] Division of Infectious Diseases, University of Rochester Medical Center, 601 Elmwood Avenue, Box 689, Rochester, NY 14642, USA
* Corresponding author.
E-mail address: shon@tuftsmedicalcenter.org

Cardiol Clin 40 (2022) 45–54
https://doi.org/10.1016/j.ccl.2021.08.004
0733-8651/22/© 2021 Elsevier Inc. All rights reserved.

Table 1
Clinical classification of pulmonary hypertension (6th World Symposium on pulmonary hypertension)

1 PAH	1.1 Idiopathic PAH
	1.2 Heritable PAH
	1.3 Drug- and toxin-induced PAH
	1.4 PAH associated with:
	1.4.1 Connective tissue disease
	1.4.2 HIV infection
	1.4.3 Portal hypertension
	1.4.4 Congenital heart disease
	1.4.5 Schistosomiasis
	1.5 PAH long-term responders to calcium channel blockers
	1.6 PAH with overt features of venous/capillaries (PVOD/PCH) involvement
	1.7 Persistent PH of the newborn syndrome
2 PH due to left heart disease	2.1 PH due to heart failure with preserved LVEF
	2.2 PH due to heart failure with reduced LVEF
	2.3 Valvular heart disease
	2.4 Congenital/acquired cardiovascular conditions leading to postcapillary PH
3 PH due to lung disease and/or hypoxia	3.1 Obstructive lung disease
	3.2 Restrictive lung disease
	3.3 Other lung diseases with mixed restrictive/obstructive pattern
	3.4 Hypoxia without lung disease
	3.5 Developmental lung disorders
4 PH due to pulmonary artery obstructions	4.1 Chronic thromboembolic PH
	4.2 Other pulmonary artery obstructions
5 PH due to unclear and/or multifactorial mechanisms	5.1 Hematologic disorders
	5.2 Systemic and metabolic disorders
	5.3 Others
	5.4 Complex congenital heart disease

Abbreviations: LVEF, left ventricular ejection fraction; PAH, pulmonary arterial hypertension; PCH, pulmonary capillary hemangiomatosis; PH, pulmonary hypertension; PVOD, pulmonary veno-occlusive disease.

Adapted from Simonneau G, Montani D, Celermajer DS, Denton CP, Gatzoulis MA, Krowka M, Williams PG, Souza R. Haemodynamic definitions and updated clinical classification of pulmonary hypertension. Eur Respir J. 2019 Jan 24;53(1):1801913. Reproduced with permission of the © ERS 2021; DOI: 10.1183/13993003.01913-2018 Published 24 January 2019.

and,[5] unfortunately, the virus developed resistance to a single agent; it was not until 1996 that the AIDS Clinical Trials Group study showed that highly active antiretroviral therapy (HAART also called ART) could inhibit viral replication at different sites by using 3 antiviral agents and could prevent the development of resistance.[6] As therapies based on this principle have expanded and improved, HIV has been transformed into chronic disease. As such, as the HIV population ages, they will develop other comorbidities, including cardiovascular diseases.[7,8]

According to the most recent reports from the Center for Disease Control (CDC) in 2018, there were approximately 1.2 million people living with HIV in the United States. As more is learned about HIV and advancements are made in therapies, the life expectancy of HIV-infected patients on uninterrupted ART has nearly matched that of non–HIV-infected patients. Current practice is to start ART as soon as a patient is diagnosed.[9] As people with HIV live longer, their care becomes more complex because of the development of many comorbidities associated with advanced age. Chronic conditions such as cardiac, pulmonary, and metabolic diseases become more frequent, including human immunodeficiency virus-associated pulmonary arterial hypertension (HIV-PAH). In addition to these comorbidities, interactions between ART and therapies to treat HIV-PAH and other conditions become more numerous and difficult to manage.[9]

HIV-PAH was first described in 1987 by Kim and Factor.[10] In 1991, a Swiss study of 1200 patients with untreated HIV suggested a prevalence of HIV-PAH of 0.5% among this population with respiratory symptoms of unclear etiology; however, the true prevalence may be higher because patients with asymptomatic were excluded.[11] Subsequent studies, including both transthoracic echocardiogram (TTE) and diagnostic confirmation with RHC, found similar prevalence rates, even after the introduction of ART.[12,13] With that said, patients with HIV with higher viral load and lower CD-4 cell counts do have worse outcomes than patients with non–HIV.[14] Although a prevalence of 1 in 200 patients seems low, it is still 100 to 1000 times greater than in the non–HIV-infected population.[13]

PATHOPHYSIOLOGY

The precise pathophysiology of HIV-PAH is unknown, but like many other diseases that are not well understood, it is thought to be multifactorial. It is hypothesized that mechanisms include chronic inflammation, protein Gp120, transactivator of transcription(Tat) protein negative factor (nef) and genetic predisposition determined by HLA-DR6 and HLA-DR52 frequency (**Fig. 1**).

We do know, however, that the pathophysiology of pulmonary hypertension in patients with HIV is not related to the direct infection of the HIV to the pulmonary vascular cells, as HIV material is not found in the pulmonary vasculature.[15] Moreover, the development of HIV-PAH is independent of the CD4 count, the HIV viral load, or history of

previous opportunistic infections; however, it does seem related to the length of HIV infection.

Chronic Inflammation

HIV infection is known to be a chronic inflammatory state.[16] Chronic inflammation is associated with the inhibition of nitric oxide (NO) synthase which increases NO signaling causing endothelial dysfunction and smooth muscle proliferation that is, linked to the development of PAH.[17]

Gp120

Gp 120 is an HIV surface glycoprotein which by binding with the CD4 lymphocyte glycoprotein, initiates the process which allows the entry of the HIV into the host cell.[18] This glycoprotein has also been related to the pathophysiology of PAH through 2 pathways: chronic inflammation and endothelin-1 secretion. Gp120 stimulates the proinflammatory cytokine cascade[19] which has proliferative effects on vascular smooth muscle causing concentric intimal fibrosis, medial hypertrophy, and plexiform lesions, findings similar to the histology of group 1 patients with PAH who are not HIV infected. Gp120 is also known to stimulate the secretion of endothelin-1 in the lung endothelium which causes vasoconstriction and increases apoptosis which leads to intimal fibrosis.[15]

Transactivator of Transcription

HIV-infected cells secrete a Tat protein which is required for viral transcription.[20] In-vitro studies

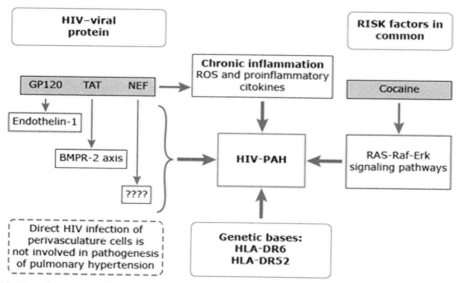

Fig. 1. HIV-PAH pathogenesis. (*From* Correale M, Palmiotti GA, Lo Storto MM, et al. HIV-associated pulmonary arterial hypertension: from bedside to the future. Eur J Clin Invest 2015; 45(5):515-28.)

have shown that Tat protein suppresses the bone morphogenic protein receptor-2 (BMPR-2) gene expressed by human macrophages.[21] BMPR-2 is part of the transforming growth factor (TGF) pathway which regulates smooth muscle cell growth and proliferation.[22] This finding is similar to some patients with heritable PAH who have lost the function of BMPR-2 through genetic mutations. Exogenous Tat can also stimulate the release of endothelial cell-mediated growth factor and production of reactive O_2 species. This process further alters the endothelial function which could lead to the development of PAH.[23]

Negative Factor

Nef is a protein encoded by HIV as part of host cell signaling[24]; it has been found in the endothelium of pulmonary and vascular cell types of patients with HIV-PAH.[25] Increased HIV-Nef gene polymorphisms have been reported in patients with HIV-PAH, compared patients with HIV that do not have PAH.[26] In vitro studies have shown that Nef promotes angiogenesis in other vascular diseases such as Kaposi sarcoma.[27]

Genetic Bases: HLA-DR6, HLA-DR52

There is a report of increased frequency of HLA-DR6 (-DRB1*1301/2 subtypes) and of HLA-DR52 (DRB3*0301 subtype), in patients with HIV with PAH and this finding suggests that there is a genetic susceptibility that predisposes to HIV-PAH.[28]

DIAGNOSIS
Clinical Presentation

In most patients, the diagnosis of HIV is already present when signs and symptoms suggestive of pulmonary hypertension arise. Rarely, HIV is discovered during the routine evaluation for pulmonary hypertension. Diagnosis can occur at any stage of HIV infection, both early and late stages.[29]

Independent risk factors associated with pulmonary hypertension in patients with HIV include female sex, history of intravenous drug use, detectable viral load as well as chronic hepatitis C infection. However, no correlation has been observed between age, duration of infection, and CD4 count with the development or severity of pulmonary hypertension in patients with HIV.[30]

The clinical presentation of HIV-PAH can prove challenging as it mimics many other cardiopulmonary diseases. The most common symptoms are dyspnea (85%), lower extremity edema (30%), nonproductive cough (19%), fatigue (13%), syncope or presyncope (12%), and chest pain (7%).[31] Most of the symptoms seen in patients with HIV-PAH reflect right ventricular dysfunction and manifest with exercise intolerance. The dyspnea on exertion, eventually, progresses to dyspnea with minimal activity to finally dyspnea even at rest. Symptoms of HIV-PAH are indistinguishable from those of other forms of pulmonary hypertension. However, a more recent study showed that the time interval between the onset of symptoms and diagnosis is much shorter in patients with HIV (6 months) than those with idiopathic PAH (2.5 years),[32] possibly reflecting the closer monitoring of HIV-infected patients.

Certain findings on physical examination are commonly seen in patients with pulmonary hypertension regardless of etiology. These include an increase in the pulmonic component of the second heart sound (P2), a right-sided S3 gallop, murmurs of tricuspid and pulmonic regurgitation, and increased jugular venous pressure and peripheral edema.[31] It is important to recognize these findings and initiate appropriate evaluation for pulmonary hypertension. As patients with HIV-PAH may have chronic pulmonary and cardiac diseases that contribute to the symptoms of dyspnea and heart failure, a complete evaluation is required to identify all etiologies contributing to an elevated pulmonary artery pressure.[33]

Diagnostic Testing

Initial diagnostic testing includes routine examinations such as electrocardiograms, radiographs, and pulmonary function tests. Electrocardiograms may show right axis deviation, right atrial abnormalities (tall prominent P waves in leads II, III, aVF), right ventricular hypertrophy, and/or right ventricular strain (complete or incomplete right bundle branch block) or sinus tachycardia.[34] Chest radiograph frequently shows prominent pulmonary arteries (71%–90%) with enlarged hilar vessels (80%), decrease in peripheral vasculature described as pruning (51%), and cardiomegaly (72%).[34] Pulmonary function tests are commonly obtained in the setting of dyspnea and most frequently reveal a decrease in diffusing capacity for carbon monoxide in patients with pulmonary hypertension.[34] Arterial blood gases if obtained commonly demonstrate hypoxemia and respiratory alkalosis (hypocapnia).[34]

Until recently, echocardiography has not been used to screen HIV-infected patients without clinical suspicion of PAH. However, since recommendations were updated at the 2018 6th World Symposium of Pulmonary Hypertension, it is now standard of care for the echocardiographic screening of HIV-infected patients with one of the following risk factors: female sex, intravenous drug use/cocaine or methamphetamine use, hepatitis C virus infection, origin from a high-prevalence country, known Nef or Tat HIV proteins, and US African American patients independent of symptoms.[35] The most frequent findings on TTE include: systolic flattening of interventricular septum, right atrial and right ventricular enlargement, and tricuspid regurgitation. Pulmonary arterial systolic pressure (PASP) can be estimated on TTE by measuring Doppler flow through the tricuspid valve, specifically the tricuspid regurgitant jet velocity (TRV). The pressure gradient between the right atrium and right ventricle is then calculated based on the Bernoulli's equation and added to the estimated right atrial pressure (RAP).[36] A TRV ≥2.8 m.s-1, ePASP greater than 35 mm Hg in young adults or greater than 40 mm Hg in older adults, and/or abnormal RV size, wall thickness and function suggest pulmonary hypertension, although the absence of these findings does not rule out the diagnosis.[37] Other echocardiographic measurements used to extrapolate information on right-sided cardiac pressures include pulmonary artery acceleration time, which is the interval between the onset of systolic pulmonary arterial flow and peak flow velocity measured by pulsed-wave Doppler analysis, as well as the morphology of right ventricular outflow tract velocity envelopes as midsystolic flow deceleration and notching have correlated with higher pulmonary artery pressures, higher PVR, and worse outcomes.[38–40]

Although TTE is a helpful noninvasive test for screening and can reveal other secondary causes of pulmonary hypertension such as valvular disease or congenital heart disease, Doppler estimates of PASP are inaccurate when compared with the gold standard of direct hemodynamic measurements by RHC. In the general PAH population, studies have shown estimated PASP to be inaccurate by TTE measurements in 48% cases when compared with invasive hemodynamic measurements.[41] In the HIV patient population, 1 in 3 patients with a diagnosis of HIV-PAH were missed due to inaccurate TTE-based ePASP measurements when compared with invasive hemodynamic measurements.[42] Thus, RHC remains the gold standard for diagnosis of pulmonary hypertension and measurement of hemodynamic values.

For the diagnosis of pulmonary hypertension, measurements obtained during RHC must include pulmonary arterial pressure (PAP), cardiac output (CO), and pulmonary artery wedge pressure (PAWP), such that PVR and cardiac index (CI) can be calculated. These calculated indices are important for a complete and comprehensive

understanding of the severity of pulmonary hypertension, as the mean PAP in isolation is inadequate to make a diagnosis or assess prognosis. As the right ventricle fails, the inability to generate a normal CO will result in a lower PAP (**Fig. 2**). Routine vasodilator testing is not recommended in patients with suspected HIV-PAH because vasodilator responsiveness is rarely found in patients with HIV-PAH.

Once the patient is diagnosed with PAH (mean PAP >20 mm Hg with a PAWP ≤15 mm Hg and a PVR ≥3 Wood units), evaluation should exclude other etiologies. Patients with HIV-associated PH should have a ventilation/perfusion (V/Q) scan to rule out thromboembolic disease and testing to evaluate for congenital or acquired valvular or myocardial disease, connective tissue disease, or parasitic disease affecting the lungs. Particularly in patients with HIV infection, pulmonary hypertension has been observed in intravenous drug users who inject crushed pills contaminated with foreign particles (particularly talc), as well as drugs/toxins known to be associated with pulmonary hypertension such as cocaine and methamphetamine. Risk factors for HIV such as polysubstance use also portend risk for hepatitis and liver disease with portal hypertension, thus it is not uncommon to find patients with HIV infection and liver disease developing portopulmonary hypertension. However, there are hemodynamic parameters that help differentiate portopulmonary hypertension from HIV-associated pulmonary hypertension, such as high CO in the former.[43] Hypoxemia due to *Pneumocystis jirovecii* pneumonia, lymphocytic interstitial pneumonia, nonspecific interstitial pneumonia, and cytomegalovirus pneumonia is frequently seen in patients with HIV and may contribute to pulmonary hypertension.

TREATMENT
General Human Immunodeficiency Virus Treatments

The cornerstone of treatment for compliant HIV patients as recommended by IDSA HIV guidelines is ART independent of CD4 count or viral load, as it has shown to improve survival, decrease comorbidities, and decrease transmission of HIV. Nevertheless, the impact of ART on HIV-PAH hemodynamics and outcomes remains controversial.

Antiretroviral Therapy and Its Relation to Pulmonary Arterial Hypertension

Some studies have suggested improved outcomes in patients treated with ART including reduced incidence of PAH in these patients.[44,45]

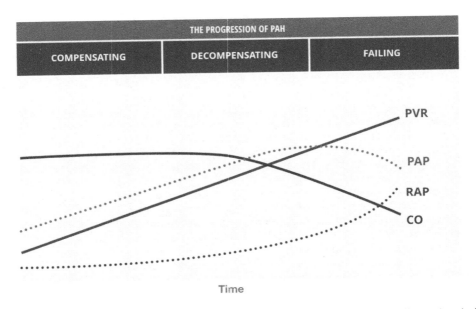

Fig. 2. Hemodynamic parameters in the progression of pulmonary hypertension. (*From* Hill NS. Historical perspective and classification. In: Hill NS, ed. Pulmonary Hypertension Therapy. Armonk, NY: Summit Communications, LLC; 2006:9.)

A small retrospective echocardiography study of 47 patients followed for 3 days to 10.5 years (median duration 2.7 years) showed that those who received ART had a decrease in the RVSP-RAP gradient of 21 mm Hg; in contrast, patients who did not receive ART had an increase of 25 mm Hg.[44] However, the lack of direct hemodynamic studies with RHC measurements significantly limits previously published studies. When RHC was used for evaluation, ART was associated with improvement in 6-min walk distance, but no significant improvement in hemodynamics without targeted PAH treatments.[46] Furthermore, a large prospective French cohort study demonstrated that the prevalence of HIV-PAH remained unchanged after treatment with ART became routine for patients with HIV, suggesting that ART does not affect the development of HIV-PAH.[13]

PAH-Directed Therapy

General principles of managing pulmonary hypertension apply to patients with HIV-PAH including encouraging exercise as tolerated, counseling against smoking and pregnancy, oxygen supplementation for hypoxemia, and diuretics for volume overload. Positive responses to vasoreactivity testing in patients with HIV-PAH have been rare, and thus calcium channel blockers should be judiciously used in select patients while monitoring for worsening symptoms and hemodynamics.[47] Additionally, calcium channel blockers benefit a very

small proportion of patients with HIV-PAH and can incur intolerable side effects such as hypotension and drug–drug interactions with ART such as protease inhibitors.[47,48]

Although patients with HIV are underrepresented in, or excluded from studies of PAH-directed therapy, patients with HIV-PAH respond well to PAH-specific treatments, as reports have shown normalization of hemodynamics, which is rare in other etiologies.[49] The management of pulmonary hypertension depends on the patients' symptoms, New York Heart Association (NYHA) or World Health Organization (WHO) functional class and severity of pulmonary hypertension. There are several classes of medications used to treat pulmonary hypertension including endothelin receptor antagonists, NO–cyclic guanosine monophosphate (cGMP) enhancers including phosphodiesterase inhibitors and guanylate cyclase stimulants, and prostacyclin pathway agonists.

Endothelin Receptor Antagonists

There is limited data supporting the use of endothelin receptor antagonists specifically for HIV-PAH, but bosentan, ambrisentan, and macitentan have all been shown to improve hemodynamics and exercise tolerance and prevent worsening of PH in general. Small studies including a prospective study of 16 patients with severely symptomatic (NYHA class III-IV) HIV-PAH showed that 16 weeks of bosentan improved exercise capacity as measured by 6-min walk distance (91 ± 60m, $P<.001$), functional class, mPAP (decreased by 21%), PVR (decreased by 43%), CI (increased by 39%), RV size and function, and quality of life.[50] This trend was supported in longer treatment duration in a study of 59 patients with HIV-PAH receiving bosentan more than 29 months, with improvements seen in symptoms, exercise tolerance, and hemodynamic parameters. Survival rates improved to 93%, 86%, and 66% at 1, 2, and 3 years, respectively, with the normalization of hemodynamic parameters in 10 of 59 patients.[51] In general, bosentan was observed to be safe and overall well tolerated in conjunction with ART for the treatment of HIV-PAH, albeit dosage adjustments should be considered for concomitant use of a pharmacologic boosting agent such as ritonavir or cobicistat.

Unfortunately, there is still insufficient dedicated data for newer endothelin receptor antagonists such as ambrisentan and macitentan for treating HIV-PAH. However, small numbers of patients with HIV were included in larger trials (ARIES [ambrisentan] and SERAPHIN [macitentan]) that resulted in Food and Drug Administration approval for use in PAH.[52,53] Ambrisentan and macitentan are increasingly favored over bosentan for the lower frequency of liver function test abnormalities and fewer drug interactions with ART.[54]

Nitric Oxide-Cyclic Guanosine Monophosphate Enhancers

Phosphodiesterase type 5 inhibitors include sildenafil and tadalafil. Case reports and series have suggested that sildenafil can improve dyspnea, NYHA functional class, exercise capacity, and mean PAP in HIV-PAH.[55] However, this class of medications requires careful monitoring and considerations for drug–drug interaction, as its metabolism is mediated by cytochrome P450 CYP3A4 and CYP2C9, which are inhibited by protease inhibitors and boosting agents such as ritonavir. Pharmacologic studies have shown marked increases in sildenafil levels in the setting of coadministration with indinavir, saquinavir, and ritonavir; the clinical relevance of these findings is not clear, because hypotension and other adverse effects were not observed in pharmacokinetic studies.[56] Tadalafil, in addition to convenient daily dosing, also seems to be less affected by ritonavir.[57]

Riociguat is a guanylate cyclase stimulant that both directly increases the generation of cGMP leading to subsequent vasodilation and sensitizes guanylate cyclase to endogenous NO. This medication has been approved for the treatment of Group 1 PAH and Group 4 chronic thromboembolic pulmonary hypertension (CTEPH) but has not been studied in HIV-PAH. However, drug–drug interaction studies suggest it is safe with currently available ART regimens.[58]

Prostacyclin Analogs

Prostacyclin therapies can be administered via different routes including intravenous, subcutaneous, inhaled, or oral. Systemic epoprostenol reduces PVR and PAP and improves CO in patients with HIV-PAH.[59–61] Moreover, the study by Aguilar and colleagues[62] demonstrated a durable hemodynamic and clinical response out to 4 years in these patients. Subcutaneous treprostinil has been used in HIV-PAH (n = 3) demonstrating improved exercise capacity, functional class, and PASP on echocardiography at 1 year. Inhaled iloprost has been studied in 8 patients with HIV-PAH and demonstrated acute improvement in PVR and CI with long-term improvements in hemodynamic parameters and exercise capacity.[63] In the pivotal trial of selexipag, an oral prostacyclin receptor analog, there were 10 patients with HIV-PAH (1156 patients total),[64] though their data were not separately analyzed. There are no specific data regarding oral treprostinil use in HIV-PAH.

Refractory Disease

In those patients with refractory HIV-PAH to conventional therapy, it may be reasonable to consider creating right-to-left shunts, for example, atrial septostomy as right ventricular salvage therapy. Lung transplantation, once contraindicated in these patients, is now selectively considered, albeit with strict criteria. A case series of 3 patients who underwent lung transplantation for HIV-PAH or IPF demonstrated feasibility for carefully selected patients in the setting of controlled HIV infection, but raised the concern for more common acute graft rejection.[65]

Prognosis

Since the era of advancing PAH-directed therapy and ART, mortality among patients with HIV-PAH has significantly improved from 27% to 66% mortality in the early 2000s to survival rates of 88% (1-year) and 72% (3-year) in a 2010 study of 77 patients with HIV-PAH; all received ART and 65% also received PAH-directed therapy.[31,32,44,46,66]

SUMMARY

HIV-PAH is a complication of HIV infection that results in significant morbidity and mortality.

However, early diagnosis and initiation of treatment for both HIV and PAH have resulted in dramatically improved outcomes. Although incompletely understood, HIV proteins and chronic immune activation seem to be significant mechanisms in the pathogenesis of HIV-PAH. ART and PAH-specific therapy remain the cornerstone of the management of this disease with care to avoid drug-drug interactions. Further studies, especially randomized clinical trials, are needed not only to validate current PAH-directed therapy for patients with HIV-PAH but also to better understand the pathogenic mechanisms of HIV-PAH to find optimal targets for treatment.

CLINICS CARE POINTS

- HIV-associated pulmonary arterial hypertension can occur at any stage of HIV infection, independent of CD4 count and viral load.
- Since the updated recommendations presented at the 2018 6th World Symposium of Pulmonary Hypertension, it is now standard of care for echocardiographic screening of HIV-infected patients with one of the following risk factors: female sex, intravenous drug use/cocaine or methamphetamine use, hepatitis C virus infection, origin from a high-prevalence country, known Nef or Tat HIV proteins, and African American patients in the United States, independent of symptoms.
- Right heart catheterization is the gold standard for diagnosis of pulmonary hypertension and measurement of hemodynamic values, but routine vasodilator testing is not recommended in patients with suspected HIV-PAH since vasodilator responsiveness is rarely found in patients with HIV-PAH. Because of this and the potential for significant side effects, such as hypotension and drug-drug interactions with antiretroviral therapy such as protease inhibitors, calcium channel blockers should be avoided in this population.
- The cornerstone of treatment for compliant HIV patients is antiretroviral therapy independent of CD4 count or viral load, however the impact of ART on HIV-PAH hemodynamics and outcomes remains controversial as the prevalence of HIV-PAH has remained unchanged after ART became routine treatment for patients with HIV.
- Although patients with HIV are underrepresented in, or excluded from studies of PAH-directed therapy, patients with HIV-PAH respond well to PAH-specific treatments including endothelin receptor antagonists, nitric oxide-cyclic guanosine monophosphate enhancers and prostacyclin analogues. Reports have shown normalization of hemodynamics, rare in other subgroups of PAH. However, it is important to be cognizant of drug-drug interactions between these medications and HIV medications.

DISCLOSURE

The authors have nothing to disclose.

REFERENCES

1. Dresdale DT, Schultz M, Michtom RJ. Primary pulmonary hypertension. I. Clinical and hemodynamic study. Am J Med 1951;11(6):686–705.
2. Simonneau G, Montani D, Celermajer DS, et al. Haemodynamic definitions and updated clinical classification of pulmonary hypertension. Eur Respir J 2019;53(1).
3. Luciw PA. Human immunodeficiency virus and their replication. In: Fields BN, Knippe DM, Howley PM, editors. Field virology. Philadelphia: Lippincott-Raven; 1996. p. 1881–952.
4. Centers for Disease C. A cluster of Kaposi's sarcoma and Pneumocystis carinii pneumonia among homosexual male residents of Los Angeles and Orange Counties, California. MMWR Morb Mortal Wkly Rep 1982;31(23):305–7.
5. Fischl MA, Richman DD, Grieco MH, et al. The efficacy of azidothymidine (AZT) in the treatment of patients with AIDS and AIDS-related complex. A double-blind, placebo-controlled trial. N Engl J Med 1987;317(4):185–91.
6. Collier AC, Coombs RW, Schoenfeld DA, et al. Treatment of human immunodeficiency virus infection with saquinavir, zidovudine, and zalcitabine. AIDS Clinical Trials Group. N Engl J Med 1996;334(16):1011–7.
7. Chu C, Umanski G, Blank A, et al. Comorbidity-related treatment outcomes among HIV-infected adults in the Bronx, NY. J Urban Health 2011;88(3):507–16.
8. Wada N, Jacobson LP, Cohen M, et al. Cause-specific life expectancies after 35 years of age for human immunodeficiency syndrome-infected and human immunodeficiency syndrome-negative individuals followed simultaneously in long-term cohort studies, 1984-2008. Am J Epidemiol 2013;177(2):116–25.
9. Thompson MA, Horberg MA, Agwu AL, et al. Primary care guidance for persons with human immunodeficiency virus: 2020 update by the HIV medicine association of the infectious diseases

society of America. Clin Infect Dis 2020;ciaa1391. https://doi.org/10.1093/cid/ciaa1391.

10. Kim KK, Factor SM. Membranoproliferative glomerulonephritis and plexogenic pulmonary arteriopathy in a homosexual man with acquired immunodeficiency syndrome. Hum Pathol 1987; 18(12):1293–6.

11. Speich R, Jenni R, Opravil M, et al. Primary pulmonary hypertension in HIV infection. Chest 1991; 100(5):1268–71.

12. Humbert M, Sitbon O, Chaouat A, et al. Pulmonary arterial hypertension in France: results from a national registry. Am J Respir Crit Care Med 2006; 173(9):1023–30.

13. Sitbon O, Lascoux-Combe C, Delfraissy JF, et al. Prevalence of HIV-related pulmonary arterial hypertension in the current antiretroviral therapy era. Am J Respir Crit Care Med 2008;177(1):108–13.

14. Brittain EL, Duncan MS, Chang J, et al. Increased echocardiographic pulmonary pressure in HIV-infected and -uninfected individuals in the veterans aging cohort study. Am J Respir Crit Care Med 2018;197(7):923–32.

15. Kanmogne GD, Primeaux C, Grammas P. Induction of apoptosis and endothelin-1 secretion in primary human lung endothelial cells by HIV-1 gp120 proteins. Biochem Biophys Res Commun 2005;333(4):1107–15.

16. Kamin DS, Grinspoon SK. Cardiovascular disease in HIV-positive patients. AIDS 2005;19(7):641–52.

17. Sanders KA, Hoidal JR. The NOX on pulmonary hypertension. Circ Res 2007;101(3):224–6.

18. Kwong PD, Wyatt R, Robinson J, et al. Structure of an HIV gp120 envelope glycoprotein in complex with the CD4 receptor and a neutralizing human antibody. Nature 1998;393(6686):648–59.

19. Kim J, Ruff M, Karwatowska-Prokopczuk E, et al. HIV envelope protein gp120 induces neuropeptide Y receptor-mediated proliferation of vascular smooth muscle cells: relevance to AIDS cardiovascular pathogenesis. Regul Pept 1998;75-76: 201–5.

20. Tahirov TH, Babayeva ND, Varzavand K, et al. Crystal structure of HIV-1 Tat complexed with human P-TEFb. Nature 2010;465(7299):747–51.

21. Caldwell RL, Gadipatti R, Lane KB, et al. HIV-1 TAT represses transcription of the bone morphogenic protein receptor-2 in U937 monocytic cells. J Leukoc Biol 2006;79(1):192–201.

22. Yang X, Long L, Southwood M, et al. Dysfunctional Smad signaling contributes to abnormal smooth muscle cell proliferation in familial pulmonary arterial hypertension. Circ Res 2005;96(10):1053–63.

23. Rusnati M, Presta M. HIV-1 Tat protein and endothelium: from protein/cell interaction to AIDS-associated pathologies. Angiogenesis 2002;5(3):141–51.

24. Almodovar S, Hsue PY, Morelli J, et al. Pathogenesis of HIV-associated pulmonary hypertension: potential role of HIV-1 Nef. Proc Am Thorac Soc 2011;8(3): 308–12.

25. Marecki JC, Cool CD, Parr JE, et al. HIV-1 Nef is associated with complex pulmonary vascular lesions in SHIV-nef-infected macaques. Am J Respir Crit Care Med 2006;174(4):437–45.

26. Almodovar S, Knight R, Allshouse AA, et al. Human immunodeficiency virus nef signature sequences are associated with pulmonary hypertension. AIDS Res Hum Retroviruses 2012;28(6):607–18.

27. Yan Q, Ma X, Shen C, et al. Inhibition of Kaposi's sarcoma-associated herpesvirus lytic replication by HIV-1 Nef and cellular microRNA hsa-miR-1258. J Virol 2014;88(9):4987–5000.

28. Morse JH, Barst RJ, Itescu S, et al. Primary pulmonary hypertension in HIV infection: an outcome determined by particular HLA class II alleles. Am J Respir Crit Care Med 1996;153(4 Pt 1):1299–301.

29. Mesa RA, Edell ES, Dunn WF, et al. Human immunodeficiency virus infection and pulmonary hypertension: two new cases and a review of 86 reported cases. Mayo Clin Proc 1998;73(1):37–45.

30. Quezada M, Martin-Carbonero L, Soriano V, et al. Prevalence and risk factors associated with pulmonary hypertension in HIV-infected patients on regular follow-up. AIDS 2012;26(11):1387–92.

31. Mehta NJ, Khan IA, Mehta RN, et al. HIV-Related pulmonary hypertension: analytic review of 131 cases. Chest 2000;118(4):1133–41.

32. Nunes H, Humbert M, Sitbon O, et al. Prognostic factors for survival in human immunodeficiency virus-associated pulmonary arterial hypertension. Am J Respir Crit Care Med 2003;167(10):1433–9.

33. Barnett CF, Alvarez P, Park MH. Pulmonary arterial hypertension: diagnosis and treatment. Cardiol Clin 2016;34(3):375–89.

34. Petrosillo N, Pellicelli AM, Boumis E, et al. Clinical manifestation of HIV-related pulmonary hypertension. Ann N Y Acad Sci 2001;946:223–35.

35. Frost A, Badesch D, Gibbs JSR, et al. Diagnosis of pulmonary hypertension. Eur Respir J 2019;53(1): 1801904. https://doi.org/10.1183/13993003.01904-2018.

36. Yock PG, Popp RL. Noninvasive estimation of right ventricular systolic pressure by Doppler ultrasound in patients with tricuspid regurgitation. Circulation 1984;70(4):657–62.

37. Ghio S, Mercurio V, Fortuni F, et al. A comprehensive echocardiographic method for risk stratification in pulmonary arterial hypertension. Eur Respir J 2020;56(3):2000513. https://doi.org/10.1183/13993003.00513-2020.

38. Arkles JS, Opotowsky AR, Ojeda J, et al. Shape of the right ventricular Doppler envelope predicts hemodynamics and right heart function in pulmonary hypertension. Am J Respir Crit Care Med 2011; 183(2):268–76.

39. Yared K, Noseworthy P, Weyman AE, et al. Pulmonary artery acceleration time provides an accurate estimate of systolic pulmonary arterial pressure during transthoracic echocardiography. J Am Soc Echocardiogr 2011;24(6):687–92.

40. Takahama H, McCully RB, Frantz RP, et al. Unraveling the RV ejection Doppler envelope: Insight into pulmonary artery hemodynamics and disease severity. JACC Cardiovasc Imaging 2017;10(10 Pt B):1268–77.

41. Fisher MR, Forfia PR, Chamera E, et al. Accuracy of Doppler echocardiography in the hemodynamic assessment of pulmonary hypertension. Am J Respir Crit Care Med 2009;179(7):615–21.

42. Selby VN, Scherzer R, Barnett CF, et al. Doppler echocardiography does not accurately estimate pulmonary artery systolic pressure in HIV-infected patients. AIDS 2012;26(15):1967–9.

43. Kuo PC, Plotkin JS, Johnson LB, et al. Distinctive clinical features of portopulmonary hypertension. Chest 1997;112(4):980–6.

44. Zuber JP, Calmy A, Evison JM, et al. Pulmonary arterial hypertension related to HIV infection: improved hemodynamics and survival associated with antiretroviral therapy. Clin Infect Dis 2004;38(8):1178–85.

45. Pugliese A, Isnardi D, Saini A, et al. Impact of highly active antiretroviral therapy in HIV-positive patients with cardiac involvement. J Infect 2000;40(3):282–4.

46. Degano B, Guillaume M, Savale L, et al. HIV-associated pulmonary arterial hypertension: survival and prognostic factors in the modern therapeutic era. AIDS 2010;24(1):67–75.

47. Montani D, Savale L, Natali D, et al. Long-term response to calcium-channel blockers in non-idiopathic pulmonary arterial hypertension. Eur Heart J 2010;31(15):1898–907.

48. Sitbon O, Humbert M, Jais X, et al. Long-term response to calcium channel blockers in idiopathic pulmonary arterial hypertension. Circulation 2005; 111(23):3105–11.

49. Galie N, Corris PA, Frost A, et al. Updated treatment algorithm of pulmonary arterial hypertension. J Am Coll Cardiol 2013;62(25 Suppl):D60–72.

50. Sitbon O, Gressin V, Speich R, et al. Bosentan for the treatment of human immunodeficiency virus-associated pulmonary arterial hypertension. Am J Respir Crit Care Med 2004;170(11):1212–7.

51. Degano B, Yaici A, Le Pavec J, et al. Long-term effects of bosentan in patients with HIV-associated pulmonary arterial hypertension. Eur Respir J 2009;33(1):92–8.

52. Galie N, Olschewski H, Oudiz RJ, et al. Ambrisentan for the treatment of pulmonary arterial hypertension: results of the ambrisentan in pulmonary arterial hypertension, randomized, double-blind, placebo-controlled, multicenter, efficacy (ARIES) study 1 and 2. Circulation 2008;117(23):3010–9.

53. Pulido T, Adzerikho I, Channick RN, et al. Macitentan and morbidity and mortality in pulmonary arterial hypertension. N Engl J Med 2013;369(9):809–18.

54. Ben-Yehuda O, Pizzuti D, Brown A, et al. Long-term hepatic safety of ambrisentan in patients with pulmonary arterial hypertension. J Am Coll Cardiol 2012;60(1):80–1.

55. Barnett CF, Machado RF. Sildenafil in the treatment of pulmonary hypertension. Vasc Health Risk Manag 2006;2(4):411–22.

56. Muirhead GJ, Wulff MB, Fielding A, et al. Pharmacokinetic interactions between sildenafil and saquinavir/ritonavir. Br J Clin Pharmacol 2000;50(2):99–107.

57. Garraffo R, Lavrut T, Ferrando S, et al. Effect of tipranavir/ritonavir combination on the pharmacokinetics of tadalafil in healthy volunteers. J Clin Pharmacol 2011;51(7):1071–8.

58. DeJesus E, Saleh S, Cheng S, et al. Pharmacokinetic interaction of riociguat and antiretroviral combination regimens in HIV-1-infected adults. Pulm Circ 2019;9(2). 2045894019848644.

59. Petitpretz P, Brenot F, Azarian R, et al. Pulmonary hypertension in patients with human immunodeficiency virus infection. Comparison with primary pulmonary hypertension. Circulation 1994;89(6):2722–7.

60. Stricker H, Domenighetti G, Mombelli G. Prostacyclin for HIV-associated pulmonary hypertension. Ann Intern Med 1997;127(11):1043.

61. Aguilar RV, Farber HW. Epoprostenol (prostacyclin) therapy in HIV-associated pulmonary hypertension. Am J Respir Crit Care Med 2000;162(5):1846–50.

62. Cea-Calvo L, Escribano Subias P, Tello de Menesses R, et al. [Treatment of HIV-associated pulmonary hypertension with treprostinil]. Rev Esp Cardiol 2003;56(4):421–5.

63. Ghofrani HA, Friese G, Discher T, et al. Inhaled iloprost is a potent acute pulmonary vasodilator in HIV-related severe pulmonary hypertension. Eur Respir J 2004;23(2):321–6.

64. Sitbon O, Channick R, Chin KM, et al. Selexipag for the treatment of pulmonary arterial hypertension. N Engl J Med 2015;373(26):2522–33.

65. Kern RM, Seethamraju H, Blanc PD, et al. The feasibility of lung transplantation in HIV-seropositive patients. Ann Am Thorac Soc 2014;11(6):882–9.

66. Opravil M, Sereni D. Natural history of HIV-associated pulmonary arterial hypertension: trends in the HAART era. AIDS 2008;22(Suppl 3):S35–40.

Pulmonary Hypertension in Adults with Congenital Heart Disease

Sarah A. Goldstein, MD, Richard A. Krasuski, MD*

KEYWORDS

- Adult congenital heart disease • Advanced medical therapy • Clinical management
- Eisenmenger syndrome • Pulmonary arterial hypertension

KEY POINTS

- Pulmonary arterial hypertension (PAH) related to congenital heart disease (CHD) is the result of pulmonary vascular remodeling due to chronic systemic-to-pulmonary shunting and is associated with increasing morbidity, mortality, and functional limitation.
- Eisenmenger syndrome is the most severe phenotype of PAH-CHD and is characterized by severe pulmonary vascular resistance elevation and shunt reversal (pulmonary-to-systemic shunting), leading to systemic cyanosis and various complications.
- Treatment strategies typically focus on medical management, although select patients with large shunts who have not yet developed severe PAH may be appropriate for either surgical or percutaneous defect closure.
- Women of childbearing age with PAH-CHD should be counseled about the risks of pregnancy and appropriate contraceptive strategies.
- Lung or heart-lung transplantation should be considered in patients with advanced disease.

INTRODUCTION

In 1897, Dr Victor Eisenmenger[1] published a post-mortem examination of a patient with a ventricular septal defect (VSD), cyanosis since childhood, clubbing of the fingers and toes, polycythemia, and evidence of right heart failure. Although he did not at the time deduce that this patient's cyanosis was related to increased pulmonary vascular resistance (PVR) leading to right-to-left shunting, his publication represented the first description of pulmonary arterial hypertension (PAH) associated with congenital heart disease (CHD). It was not until more than 50 years later, in 1951, that Dr Paul Wood published the first case series of 5 patients with bidirectional shunt lesions who had pulmonary artery pressures at systemic levels.[2,3] In 1951, Dr Paul Wood published a textbook that used the term, *Eisenmenger syndrome* (ES), likely for the first time. He described ES as "pulmonary arterial hypertension with a reversed shunt."[3] Since that time, it has become well recognized that chronically increased flow and transmitted pressures to the pulmonary circulation resulting from chronic left-to-right shunting induces pulmonary vascular remodeling and in some cases leads to PAH. It is now recognized, however, that the pathophysiology of PAH-CHD likely is more complicated than just this process. In contemporary cohorts, PAH affects 5% to 10% of adults with CHD and is associated with significant morbidity, mortality, and functional limitation.[4–7] Women are affected more commonly by PAH-CHD and risk increases with

Dr R.A. Krasuski has received honoraria from Actelion Pharmaceuticals and research grants from Actelion Pharmaceuticals, Edwards Lifesciences, Corvia, CryoLife, and the Adult Congenital Heart Association. Dr S.A. Goldstein has nothing to disclose.

Section of Adult Congenital Heart Disease, Division of Cardiology, Duke University Medical Center, Box 3331, Durham, NC 27710, USA

* Corresponding author. Duke University Medical Center, Box 3331, Durham, NC 27710.

E-mail address: richard.krasuski@duke.edu

increasing biological age and the age when defect closure occurred.[5] This review describes the pathophysiology of PAH-CHD, discusses the definition and classification of PAH-CHD, outlines how PAH-CHD is diagnosed, and summarizes current management strategies.

PATHOPHYSIOLOGY OF PULMONARY ARTERIAL HYPERTENSION ASSOCIATED WITH CONGENITAL HEART DISEASE

PAH-CHD develops as a consequence of intracardiac or extracardiac systemic-to-pulmonary shunts that lead to volume and/or pressure overload of the pulmonary circulation and subsequent pulmonary vascular remodeling over time. Early in this process, pulmonary vascular remodeling can be stabilized or reversed if the shunt lesion is closed either through surgical or percutaneous intervention. If the shunt is not addressed, however, adverse pulmonary vascular changes can become irreversible. Once present, PAH-CHD typically progresses over time, sometimes causing severe elevation in PVR that exceeds that of the systemic circulation and results in pulmonary-to-systemic (right-to-left) shunting with hypoxemia and central cyanosis.

The pathologic process underlying the development of PAH-CHD is similar to that observed in other forms of class 1 PH. Persistent volume and pressure overload of the pulmonary vascular system lead to increased shear stress and arterial endothelial damage. Endothelial damage is associated with degeneration of the extracellular matrix and release of vasoactive mediators, such as fibroblast growth factor, angiopoietin-1, and transforming growth factor ß. When pathologically upregulated, these growth factors induce smooth muscle hypertrophy and proliferation.[8] Endothelial dysfunction also leads to platelet adherence and activation, cytokine release and activation of local inflammatory cascades, and an imbalance of vasoactive mediators that favors vasoconstriction.[8–10] Long-standing PAH is associated with pulmonary arterial fibrosis that results in decreased pulmonary artery diameter and further increase in pulmonary artery pressure and PVR over time.[11]

DEFINITION AND CLASSIFICATION OF PULMONARY ARTERIAL HYPERTENSION ASSOCIATED WITH CONGENITAL HEART DISEASE

PAH is defined by the 6th World Symposium on Pulmonary Hypertension as a mean pulmonary artery pressure greater than 20 mm Hg in the setting of a pulmonary artery wedge pressure less than or equal to 15 mm Hg and PVR greater than or equal to 3 Wood units (WU).[12] Pulmonary hypertension (PH) has been categorized into 5 groups based on the World Health Organization classification system (**Table 1**). PAH-CHD is included in group 1. PH in CHD can result from several different etiologies, spanning all 5 PH groups. Although PAH-CHD appears to have the greatest impact on morbidity and mortality, awareness of and differentiation from the other classes are essential in providing the most appropriate clinical management.

The most common etiology of PH in CHD is related to diseases of the left heart, categorized as group 2 disease. Patients with CHD are unique, because they may have a systemic right ventricle (as in congenitally corrected transposition of the great arteries) or single-ventricle physiology (as in a Fontan-palliated anatomy). As such, referring to the *systemic ventricle* and *subpulmonary ventricle* (as subsequently is done in this review) provides greater clarity than describing right-sided or left-sided cardiac chambers. Systolic or diastolic function of the systemic ventricle or abnormalities in the aortic or systemic atrioventricular valves can lead to elevated pulmonary capillary wedge pressure and secondary elevation of the pulmonary arterial pressure. The PVR in such cases usually is less than 3 WU, differentiating this cause of elevated pulmonary pressure from other causes. In some cases, there can be mixed disease, in which the pulmonary capillary wedge pressure is elevated, but the pulmonary arterial pressure is elevated disproportionately. These can be among the most challenging patients to manage, due to their predilection toward pulmonary edema with targeted PAH therapies. In general, management of systemic ventricular etiologies of PH should precede any attempt to target the pulmonary arterial component.

Patients with CHD often are subjected to multiple sternotomies and thoracotomies related to surgical interventions, resulting in restrictive lung disease. This also can lead to PH, categorized as group 3 disease. Finally, patients with CHD may develop thromboembolic disease, which can lead to group 4 disease and/or can have concomitant systemic disease that leads to group 5 disease. The most complex forms of PAH-CHD have been classified as group 5. These include segmental forms of PAH (discussed later) and single-ventricle anatomy. Although the absence of a subpulmonary ventricle in Fontan-palliated patients precludes the development of high pulmonary pressures, the presence of increased PVR is a well-known cause of categorized as

Table 1
Classification of pulmonary arterial hypertension based on the 6th World Symposium on Pulmonary Hypertension

Pulmonary Hypertension Class	Etiologies
Class 1	PAH • CHD • Idiopathic • Heritable • Drug or toxin induced • Persistent PH of the newborn • Pulmonary veno-occlusive disease • Connective tissue diseases • Human immunodeficiency virus infection • Portal hypertension • Schistosomiasis • Chronic hemolytic anemia
Class 2	PH caused by left heart disease • Systolic dysfunction • Diastolic dysfunction • Valvular heart disease
Class 3	PH caused by lung disease or hypoxia • Chronic obstructive lung disease • Interstitial lung disease • Mixed restrictive/obstructive lung disease • Sleep-disordered breathing • Chronic exposure to high altitude
Class 4	Chronic thromboembolic PH

Class 5	PH with unclear multifactorial mechanisms
	• Hematologic disorders
	  ○ Myeloproliferative disorders, splenectomy
	• Systemic disorders
	  ○ Sarcoidosis, Langerhans cell histiocytosis
	• Metabolic disorders
	  ○ Glycogen storage disease
	  ○ Gaucher disease
	  ○ Thyroid disorders
	• Others
	  ○ Tumoral obstruction
	  ○ Fibrosing mediastinitis
	  ○ Chronic renal failure on dialysis

Fontan failure. Whether targeted PAH therapies are beneficial for such patients remains under active investigation. Further discussion of groups 2 to 5 PH is beyond the scope of this review.

PAH-CHD has been categorized into 4 clinical subgroups: ES, PAH associated with persistent systemic-to-pulmonary shunts, PAH with small/coincidental shunts, and PAH persisting or developing after defect closure (**Table 2**).[13] This classification system defines underlying etiology and physiology and assists in identifying targeted treatment options.

Eisenmenger Syndrome

ES is the most severe phenotype of PAH-CHD. It results from large systemic-to-pulmonary (left-to-right) shunts and is characterized by severe elevation of PVR, such that there is shunt reversal (right-to-left shunting) or bidirectional shunting that results in hypoxia and central cyanosis. Chronic, and sometimes severe, cyanosis is a distinct manifestation of ES among patients with PAH-CHD and unrepaired or partially repaired defects and is associated with multisystem sequelae, including erythrocytosis, thrombocytopenia, coagulation abnormalities, thrombosis, susceptibility to infection, cerebrovascular events (ischemic, embolic, and hemorrhagic), right heart failure, and early death.[9] Despite earlier detection of CHD and advances in pediatric surgical and medical interventions for shunt lesions that have led to decreased prevalence of ES, this disease process remains prevalent among adults with CHD and requires a multidisciplinary approach to management.

Overall, patients with ES are considered to have a better prognosis than other forms of PAH.[14,15] The presence of a right-to-left shunt allows for pressure unloading of the right ventricle and maintains cardiac output, although at the expense of cyanosis. Additionally, in some patients with congenital systemic-to-pulmonary shunts, the right ventricle does not remodel after birth and maintains the adaptive hypertrophy present as a result of fetal circulation, thus allowing better tolerance of elevated pulmonary arterial pressure over time.[16] This phenomenon seems to occur more commonly in patients with post-tricuspid shunts (eg, VSD) as opposed to patients with pre-tricuspid shunts (eg, atrial septal defect), in whom the right ventricular response to PAH more closely resembles that of patients with idiopathic PAH. The presence of a pre-tricuspid shunt has been demonstrated to be an independent predictor of early death in patients with ES.[17] Despite this, long-term prognosis remains poor compared with patients with congenital shunt lesions without PAH. Based on registry data, 5-year survival from the time of diagnosis ranges between 74% and 81%, whereas long-term survival is lower (64% at 7 years and 57% at 10 years).[18–20]

Table 2
Clinical classification of pulmonary arterial hypertension with congenital heart disease[19]

ES	• Large left-to-right shunt that leads to severe elevation in PVR and shunt reversal • Characterized by hypoxia and central cyanosis
Persistent left-to-right shunt	• Moderate to large left-to-right shunt resulting in increased PVR • May or may not be correctable/reversible
Coincidental CHD	• Elevation of PVR is out of proportion to the magnitude of shunt and the size of the congenital heart lesion. • The CHD is unlikely to be directly responsible for the develop of PAH.
Postinterventional	• PAH that either persists after shunt closure or develops months or years after the intervention

Chronic cyanosis is associated with secondary erythrocytosis, a physiologic adaptive measure to augment oxygen transport and delivery. Erythrocytosis has effects on multiple other organ systems and predisposes patients to hyperviscosity syndrome, hemostatic abnormalities leading to increased risk for both bleeding and clotting, iron deficiency, hyperuricemia, and cholelithiasis.

Pulmonary Arterial Hypertension Associated with Persistent Systemic-to-Pulmonary Shunts

Patients with moderate to large left-to-right shunts may have PAH without progressing to ES. In these patients, the PVR is mildly to moderately elevated; thus, systemic-to-pulmonary shunting predominates, and cyanosis is not present at rest. Early identification of patients with PAH-CHD and persistent systemic-to-pulmonary shunts is important because shunt closure potentially can halt or reverse the progression of pulmonary vascular disease.

Pulmonary Arterial Hypertension with Small/Coincidental Shunts

PAH with small/coincidental shunts form of PAH-CHD is diagnosed in patients with markedly elevated PVR despite the presence of only very small shunt lesions. In this class of PAH-CHD,

the severity of PAH is considered out of proportion to the size of the left-to-right shunt. Consideration of other underlying causes of PAH, therefore, is strongly recommended. The prognosis associated with PAH with small/coincidental shunts is similar to that seen in patients with idiopathic PAH.[15,21]

Pulmonary Arterial Hypertension after Defect Closure

PAH after defect closure is relatively rare, with contemporary data suggesting a prevalence of 3% among patients with corrected, simple shunt lesions.[22] This group consists of 2 PAH-CHD phenotypes: those who with persistent PAH despite defect closure and those who develop PAH many years after defect closure. The former most likely occurs in the setting of late diagnosis and shunt intervention. The pathophysiology underlying the development of PAH in the latter phenotype remains unclear, although genetic predisposition has been hypothesized.[9] Clinical characteristics that predict development or persistence of PAH following defect closure include type of defect (complete atrioventricular septal defect, sinus venosus defect, large defect, or concomitant moderate or high complexity congenital heart defects), ratio of pulmonary-to-ystemic blood flow (Qp:Qs) greater than or equal to 3 or pulmonary artery systolic pressure greater than 40 mm Hg prior to closure, presence of an associated genetic syndrome, older age at repair, and female sex.[23] The prognosis associated with this form of PAH-CHD is considered particularly poor, with a clinical phenotype that often is aggressive.[15,21,22]

Segmental Pulmonary Arterial Hypertension

Segmental PAH is diagnosed when segments of the pulmonary vasculature, as opposed to the entire pulmonary vascular bed, are affected by pulmonary vascular remodeling and elevated PVR. This form of PAH-CHD occurs when there is increased blood flow to localized portions of the lung. Some examples of underlying etiologies that can cause segmental PAH include a large left-to-right shunt with peripheral pulmonary artery stenosis (either occurring natively or due to branch pulmonary artery banding), absence or atresia of a single pulmonary artery, anomalous pulmonary artery from the aorta feeding a single lung segment, and surgical shunts, such as the Waterston shunt or Potts shunt, that may supply only part of the pulmonary vasculature. Each portion of the involved pulmonary vasculature may be affected by PAH of differing severity. Symptoms typically are related to the severity of ventilation-perfusion mismatch and the degree of right ventricular dysfunction.[24]

DIAGNOSIS
Clinical History and Presenting Symptoms

A diagnosis of PAH-CHD requires a high degree of clinical suspicion, because presenting symptoms typically are nonspecific. Exertional dyspnea and fatigue are the most common presenting symptoms but also can result from arrhythmia, heart failure, and/or deconditioning in patients with CHD. Exertional syncope also can occur and typically is a marker of severe disease with increased associated mortality. Patients also may experience chest pain, which can be ischemic in nature as a result of a hypertrophied right ventricle with increased metabolic demands, elevated right ventricular end diastolic pressure resulting in reduced coronary perfusion, hypoxia, or extrinsic compression of the left main coronary artery by a dilated pulmonary artery.[25,26] Suggestive physical examination findings include an accentuated P_2, a right ventricular heave, elevated jugular venous pulsation and signs of right heart failure. Patients with CHD who report any of these symptoms or have relevant physical examination findings (**Fig. 1**) should undergo further evaluation for the presence of PAH. The more extreme physical characteristics of a patient with ES are illustrated in **Fig. 2**.

Diagnostic Testing

In patients with CHD in whom there is concern for PAH, transthoracic echocardiography (TTE) is an important initial diagnostic testing modality. Ideally, TTE should be completed by a performing sonographer and interpreting cardiologist with expertise in CHD. In addition to being used to assess the location and size of underlying congenital cardiac defects, TTE can be used to estimate the right ventricular systolic pressure, which, in the absence of pulmonary stenosis, approximates the pulmonary artery pressure. TTE also is useful in assessing right ventricular dysfunction. Although not an integral part of the diagnostic evaluation for PAH, cardiac magnetic resonance imaging also may be useful to better determine the size and location of the congenital defect, the direction and quantity of shunting, and, when appropriate, the feasibility of percutaneous defect closure.

Right heart catheterization (RHC) is the gold standard for establishing the diagnosis of PAH. As discussed previously, patients with CHD may have other reasons for pulmonary artery or right ventricular systolic pressure elevation, such as left heart disease with elevated left-sided filling pressures, pulmonary artery or vein stenosis, subpulmonary ventricular outflow or pulmonary valve stenosis, and thromboembolic disease. In some of these patients, use of vasodilator therapy, the hallmark of PAH treatment, may be harmful. RHC also is instrumental in establishing the magnitude of right-to-left and left-to-right shunting, which is reported as Qp:Qs. Additionally, a vasodilator challenge during RHC can be helpful in assessing prognosis and predicting response to targeted medical therapy.

Assessment of exercise tolerance also has important prognostic value in patients with PAH. When chronically managing patients with PAH-CHD, the 6-minute walk distance (6MWD) is used most commonly and can assess baseline functional status as well as serial improvement with targeted medical therapy.[27–29]

MANAGEMENT

Patients with PAH-CHD should be managed at centers with multidisciplinary expertise, including CHD and PAH specialists, CHD imaging experts, cardiovascular surgery, congenital heart interventionalists, and advanced heart failure/transplant teams. The primary management strategy for most patients with PAH-CHD is medical therapy, although defect closure may be considered in select cases of PVR elevation that is not severe and still may be reversible (**Fig. 3**). Invasive hemodynamic assessment with cardiac catheterization is recommended prior to initiation of medical therapy or consideration of surgical or transcatheter intervention in all patients with PAH-CHD to confirm the diagnosis, evaluate safety of medical therapy, and determine suitability of defect closure.[23] The most appropriate management strategy depends on the direction and magnitude of shunting and severity of PAH.

Defect Closure

In appropriate patients with PAH-CHD, defect closure can halt the progression of PAH and, in some cases, lead to reversal of disease. Multiple studies have demonstrated a decrease in prevalence of PAH following ASD closure as well as a reduction in pulmonary arterial pressure.[30] Shunt closure is not appropriate in all patients, however. Among patients with ES who have PVR elevation such that there is significant right-to-left shunting, defect closure is contraindicated. In these patients, the right-to-left shunt serves as a relief valve, allowing blood to reach the left heart and systemic circulation despite the presence of very elevated PVR, albeit at the expense of systemic desaturation. The defect also serves to reduce right ventricular afterload and therefore

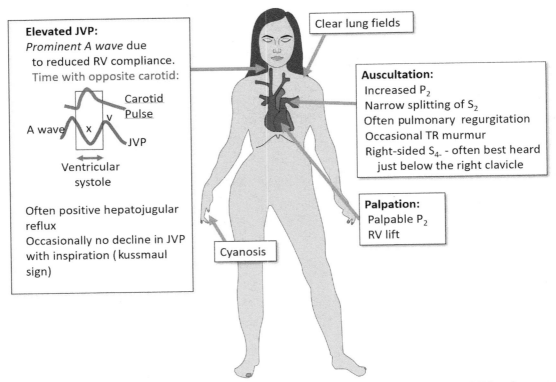

Fig. 1. Physical manifestations and common examination findings in a patient with PAH-CHD. JVP, jugular venous pulsation; RV, right ventricle; TR, tricuspid regurgitation.

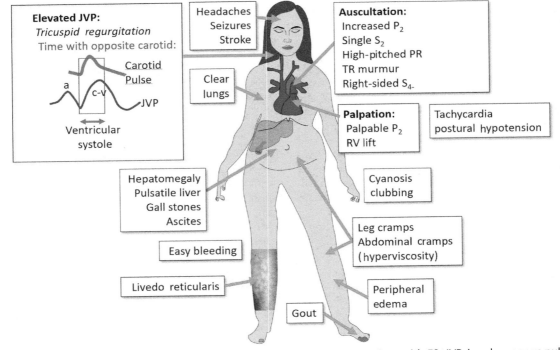

Fig. 2. Physical manifestations and common examination findings in a patient with ES. JVP, jugular venous pulsation; PR, pulmonary regurgitation; RV, right ventricle; TR, tricuspid regurgitation.

Treatment Algorithm for CHD Patients with PAH

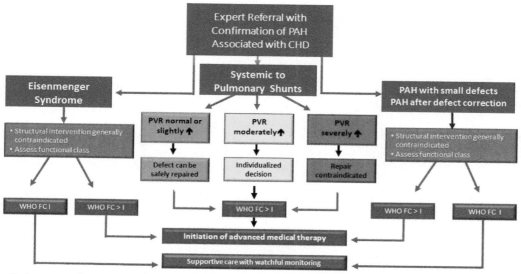

Fig. 3. A proposed treatment algorithm for patients with PAH-CHD arranged by subtype. For patients with unrepaired or residual shunts, defect correction should be considered, depending on the PVR. Larger left-to-right shunts with lower PVR should be closed, whereas smaller net left-to-right shunts with higher resistance should not be, because closure could be detrimental. For cases between these extremes, assessing response to vasodilators or reassessing hemodynamics during temporary balloon occlusion in the catheterization laboratory can be helpful. For patients with ES and corrected or small shunts, advanced medical therapies should be initiated in the presence of associated symptoms. FC, functional class; WHO, World Health Organization. (*Adapted from* Fathallah M, Krasuski RA. A Multifaceted Approach to Pulmonary Hypertension in Adults With Congenital Heart Disease. Prog Cardiovasc Dis. 2018 Sep-Oct;61(3-4):320-327.)

preserve right ventricular function. Closure of the defect may precipitate right heart failure and lead to cardiovascular collapse and death. In patients with desaturation with exertion suggestive of right-to-left shunting with exercise, device closure similarly is not recommended. Although assessment of upper extremity saturation is sufficient in patients with an atrial septal defect or VSD, it is important to assess for lower extremity hypoxia in patients with a patent ductus arteriosus, because the shunt may be located distal to the upper extremity blood supply. Finally, in patients with small/coincidental shunts, closure is not recommended, because it is unlikely to have an impact on the trajectory of PAH and potentially could be harmful if it is serving as a pressure relief valve for the right ventricle.

Some patients with a large shunt who have PAH but have not yet developed ES may benefit from defect closure. The 2018 American College of Cardiology/American Heart Association (ACC/AHA) Guideline for the Management of Adults with Congenital Heart Disease recommends surgical or percutaneous closure of large defects in patients with mildly or moderately elevated PVR who have

evidence of significant left-to-right shunting. Specifically, defect closure is recommended only in patients with PVR less than one-third of systemic vascular resistance (SVR), pulmonary artery systolic pressure less than 50% systemic systolic pressure, and Qp:Qs greater than or equal to 1.5:1.[23]

The 2020 European Society of Cardiology Guidelines for the Management of Adult Congenital Heart Disease present a slightly different algorithm for selecting patients with PAH-CHD who may benefit from defect closure. The concept of treat to close, in which some patients with PAH-CHD initially ineligible for defect closure may become eligible with targeted PAH treatment, also is introduced. Shunt closure without preceding treatment of PAH is recommended in patients with a large shunt, PVR less than 5 WU, and Qp:Qs greater than 1.5. Among patients with PVR greater than 5 WU, a trial of PAH targeted medical therapy is recommended followed by reassessment of invasive hemodynamics. If after treatment the PVR is less than 5 WU and the Qp:Qs is greater than 1.5, defect closure with fenestration may be considered.[31]

Targeted Medical Therapy

For those patients with PAH-CHD and a large shunt in whom device closure is not recommended, medical therapy is the mainstay of management. Targeted medical therapy provides survival benefit in patients with ES and likely also in other forms of PAH-CHD.[32,33] Oral medications targeting the endothelin-1 receptor and the nitric oxide pathway as well as oral, parenteral, and inhaled formulations that target the prostacyclin pathway are commercially available. Although medical therapy typically is well tolerated in patients with pre-tricuspid shunts, those with post-tricuspid shunts require close clinical observation, because therapy can lead to left ventricular volume overload and left heart failure related to increased left-to-right shunting.

Endothelin-1 receptor antagonists work by blocking the binding of endothelin-1, a potent vasoconstrictor that is overproduced in the pulmonary vasculature in patients with PAH, to its receptor. Bosentan, a drug in this class, is the most extensively studied targeted PAH therapy for patients with CHD. Both short-term and long-term observational studies have demonstrated safety and tolerability of bosentan among patients with PAH-CHD, while also showing hemodynamic benefits and improvement in 6MWD.[34–40] The Bosentan Randomized Trial of Endothelin Antagonist Therapy-5 (BREATHE-5) was the first multicenter, double-blind, randomized, placebo-controlled trial studying the benefits and safety of bosentan use in patients with PAH-CHD.[41] In this study, 54 patients with ES and advanced functional class were randomized to bosentan or placebo for 16 weeks. Those with patent ductus arteriosus, complex CHD, and/or concomitant treatment with other PAH medications were excluded. During the study period, 6MWD improved by 12% among patients treated with bosentan and decreased by 3% with placebo. Bosentan led to statistically significant reductions in PVR (9.3% reduction vs 5.4% increase with placebo) and mean pulmonary artery pressure (decreased by 5 mm Hg with treatment vs 0.5–mm Hg increase with placebo) and improved functional status. An open-label extension of BREATHE-5 followed 37 patients to 40 weeks of therapy and demonstrated sustained improvements in exercise and functional capacity.[42] Based on these data, current ACC/AHA guidelines recommend bosentan as first-line medical therapy in patients with PAH-CHD who are not eligible for defect closure.[23]

A second randomized controlled trial examining the use of a newer endothelin-1 receptor antagonist, macitentan, did not replicate the results of BREATHE-5. The Macitentan in Eisenmenger Syndrome to Explore Exercise Capacity (MAESTRO) study included 226 patients with ES and moderately to severely reduced functional status treated with macitentan or placebo for 16 weeks.[43] In addition to being a larger study that included patients with less severe PAH, MAESTRO included a more heterogeneous population of patients because it did not exclude those with severe congenital cardiac lesions or patients receiving other PAH therapies. MAESTRO failed to show a superior treatment effect of macitentan over placebo with respect to 6MWD or functional class, although the N-terminal fragment of the prohormone brain natriuretic peptide (NT-proBNP) levels were reduced and a hemodynamic substudy of 39 patients showed a reduction in indexed PVR.

Phosphodiesterase-5 (PDE-5) inhibitors, another targeted medication class used to treat PAH, function by blocking the action of PDE-5, an enzyme involved in the breakdown of nitric oxide. PDE-5 is present in high concentrations in the lung vasculature and is up-regulated in patients with PAH. The use of PDE-5 inhibitors, including sildenafil and tadalafil, has led to improvements in 6MWD and functional status among patients with PAH-CHD in observational studies.[44,45] The benefit of sildenafil also has been examined as an adjunctive therapy to bosentan in patients with PAH-CHD. One observational study evaluated bosentan-sildenafil combination therapy among patients who failed to respond to bosentan monotherapy.[46] After 6 months of combination therapy, there was a significant improvement in functional status, 6MWD, and hemodynamics. A randomized controlled trial assessing the effect of adding sildenafil after 9 months of treatment with bosentan did not demonstrate significant clinical improvements, although resting oxygen saturation did increase.[47] Guidelines currently recommend using PDE-5 inhibitors in patients with PAH-CHD without symptomatic improvement on single-drug therapy.[23]

Randomized, placebo-controlled studies focused on PAH-CHD are listed in **Table 3**. All these studies were conducted in ES. There are few data on the medical treatment of PAH-CHD with a coincidental shunt and patients with PAH-CHD after shunt closure. Most large, randomized studies of drug therapy in PAH have included a small subset of patients with repaired shunts. The largest such substudy examined the use of selexipag, a medication that selectively activates the prostacyclin receptor, thus inducing vasodilation and inhibiting proliferation of vascular smooth muscle cells. In the published post hoc secondary analysis of GRIPHON, a multicenter, double-blind,

Table 3
Randomized controlled trials investigating medical therapy in PAH-CHD

Study	Year	Drug (Class)	Population	N	Functional Class, % (II/III/IV)	Findings
BREATHE-5	2006	Bosentan (ERA)	ES	54	0/100/0	⇓ Indexed PVR ⇓ Mean PAP ⇑ 6MWD
Unnamed	2006	Sildenafil (PDE-5 inhibitor)	ES	10	30/60/10	⇓ Functional class ⇓ Mean PAP ⇑ 6MWD
Unnamed	2010	Bosentan (ERA) + sildenafil (PDE-5 inhibitor)	ES	21	43/48/5	⇑ Resting saturation ⇔ 6MWD
Unnamed	2011	Tadalafil (PDE-5 inhibitor)	ES	28	79/21/0	⇓ Functional class ⇑ 6MWD ⇓ PVR
MAESTRO	2017	Macitentan (ERA)	ES	226	60/40/0	⇓ Indexed PVR ⇓ NT-proBNP ⇔ Functional class ⇔ 6MWD

Abbreviations: ERA, endothelin receptor antagonist; PAP, pulmonary artery pressure.
A summary of randomized controlled trials investigating the effects of targeted advanced medical therapy in patients with pulmonary arterial hypertension with congenital heart disease. Studies are listed in chronologic order.

placebo-controlled study of the safety and efficacy of selexipag on morbidity and mortality in patients with PAH, patients with PAH-CHD after defect closure who were treated with selexipag experienced a lower combined endpoint of morbidity and mortality compared with those treated with placebo.[48] In general, given the similarities in disease progression and severity, it is recommended that patients with PAH-CHD with a coincidental shunt and PAH-CHD after shunt closure be treated with the same therapies used to treat idiopathic PAH.[9]

There also is a paucity of data dictating the appropriate medical management of patients with segmental PAH-CHD. Very small observational studies have demonstrated safety as well as improvements in 6MWD, symptoms, and hemodynamics with the use of both bosentan and sildenafil.[49–52] Other case reports, however, have noted worsening hypoxemia attributed to more pronounced ventilation/perfusion mismatching.[53,54] Patients with segmental PAH-CHD, should be followed closely after initiation of advanced medical therapies.

Organ Transplantation

Determining appropriate timing for when to consider organ transplantation in patients with ES and other forms of PAH-CHD can be difficult. Although some forms of PAH-CHD seem to mimic the expected disease progression seen in idiopathic PAH, those with ES and PAH-CHD with an uncorrected, large shunt appear to have a more unpredictable clinical course. Some patients can have prolonged survival before symptomatic deterioration or end-organ dysfunction occurs related to chronic hypoxia, whereas others deteriorate more rapidly.[55] Most patients with PAH-CHD who progress to end-stage disease require heart-lung transplantation. Discussion of the intricacies involved in the decision for lung transplant with congenital defect repair versus dual organ transplant is outside of the scope of this review. Early post-transplant mortality is higher among patients with PAH-CHD compared with other transplant recipients, but after the immediate post-transplant period PAH-CHD patients experience excellent clinical outcomes.[56]

Palliative Care

Palliative care is an important pillar of the management of patients with PAH-CHD and should be considered in patients with symptom burden such that their quality of life is affected. Primarily due to the young age of many patients with PAH-CHD, it is common to postpone discussions about palliative care and end-of-life decisions until all other treatment modalities have been exhausted. International guidelines, however, suggest that physicians caring for patients with PAH-CHD should be proactive in discussing advanced directives and end-of-life issues.

Additionally, following the initiation of end-of-life discussions by PAH-CHD specialists, referral to palliative care specialists should be considered early in the disease process alongside parallel multidisciplinary disease management and treatment with PAH therapies. Early palliative care involvement not only is helpful for symptom management but also can provide physical, psychological, and social support for patients and their families.[57] Timing of palliative care referral and services provided by palliative care specialists should be individualized to each patient's symptomatic and psychosocial needs.

PREGNANCY AND CONTRACEPTION

During pregnancy and the postpartum period, the maternal cardiovascular system must undergo profound and dynamic changes to support fetal growth and development that include increased cardiac output and circulating blood volume, decreased SVR and PVR, and increased heart rate. Although well tolerated in healthy women, these changes can be associated with catastrophic outcomes, including death, among patients with PAH. In the setting of PAH, the pulmonary vasculature already is maximally dilated and cannot undergo the necessary decrease in vascular resistance to permit the increased cardiac output that is needed during pregnancy. Additionally, patients with right heart dilation and failure typically are unable to tolerate the increased volume load that occurs during pregnancy and delivery. Related to this, patients with PAH are at risk for right heart failure, decreased cardiac output, PH crisis, hypotension, hypoperfusion, and end-organ compromise related to pregnancy. Contemporary observational studies report a 16% to 30% pregnancy-related mortality rate among women with PAH.[58–60] Although increased severity of PAH is associated more strongly with risk of death, patients with any degree of PAH are at increased risk for adverse outcomes.[59] The offspring of women with PAH also are affected, with increased rates of fetal and neonatal mortality, particularly in the setting maternal hypoxia, reduced cardiac output, and preterm delivery. As such, professional society guidelines recommend that women with PAH be counseled to avoid pregnancy, and termination should be discussed when pregnancy occurs.[61]

Among patients with PAH-CHD, those with ES experience particularly high mortality associated with pregnancy (20%–50%).[62] In patients with ES, the pregnancy-related reduction in SVR can lead to increased right-to-left shunting and decreased pulmonary blood flow that results in increased cyanosis, low cardiac output, and increased risk of paradoxic embolism in the setting of the hypercoagulability that occurs during pregnancy. Fetal and neonatal outcomes also are poor among offspring of mothers with ES, with 65% of pregnancies complicated by preterm delivery, 37% by small-for-gestational-age infants, and 28% by offspring death.[63] Avoidance of pregnancy is extremely important in these patients, because even the termination procedure itself can pose significant maternal risk.[61]

Counseling regarding safe and reliable contraception options should be pursued with all women of childbearing age with CHD but particularly in those with PAH-CHD. Combined hormonal contraception (ie, estrogen-containing oral contraceptive pill) use is associated with increased risk for thromboembolic events and, therefore, is not recommended in patients with PAH, cyanosis, or the potential for right-to-left shunting. Long-term reversible contraceptive methods that do not contain estrogen (levonorgestrel intrauterine device, copper intrauterine device, and tonogestrel subdermal implant) have a less than 1% failure rate and are favored in women with PAH-CHD.[64] The copper intrauterine device can be associated with heavier menstrual bleeding in some women and thus may be poorly tolerated in patients with PAH-CHD who are treated with anticoagulation or those with hemostatic derangements related to ES.

Patients with PAH-CHD who become pregnant and decide against termination should be managed at a multidisciplinary tertiary care center with experienced CHD, PAH, advanced heart failure, and cardiothoracic surgery specialists. Medical therapy is limited to phosphodiesterase inhibitors and prostanoids. Bosentan and other endothelin-1 receptor antagonists are thought to be teratogenic based on mouse data and, therefore, are contraindicated during pregnancy. Patients with PAH-CHD should be monitored closely throughout pregnancy with serial TTE and RHC when there is diagnostic uncertainty or invasive hemodynamic information is needed to make difficult therapeutic decisions. A detailed delivery plan, including timing of delivery, mode of delivery, and anesthetic plan, should be determined early in pregnancy in a multidisciplinary setting. Women are at highest risk for cardiovascular decompensation in the postpartum period, and most patients with PAH-CHD should be monitored in an intensive care setting, possibly with invasive hemodynamic monitoring, following delivery for close volume management and support of right ventricular function.[65] Patients with PAH remain at elevated risk for cardiovascular complications for many months after delivery and thus require close follow-up after discharge.[61] Counseling about contraception and the risks of future pregnancies should be completed prior to discharge from the delivery hospitalization.

SUMMARY

PAH-CHD is a common complication seen in patients with CHD and is associated with increased morbidity and mortality. In patients with a large defect who have not yet developed ES physiology, surgical or percutaneous defect closure is the preferred treatment and may prevent progression to severe PAH. Although recent randomized controlled trials have begun to identify safe and effective targeted medical therapies in patients with PAH-CHD, more research is needed to determine the optimal treatment strategy. Lung or heart-lung transplantation should be considered in patients with advanced disease. Early involvement of palliative care specialists is recommended. Women of childbearing age with PAH-CHD should be counseled proactively about the risks of pregnancy and appropriate contraceptive strategies.

CLINICS CARE POINTS

- A diagnosis of PAH-CHD requires a high degree of clinical suspicion as presenting symptoms are non-specific.
- Right heart catheterization is the gold standard for establishing the diagnosis of PAH-CHD.
- Defect closure is contraindicated in patients with ES.
- Defect closure is recommended in patients with PVR < 1/3 of SVR, PAP < 50% systemic systolic pressure and Qp:Qs >/= 1.5:1.
- For patients with PAH-CHD and a large shunt in whom device closure is not recommended, medical therapy is the mainstay of management.
- Avoidance of pregnancy is recommended among patients with ES due to a high risk of maternal and fetal mortality.

ACKNOWLEDGMENTS

The authors would like to acknowledge the fantastic artwork and inspirational mentorship of Dr Thomas M. Bashore of Duke University Medical Center.

REFERENCES

1. Eisenmenger V. Die angeborenen defekte der kammerscheidewand des herzens. Z Klin Med 1897; 32:1–28.
2. Wood P. The Eisenmenger syndrome: i. Br Med J 1958;2:701.
3. Partin C. The evolution of Eisenmenger's eponymic enshrinement. Am J Cardiol 2003;92:1187–91.
4. Duffels MG, Engelfriet PM, Berger RM, et al. Pulmonary arterial hypertension in congenital heart disease: an epidemiologic perspective from a Dutch registry. Int J Cardiol 2007;120:198–204.
5. van Riel AC, Schuuring MJ, van Hessen ID, et al. Contemporary prevalence of pulmonary arterial hypertension in adult congenital heart disease following the updated clinical classification. Int J Cardiol 2014;174:299–305.
6. Diller G-P, Dimopoulos K, Okonko D, et al. Exercise intolerance in adult congenital heart disease: comparative severity, correlates, and prognostic implication. Circulation 2005;112:828–35.
7. Lowe BS, Therrien J, Ionescu-Ittu R, et al. Diagnosis of pulmonary hypertension in the congenital heart disease adult population: impact on outcomes. J Am Coll Cardiol 2011;58:538–46.
8. Du L, Sullivan CC, Chu D, et al. Signaling molecules in nonfamilial pulmonary hypertension. N Engl J Med 2003;348:500–9.
9. Brida M, Nashat H, Gatzoulis MA. Pulmonary arterial hypertension: closing the gap in congenital heart disease. Curr Opin Pulm Med 2020;26:422–8.
10. Diller GP, van Eijl S, Okonko DO, et al. Circulating endothelial progenitor cells in patients with Eisenmenger syndrome and idiopathic pulmonary arterial hypertension. Circulation 2008;117:3020–30.
11. Heath D, Edwards JE. The pathology of hypertensive pulmonary vascular disease; a description of six grades of structural changes in the pulmonary arteries with special reference to congenital cardiac septal defects. Circulation 1958;18:533–47.
12. Simonneau G, Montani D, Celermajer DS, et al. Haemodynamic definitions and updated clinical classification of pulmonary hypertension. Eur Respir J 2019;53:1801913.
13. Galiè N, Humbert M, Vachiery JL, et al. 2015 ESC/ERS guidelines for the diagnosis and treatment of pulmonary hypertension: the Joint task force for the diagnosis and treatment of pulmonary hypertension of the European Society of Cardiology (ESC) and the European Respiratory Society (ERS): Endorsed by: Association for European Paediatric and Congenital Cardiology (AEPC), International Society for Heart and Lung Transplantation (ISHLT). Eur Heart J 2016;37:67–119.
14. Kaemmerer H, Gorenflo M, Huscher D, et al. Pulmonary hypertension in adults with congenital

heart disease: Real-World data from the International COMPERA-CHD registry. J Clin Med 2020; 9:1456.

15. Manes A, Palazzini M, Leci E, et al. Current era survival of patients with pulmonary arterial hypertension associated with congenital heart disease: a comparison between clinical subgroups. Eur Heart J 2014; 35:716–24.

16. Hopkins WE. The remarkable right ventricle of patients with Eisenmenger syndrome. Coron Artery Dis 2005;16:19–25.

17. Kempny A, Hjortshøj CS, Gu H, et al. Predictors of death in contemporary adult patients with Eisenmenger syndrome: a multicenter study. Circulation 2017;135:1432–40.

18. Hurdman J, Condliffe R, Elliot CA, et al. ASPIRE registry: assessing the Spectrum of Pulmonary hypertension Identified at a REferral centre. Eur Respir J 2012;39:945–55.

19. Barst RJ, Ivy DD, Foreman AJ, et al. Four- and seven-year outcomes of patients with congenital heart disease-associated pulmonary arterial hypertension (from the REVEAL Registry). Am J Cardiol 2014;113:147–55.

20. Diller GP, Körten MA, Bauer UM, et al. Current therapy and outcome of Eisenmenger syndrome: data of the German National Register for congenital heart defects. Eur Heart J 2016;37:1449–55.

21. Simonneau G, Gatzoulis MA, Adatia I, et al. Updated clinical classification of pulmonary hypertension. J Am Coll Cardiol 2013;62:D34–41.

22. Lammers AE, Bauer LJ, Diller GP, et al. Pulmonary hypertension after shunt closure in patients with simple congenital heart defects. Int J Cardiol 2020;308:28–32.

23. Stout KK, Daniels CJ, Aboulhosn JA, et al. 2018 AHA/ACC Guideline for the Management of Adults With Congenital Heart Disease: A Report of the American College of Cardiology/American Heart Association Task Force on Clinical Practice Guidelines. Circulation 2019;139(14):e698–800. https://doi.org/10.1161/CIR.0000000000000603.

24. Dimopoulos K, Diller GP, Opotowsky AR, et al. Definition and management of segmental pulmonary hypertension. J Am Heart Assoc 2018;7:e008587.

25. Galiè N, Saia F, Palazzini M, et al. Left main coronary artery compression in patients with pulmonary arterial hypertension and Angina. J Am Coll Cardiol 2017;69:2808–17.

26. Constantine A, Dimopoulos K, Opotowsky AR. Congenital heart disease and pulmonary hypertension. Cardiol Clin 2020;38:445–56.

27. Paciocco G, Martinez FJ, Bossone E, et al. Oxygen desaturation on the six-minute walk test and mortality in untreated primary pulmonary hypertension. Eur Respir J 2001;17:647–52.

28. Miyamoto S, Nagaya N, Satoh T, et al. Clinical correlates and prognostic significance of six-minute walk test in patients with primary pulmonary hypertension. Comparison with cardiopulmonary exercise testing. Am J Respir Crit Care Med 2000;161: 487–92.

29. Wensel R, Opitz CF, Anker SD, et al. Assessment of survival in patients with primary pulmonary hypertension: importance of cardiopulmonary exercise testing. Circulation 2002;106:319–24.

30. Zwijnenburg RD, Baggen VJM, Geenen LW, et al. The prevalence of pulmonary arterial hypertension before and after atrial septal defect closure at adult age: a systematic review. Am Heart J 2018;201: 63–71.

31. Baumgartner H, De Backer J, Babu-Narayan SV, et al. 2020 ESC guidelines for the management of adult congenital heart disease: the task force for the management of adult congenital heart disease of the European society of Cardiology (ESC). Endorsed by: association for European Paediatric and congenital Cardiology (AEPC), International society for adult congenital heart disease (ISACHD). Eur Heart J 2020;42:563–645.

32. Dimopoulos K, Inuzuka R, Goletto S, et al. Improved survival among patients with Eisenmenger syndrome receiving advanced therapy for pulmonary arterial hypertension. Circulation 2010;121:20–5.

33. He B, Zhang F, Li X, et al. Meta-analysis of randomized controlled trials on treatment of pulmonary arterial hypertension. Circ J 2010;74:1458–64.

34. Ibrahim R, Granton JT, Mehta S. An open-label, multicentre pilot study of bosentan in pulmonary arterial hypertension related to congenital heart disease. Can Respir J 2006;13:415–20.

35. Gatzoulis MA, Rogers P, Li W, et al. Safety and tolerability of bosentan in adults with Eisenmenger physiology. Int J Cardiol 2005;98:147–51.

36. D'Alto M, Vizza CD, Romeo E, et al. Long term effects of bosentan treatment in adult patients with pulmonary arterial hypertension related to congenital heart disease (Eisenmenger physiology): safety, tolerability, clinical, and haemodynamic effect. Heart 2007;93:621–5.

37. Benza RL, Rayburn BK, Tallaj JA, et al. Efficacy of bosentan in a small cohort of adult patients with pulmonary arterial hypertension related to congenital heart disease. Chest 2006;129:1009–15.

38. Kotlyar E, Sy R, Keogh AM, et al. Bosentan for the treatment of pulmonary arterial hypertension associated with congenital cardiac disease. Cardiol Young 2006;16:268–74.

39. Schulze-Neick I, Gilbert N, Ewert R, et al. Adult patients with congenital heart disease and pulmonary arterial hypertension: first open prospective multicenter study of bosentan therapy. Am Heart J 2005;150:716.

40. Diller GP, Dimopoulos K, Kaya MG, et al. Long-term safety, tolerability and efficacy of bosentan in adults

with pulmonary arterial hypertension associated with congenital heart disease. Heart 2007;93:974–6.

41. Galiè N, Beghetti M, Gatzoulis MA, et al. Bosentan therapy in patients with Eisenmenger syndrome: a multicenter, double-blind, randomized, placebo-controlled study. Circulation 2006;114:48–54.

42. Gatzoulis MA, Beghetti M, Galiè N, et al. Longer-term bosentan therapy improves functional capacity in Eisenmenger syndrome: results of the BREATHE-5 open-label extension study. Int J Cardiol 2008;127: 27–32.

43. Gatzoulis MA, Landzberg M, Beghetti M, et al. Evaluation of macitentan in patients with Eisenmenger syndrome. Circulation 2019;139:51–63.

44. Zeng WJ, Lu XL, Xiong CM, et al. The efficacy and safety of sildenafil in patients with pulmonary arterial hypertension associated with the different types of congenital heart disease. Clin Cardiol 2011;34: 513–8.

45. Mukhopadhyay S, Sharma M, Ramakrishnan S, et al. Phosphodiesterase-5 inhibitor in Eisenmenger syndrome: a preliminary observational study. Circulation 2006;114:1807–10.

46. D'Alto M, Romeo E, Argiento P, et al. Bosentan-sildenafil association in patients with congenital heart disease-related pulmonary arterial hypertension and Eisenmenger physiology. Int J Cardiol 2012; 155:378–82.

47. Iversen K, Jensen AS, Jensen TV, et al. Combination therapy with bosentan and sildenafil in Eisenmenger syndrome: a randomized, placebo-controlled, double-blinded trial. Eur Heart J 2010;31:1124–31.

48. Beghetti M, Channick RN, Chin KM, et al. Selexipag treatment for pulmonary arterial hypertension associated with congenital heart disease after defect correction: insights from the randomised controlled GRIPHON study. Eur J Heart Fail 2019;21:352–9.

49. Schuuring MJ, Bouma BJ, Cordina R, et al. Treatment of segmental pulmonary artery hypertension in adults with congenital heart disease. Int J Cardiol 2013;164:106–10.

50. Lim ZS, Vettukattill JJ, Salmon AP, et al. Sildenafil therapy in complex pulmonary atresia with pulmonary arterial hypertension. Int J Cardiol 2008;129: 339–43.

51. Yamamura K, Nagata H, Ikeda K, et al. Efficacy of bosentan therapy for segmental pulmonary artery hypertension due to major aortopulmonary collateral arteries in children. Int J Cardiol 2012;161:e1–3.

52. Apostolopoulou SC, Vagenakis G, Rammos S. Pulmonary vasodilator therapy in tetralogy of Fallot with pulmonary atresia and major aortopulmonary collaterals: case series and review of literature. Cardiol Young 2017;27:1861–4.

53. Yasuhara J, Yamagishi H. Pulmonary arterial hypertension associated with tetralogy of Fallot. Int Heart J 2015;56(Suppl):S17–21.

54. Grant EK, Berger JT. Use of pulmonary hypertension medications in patients with tetralogy of Fallot with pulmonary atresia and multiple aortopulmonary collaterals. Pediatr Cardiol 2016;37:304–12.

55. Daliento L, Somerville J, Presbitero P, et al. Eisenmenger syndrome. Factors relating to deterioration and death. Eur Heart J 1998;19:1845–55.

56. Stoica SC, McNeil KD, Perreas K, et al. Heart-lung transplantation for Eisenmenger syndrome: early and long-term results. Ann Thorac Surg 2001;72: 1887–91.

57. Constantine A, Condliffe R, Clift P, et al. Palliative care in pulmonary hypertension associated with congenital heart disease: systematic review and expert opinion. ESC Heart Fail 2021;8(3):1901–14.

58. Mandalenakis Z, Rosengren A, Skoglund K, et al. Survivorship in children and young adults with congenital heart disease in Sweden. JAMA Intern Med 2017;177:224–30.

59. Sliwa K, van Hagen IM, Budts W, et al. Pulmonary hypertension and pregnancy outcomes: data from the registry of pregnancy and cardiac disease (RO-PAC) of the European society of Cardiology. Eur J Heart Fail 2016;18:1119–28.

60. Meng ML, Landau R, Viktorsdottir O, et al. Pulmonary hypertension in pregnancy: a report of 49 cases at four tertiary North American Sites. Obstet Gynecol 2017;129:511–20.

61. Regitz-Zagrosek V, Roos-Hesselink JW, Bauersachs J, et al. 2018 ESC guidelines for the management of cardiovascular diseases during pregnancy: the task force for the management of cardiovascular diseases during pregnancy of the European Society of Cardiology (ESC). Eur Heart J 2018;39:3165–241.

62. Duan R, Xu X, Wang X, et al. Pregnancy outcome in women with Eisenmenger's syndrome: a case series from west China. BMC Pregnancy Childbirth 2016; 16:356.

63. Drenthen W, Pieper PG, Roos-Hesselink JW, et al. Outcome of pregnancy in women with congenital heart disease: a literature review. J Am Coll Cardiol 2007;49:2303–11.

64. Lindley KJ, Bairey Merz CN, Davis MB, et al. Contraception and Reproductive Planning for women with cardiovascular disease: JACC focus Seminar 5/5. J Am Coll Cardiol 2021;77:1823–34.

65. Weiss BM, Zemp L, Seifert B, et al. Outcome of pulmonary vascular disease in pregnancy: a systematic overview from 1978 through 1996. J Am Coll Cardiol 1998;31:1650–7.

Left Heart Disease-Related Pulmonary Hypertension

Ayedh K. Alamri, MBBS[a], Christy L. Ma, PA-C[b], John J. Ryan, MD[b],*

KEYWORDS

- Hemodynamics • Heart failure • Diastolic dysfunction • Postcapillary • Precapillary

KEY POINTS

- Pulmonary hypertension secondary to left-sided heart disease is the most common type of pulmonary hypertension.
- The presence of pulmonary hypertension in patients with heart failure is associated with worse outcomes.
- Multiple treatments have been studied for Group 2 Pulmonary Hypertension with no significant benefits shown to date.

INTRODUCTION

Pulmonary hypertension (PH) is defined as an elevated pulmonary artery (PA) pressure during right heart catheterization. Since the First World Symposium on Pulmonary Hypertension in 1973 the diagnostic cutoff was a mean pulmonary arterial pressure (mPAP) 25 mm Hg or more at rest during right heart catheterization; however, within the last few years this was updated to be mPAP greater than 20 mm Hg at rest.[1]

PH is classified into 5 World Health Organization groups with the main purpose of classifying PH into diseases with similar mechanisms, presentation, hemodynamics, and management (**Box 1**).

PH due to left heart disease (LHD; group 2 PH) is a common complication of heart failure with reduced ejection fraction (HFrEF) and heart failure with preserved ejection fraction (HFpEF) and is often related to disease severity and duration of these diseases.[2] PH due to LHD is associated with negative impact on outcomes in addition to worse symptoms and exercise capacity. Patients with group 2 PH are more likely to be female and be older in age, with hypertension and features of metabolic syndrome.[3–6]

The prevalence of PH in patients with LHD cannot be estimated properly for multiple reasons, including that most of the studies are community based, with different diagnostic criteria and variable hemodynamic or echocardiographic results reported. However, based on published estimates both the incidence and prevalence of PH are increasing, with annual incidence increasing from 24.1 of 100,000 population in 2003 to 28.7 of 100,000 population in 2012. Prevalence has increased from 99.8 of 100,000 population in 1993 to 127.3 of 100,000 population in 2012. Of note, group 2 PH is the most common type of PH, reported alone in 34.2% of patients with PH.[7]

Right heart catheterization remains the gold standard for the diagnosis of PH.[8] Current hemodynamic definitions for PH are as follows:

- Precapillary PH: mPAP greater than 20 mm Hg, pulmonary artery wedge pressure (PAWP) 15 mm Hg or less, and pulmonary vascular resistance (PVR) 3 wood units (WU) or greater.
- Postcapillary PH: mPAP greater than 20 mm Hg, PAWP greater than 15 mm Hg, and PVR less than 3 WU.

a Department of Medicine, University of Utah, University of Utah School of Medicine, 30 North 1900 East, Room 4C116, Salt Lake City, UT 84132, USA; b Division of Cardiovascular Medicine, Department of Medicine, University of Utah, University of Utah School of Medicine, 30 North 1900 East, Room 4A100, Salt Lake City, UT 84132, USA
* Corresponding author. University of Utah Health, 30 North 1900 East, Room 4A100, Salt Lake City, UT 84132.
E-mail address: john.ryan@hsc.utah.edu

Cardiol Clin 40 (2022) 69–76
https://doi.org/10.1016/j.ccl.2021.08.007

Box 1
Classification of pulmonary hypertension

1 PAH

1.1 Idiopathic PAH

1.2 Heritable PAH

1.3 Drug- and toxin-induced PAH (**Table 2**)

1.4 PAH associated with: connective tissue disease, HIV infection, portal hypertension, congenital heart disease, and schistosomiasis.

1.5 PAH long-term responders to calcium channel blockers

1.6 PAH with overt features of venous/capillaries (PVOD/PCH) involvement

1.7 Persistent PH of the newborn syndrome

2 PH due to left heart disease

2.1 PH due to heart failure with preserved LVEF

2.2 PH due to heart failure with reduced LVEF

2.3 Valvular heart disease

2.4 Congenital/acquired cardiovascular conditions leading to postcapillary PH

3 PH due to lung disease and/or hypoxia

3.1 Obstructive lung disease

3.2 Restrictive lung disease

3.3 Other lung disease with mixed restrictive/obstructive pattern

3.4 Hypoxia without lung disease

3.5 Developmental lung disorders

4 PH due to pulmonary artery obstructions

4.1 Chronic thromboembolic PH

4.2 Other pulmonary artery obstructions

5 PH with unclear and/or multifactorial mechanisms

5.1 Hematological disorders

5.2 Systemic and metabolic disorders

5.3 Others

5.4 Complex congenital heart disease

Abbreviations: PAH, pulmonary arterial hypertension; PCH, pulmonary capillary hemangiomatosis; PVOD, pulmonary veno-occlusive disease, LVEF, left ventricular ejection fraction.

6th World Symposium on Pulmonary Hypertension, Nice, France, 2018.

Adapted from Simonneau G, Montani D, Celermajer DS, Denton CP, Gatzoulis MA, Krowka M, Williams PG, Souza R. Haemodynamic definitions and updated clinical classification of pulmonary hypertension. Eur Respir J. 2019 Jan 24;53(1):1801913. Reproduced with permission of the © ERS 2021; DOI: 10.1183/13993003.01913-2018 Published 24 January 2019.

- Combined precapillary and postcapillary PH (Cpc-PH) if mPAP greater than 20 mm Hg, PAWP greater than 15 mm Hg, and PVR 3 WU or greater, with Cpc-PH being the most challenging to diagnose and treat.[9]

Risk score or predictive tools have been developed to help differentiate between group 1 (pulmonary arterial hypertension [PAH]) and group 2 PH.[2] Some features associated with high pretest probability for group 2 PH include advanced age, cardiovascular risk factors, history of atrial fibrillation, structural heart disease, echocardiographic findings including left atrial dilation, as well as MRI and cardiopulmonary exercise tolerance test abnormalities (**Table 1**).[2,10] Jansen and colleagues[11] have developed a noninvasive tool, referred to as the OPTICS risk score, which accurately predicts the presence of PH due to LHD and helps guide decision making for invasive testing (**Table 2**).

Pathogenesis

Group 2 PH related to LHD includes left ventricular disease such as HFrEF, HFpEF, and left-sided valvular disease.[12] In group 2 PH there is an increase in the left atrial pressure (either at rest or with exercise) that causes a retrograde congestion in the pulmonary circulation resulting in an increase in pulmonary venous pressure, pulmonary capillary wedge pressure (PCWP), and PA pressure.[13] The pathophysiology is related not only to an increase in PA pressure but also to an increase in PVR due to adaptations in the vessel walls with medical hypertrophy and intimal hyperplasia (**Fig. 1**).[13] This increase in PVR is mediated by increased vascular tone and remodeling of the pulmonary vasculature, both of which can be triggered by the imbalance between the secretion of vasoactive substance like endothelin-1 (ET-1) and vasodilative substance like nitric oxide (NO) and prostacyclin.[13]

One of the main mechanisms for the development of group 2 PH is believed to be pulmonary vascular remodeling secondary to a sustained increase in intravascular PA pressure. In response to increased afterload from elevated PCWP, the PA starts to adapt by increasing wall thickness and decreasing lumen diameter. The predominant histopathological changes in PH due to LHD include intimal fibrosis and medial hypertrophy of the PA smooth muscles.[13] These changes have also been reported in the pulmonary veins.[13] These observed changes are associated with increased pulmonary vascular tone, increased resistance, and a decreased ability for pulmonary vascular vasodilation.[13,14]

Table 1
Pretest probability for pulmonary hypertension due to left heart disease

Feature	High Probability	Intermediate Probability	Low Probability
Age	>70 y	60–70 y	<60 y
Obesity, hypertension, dyslipidaemia, glucose intolerance/ diabetes	>2 factors	1–2 factors	None
Previous cardiac intervention[a]	Yes	No	No
Atrial fibrillation	Current	Paroxysmal	No
Structural LHD	Present	No	No
ECG	LBBB or LVH	Mild LVH	Normal or signs of RV strain
Echocardiography	LA dilation; grade >2 mitral flow	No LA dilation; grade <2 mitral flow	No LA dilation; E/e' <13
CPET	Mildly elevated V'E/ V'CO2 slope; EOV	Elevated V'E/ V'CO2 slope or EOV	High V'E/V'CO2 slope; no EOV
Cardiac MRI	LA strain or LA/RA >1		No left heart abnormalities

Abbreviations: CPET, cardiopulmonary exercise testing; E/e', early mitral inflow velocity/mitral annular early diastolic velocity ratio; ECG, electrocardiography; EOV, exercise oscillatory ventilation; LA, left atrial; LBBB, left bundle branch block; LVH, left ventricular hypertrophy; RA, right atrial; RV, right ventricular; V'CO2, carbon dioxide production; V'E, minute ventilation.
[a] Coronary artery and/or valvular surgical and/or nonsurgical procedures, including percutaneous interventions.
From Vachiéry J-L, Tedford RJ, Rosenkranz S, Palazzini M, Lang I, Guazzi M, et al. Pulmonary hypertension due to left heart disease. European Respiratory Journal. 2019 Jan;53(1). Reproduced with permission of the © ERS 2021; DOI: 10.1183/13993003.01897-2018.

Table 2
OPTICS risk score calculator with points for each variable and associated probability for PH due to LHD based on the total points estimated from the score

Clinical Variable	Values									Points
Obesity	Body mass index> 30 kg/m²									22
Diabetes Mellitus	Medical history of Diabetes Mellitus									26
Atrial fibrillation	Paroxysmal or persistent									21
Dyslipidemia	Non fasting total cholesterol > 5 mmol/l; HDL-C[a] < 1.0 mmol/l; LDL-C[b] > 3mmo/l									17
Valvular surgery	Mitral, aortic and no without residual left valvular disease									56
SV1+RV6 per mm	Sum of S wave in V1 and R wave in V6 on ECG									1 x (SV1+RV6)
Left atrial dilation	Left atrial volume above 34 ml/m²									21
Total points	0	17	28	37	45	54	63	74	91	107
Probability of post capillary PH	-	0.2	0.3	0.4	0.5	0.6	0.7	0.8	0.9	0.95

Abbreviations: C, electrocardiogram; LHD, left heart disease; PH, pulmonary Hypertension.
[a] HDL- C indicates high-density lipoprotein cholesterol.
[b] LDL- C, low-density lipoprotein cholesterol .
Data from Jansen SMA, Huis in 't Veld AnnaE, Jacobs W, Grotjohan HP, Waskowsky M, van der Maten J, et al. Noninvasive Prediction of Elevated Wedge Pressure in Pulmonary Hypertension Patients Without Clear Signs of Left-Sided Heart Disease: External Validation of the OPTICS Risk Score. Journal of the American Heart Association. 2020 Aug 4;9(15).

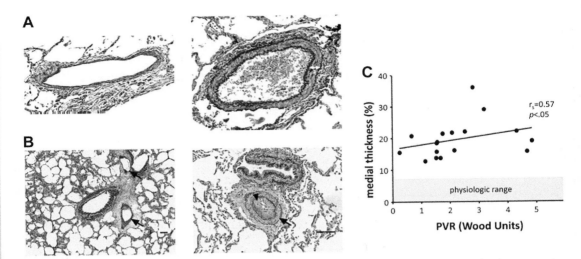

Fig. 1. Remodeling of the pulmonary vasculature in left heart disease. (A) Medial thickening of pulmonary artery, mild (left) and severe (right). (B) Normal intima and media of the pulmonary artery (arrow) (left) and pulmonary artery intima (arrowhead) and media (arrow) thickening in patients with left heart disease and pulmonary hypertension. (C) PVR in patients with heart failure and correlation to the media thickness of the pulmonary arteries. (*From* [A, C] Delgado JF, Conde E, Sá nchez V, Ló pez-Ríós F, Gó mez-Sá nchez MA, Escribano P, et al. Pulmonary vascular remodeling in pulmonary hypertension due to chronic heart failure. European Journal of Heart Failure. 2005 Oct;7(6).; and [B] Hunt JM, Bethea B, Liu X, Gandjeva A, Mammen PPA, Stacher E, et al. Pulmonary veins in the normal lung and pulmonary hypertension due to left heart disease. American Journal of Physiology-Lung Cellular and Molecular Physiology. 2013 Nov 15;305(10).)

NO plays an important role in vasodilation, anti-inflammation, and antiproliferation in the PA smooth muscle cells. NO synthesis is reduced in patients with group 2 PH, where there is also an imbalance between vasodilating and vasoconstrictive substances resulting in endothelial dysfunction.[15–18] NO affects pulmonary vascular tone through soluble guanylate cyclase (sGC), and it has been found that in HF, NO bioavailability is reduced and in turn the decrease in sGC activation leads to dysregulation of the vascular endothelium, thereby resulting in pulmonary vasoconstriction.[19] Kerem and colleagues[20] performed real-time imaging to identify endothelial dysfunction and underlying molecular mechanisms in rats after inducing left-sided heart failure by aortic banding. In areas of shear stress such as acute elevation of hydrostatic pressure or administration of acetylcholine (ACh), or histamine, there was almost complete lack of calcium response and NO synthesis in Group 2 PH[20]. Similarly, Porter and colleagues[21] showed that patients with normal PA pressures had vasodilatory response to ACh, whereas patients with group 2 PH did not.

Vasoactive peptides such as ET-1 act as potent vasoconstrictors and cause hypertrophy of PA smooth muscle cells, in addition to stimulating the production of collagen. ET-1 is predominantly produced by endothelial cells, and it is primarily expressed in pulmonary tissues. ET-1 acts on 2 types of receptors, ET_A and ET_B. The action of ET-1 on the ET_A receptor results in PH by directly increasing vascular tone. ET-1 also contributes to remodeling of the pulmonary vasculature by causing smooth muscle cell proliferation. When ET-1 acts on ET_B, which is located on smooth muscle cells and endothelial cells, it causes either vasoconstriction or vasodilation depending on the location; it also stimulates production of prostacyclin and NO, which can contribute to clearance of ET-1. However, ET_A is expressed 9 times more than ET_B, and the action of ET-1 on ET_A is more dominant to cause vasoconstriction in pulmonary tissues and in patients with heart failure.[13]

Other vasodilators such as brain natriuretic peptide (BNP), which depend on cyclic guanosine monophosphate, mediate less response on the pulmonary circulation in patients with HFrEF.[22] Decreased production of substances such as prostaglandin I2 or prostacyclin, which contributes to vasodilatation and has antiproliferative effects, is also present in patients with group 2 PH.[4,23]

Genetic factors also play a role in the development of group 2 PH. In an exploratory genetic analysis in Cpc-PH performed by Assad and colleagues,[24] the investigators found 75 shared exonic single nucleotide polymorphisms (SNPs) between Cpc-PH and PAH. These SNPs are involved in immune function, cell structure, and extracellular matrix. These SNPs were absent from isolated postcapillary PH, suggesting that Cpc-PH may be closer to PAH than to isolated postcapillary PH.

Management

The mainstay of therapy in group 2 PH is treating the underlying cause. In HFrEF, the therapeutic approach includes β-blockers and inhibition of the renin-angiotensin-aldosterone pathway with angiotensin-converting enzyme inhibitors, angiotensin receptor blockers, or angiotensin/neprilysin inhibitors, as well as the use of aldosterone antagonists.[25,26] The VICTORIA trial published in 2020 assessed the effect of the sGC stimulator vericiguat in patients with HFrEF on adequate background medical therapy and demonstrated lower cardiovascular mortality and hospitalization with vericiguat compared with placebo.[27] Because the sGC pathway impacts both the left ventricular performance and the pulmonary vasculature, this agent gives some hope that perhaps targeting group 2 PH in this manner will have potential benefit.[28] Inhibitors of the sodium-glucose cotransporter 2 (SGLT2) have increasingly been shown to be beneficial in HFrEF but to date have not been studied specifically in group 2 PH.[29]

Finding dedicated treatment of PH secondary to HFpEF remains an enigma despite increased understanding of the pathophysiology, which includes direct activation of the renin-angiotensin-

Table 3
Randomized controlled trial for pulmonary arterial hypertension-specific treatment in patients with pulmonary hypertension-left heart disease

Author/Trial	Intervention (n)	Population	End Point	Result
Shah et al,[42] 2001	Epoprostenol (201) Placebo (235)	Severe HFrEF with EF ≤ 25 and NYHA class IIIB/IV	Primary: Death Secondary: 6MWT, quality of life, and clinical status at 3 mo	Stopped prematurely for increase mortality
Liu Lcy et al,[43] 2017	Sildenafil (26) Placebo (26)	HFpEF with EF ≥ 45, mPAP > 25 and PCWP > 15. NYHA class II–IV	Quality of life, changes in echocardiography LV/RV function or dimensions, and CPECT	No difference
Hoendermis et al,[44] 2015	Sildenafil (26) Placebo (26)	HFpEF with EF ≥ 45, mPAP > 25, and PCWP > 15	mPAP, PCWP, cardiac output and peak Vo₂	No difference
SIOVAC[39]	Sildenafil (104) Placebo (96)	Patients with left-side valvular repair or replacement 1 y before	Primary: death, HF, NYHA class or quality of life Secondary: 6MWD, BNP, echocardiography	Worse outcome in the treatment group with more readmission for HF
Koller et al,[40] 2017	Bosentan (9) Placebo (11)	HFpEF with EF ≥ 50, mPAP > 25, and PCWP > 15. RV dysfunction in echocardiography	6MWD, echocardiography, estimates for PAP and RAP	Increased water retention so it was stopped and no significant changes to 6MWD, BNP, or hemodynamics
MELDOY-1[41]	Macitentan (31) Placebo (32)	HFpEF and HFrEF with EF > 35%, NYHA class II–IV and Cpc-PH with mPAP > 25 and PCWP > 15, DPG ≥7, PVR > 3.0 WU	Primary: tolerability, NYHA class and fluid retention Exploratory: NT-pro-BNP, 6MWD	More patients in treatment group got fluid retention with no changes in the exploratory outcomes

Abbreviations: 6MWD, 6-minute walk distance; CPET, cardiopulmonary exercise testing; DPG, diastolic pulmonary gradient; EF, ejection fraction; HF, heart failure; NYHA, New York Heart Association; RAP, right atrial pressure; RV, Right ventricle; VO₂; VO₂ max.

aldosterone system and increased production of neprilysin, leading to retention of fluid and increased PA pressures.[30] The focus of the treatment in HFpEF remains control of comorbidities and risk factors, with a few specific trials showing marginal benefit.[25] In the CHAMPIONS trial, continuous hemodynamic monitoring was associated with better outcomes in terms of hospitalization for both HFpEF and HFrEF.[31]

PARAGON-HF studied the angiotensin/neprilysin inhibitor combination drug sacubitril-valsartan in HFpEF. Although the study found no benefit in the overall population with HFpEF, a reduction in the primary outcome was observed in those with midrange ejection fraction (<57%).[32] The drug has subsequently received US Food and Drug Administration approval for all forms of heart failure, regardless of ejection fraction. Spironolactone similarly has a class IIb recommendation for use in HFpEF from the American College of Cardiology/American Heart Association Heart Failure Guidelines owing to positive subgroup analysis and despite the overall study results being negative.[26,33,34]

Drugs directly targeting the pulmonary vasculature that are used for treatment of group 1 PH, specifically the endothelin receptors or NO regulators, have failed to show benefit in patients with HFpEF.[2,9] sGC stimulators have not been shown to be beneficial in the HFpEF population.[35–37] SGLT inhibitors are currently being studied in HFpEF, with results from EMPEROR-Preserved and PRESERVED-HF expected over the coming year. These agents have been shown to improve diastolic function and may reduce vascular remodeling.[38]

A summary of the trials examining the use of PAH-specific treatment in patients with PH-LHD in listed in (**Table 3**). None of these studies have shown any sustained or significant clinical benefit. Furthermore, the use of some of these medications may even cause harm.[9] For example, in a trial of the phosphodiesterase 5 inhibitor sildenafil in patients with persistent group 2 PH secondary to valvular heart disease, the patients randomized to sildenafil had worse outcomes, demonstrating that off-label use of this medication in these patients should be avoided.[39] Similar findings were observed in the MELODY-1 trial, which tested the endothelin receptor blocker macitentan in patients with Cpc-PH, and showed increased fluid retention and no favorable changes in hemodynamics, exercise tolerance, or BNP.[40,41]

SUMMARY

Among all groups of PH, group 2 PH is the most common. The presence of PH in patients with LHD is associated with worse symptoms and has a negative impact on clinical outcomes.[3–6] Management remains focused on treating the underlying cause; however, there is hope that with the development of new medications, such as sGC stimulators and SGLT-2 inhibitors, targeted treatment options may soon become available.[27,29]

CLINICS CARE POINTS

- Group 2 pulmonary hypertension (PH) (PH due to left-sided heart disease) is increasing in prevalence and incidence. Group 2 PH is caused by multiple mechanisms resulting in an increase in pulmonary vascular resistance through increases in the pulmonary vascular tone and pulmonary vascular remodelling. Treating the underlying cause is the mainstay in the treatment of Group 2 PH. Multiple treatments, especially pulmonary vascular targeted medications have been studied in Group 2 PH with no clinical benefit seen.

ACKNOWLEDGMENTS

Dr Ryan and his research are supported by the Gordon family and the Reagan Foundation.

DISCLOSURE

The authors have nothing to disclose.

REFERENCES

1. Simonneau G, Montani D, Celermajer DS, et al. Haemodynamic definitions and updated clinical classification of pulmonary hypertension. Eur Respir J 2019;53(1):1801913.
2. Vachiéry J-L, Tedford RJ, Rosenkranz S, et al. Pulmonary hypertension due to left heart disease. Eur Respir J 2019;53(1):1801897.
3. Vachiéry J-L, Adir Y, Barberà JA, et al. Pulmonary hypertension due to left heart diseases. J Am Coll Cardiol 2013;62(250):D100–8.
4. Fang JC, DeMarco T, Givertz MM, et al. World health Organization pulmonary hypertension group 2: pulmonary hypertension due to left heart disease in the adult—a summary statement from the pulmonary hypertension Council of the International Society for heart and lung Transplantation. The J Heart Lung Transplant 2012;31(9):913–33.
5. Thenappan T, Shah SJ, Gomberg-Maitland M, et al. Clinical characteristics of pulmonary hypertension in patients with heart failure and preserved ejection fraction. Circ Heart Fail 2011;4(3):257–65.

6. Robbins IM, Newman JH, Johnson RF, et al. Association of the metabolic syndrome with pulmonary venous hypertension. Chest 2009;136(1):31–6.

7. Wijeratne DT, Lajkosz K, Brogly SB, et al. Increasing incidence and prevalence of World Health Organization groups 1 to 4 pulmonary hypertension. Circ Cardiovasc Qual Outcomes 2018;11(2):e003973.

8. Thenappan T, Ormiston ML, Ryan JJ, et al. Pulmonary arterial hypertension: pathogenesis and clinical management. BMJ 2018;360:j5492.

9. Maron BA, Ryan JJ. A Concerning Trend for patients with pulmonary hypertension in the Era of Evidence-based medicine. Circulation 2019;139(16):1861–4.

10. Bonderman D, Wexberg P, Martischnig AM, et al. A noninvasive algorithm to exclude pre-capillary pulmonary hypertension. Eur Respir J 2011;37(5): 1096–103.

11. Jansen SMA, Huis in 't Veld AE, Jacobs W, et al. Noninvasive prediction of elevated wedge pressure in pulmonary hypertension patients without clear Signs of left-sided heart disease: External Validation of the OPTICS risk score. J Am Heart Assoc 2020; 9(15):e015992.

12. Mayeux JD, Pan IZ, Dechand J, et al. Management of pulmonary arterial hypertension. Curr Cardiovasc Risk Rep 2021;15(1):2.

13. Breitling S, Ravindran K, Goldenberg NM, et al. The pathophysiology of pulmonary hypertension in left heart disease. Am J Physiology-Lung Cell Mol Physiol 2015;309(9):L924–41.

14. Fayyaz AU, Edwards WD, Maleszewski JJ, et al. Global pulmonary vascular remodeling in pulmonary hypertension associated with heart failure and pre-served or reduced ejection fraction. Circulation 2018;137(17):1796–810.

15. Stamler JS, Loh E, Roddy MA, et al. Nitric oxide regulates basal systemic and pulmonary vascular resistance in healthy humans. Circulation 1994;89(5): 2035–40.

16. Tousoulis D, Kampoli A-M, Tentolouris Nikolaos Papageorgiou C, et al. The role of nitric oxide on endothelial function. Curr Vasc Pharmacol 2012;10(1):4–18.

17. Kuebler WM, Uhlig U, Goldmann T, et al. Stretch activates nitric oxide production in pulmonary vascular endothelial cells in Situ. Am J Respir Crit Care Med 2003;168(11):1391–8.

18. Marti CN, Gheorghiade M, Kalogeropoulos AP, et al. Endothelial dysfunction, arterial stiffness, and heart failure. J Am Coll Cardiol 2012;60(16):1455–69.

19. Paulus WJ, Tschöpe C. A novel paradigm for heart failure with preserved ejection fraction. J Am Coll Cardiol 2013;62(4):263–71.

20. Kerem A, Yin J, Kaestle SM, et al. Lung endothelial dysfunction in congestive heart failure. Circ Res 2010;106(6):1103–16.

21. Porter TR, Taylor DO, Cycan A, et al. Endothelium-dependent pulmonary artery responses in chronic heart failure: Influence of pulmonary hypertension. J Am Coll Cardiol 1993;22(5):1418–24.

22. Melenovsky V, Al-Hiti H, Kazdova L, et al. Transpulmonary B-type natriuretic peptide uptake and cyclic guanosine monophosphate release in heart failure and pulmonary hypertension. J Am Coll Cardiol 2009;54(7):595–600.

23. Galiè N, Manes A, Branzi A. Prostanoids for pulmonary arterial hypertension. Am J Respir Med 2003; 2(2):123–37.

24. Assad TR, Hemnes AR, Larkin EK, et al. Clinical and biological insights into combined post- and pre-capillary pulmonary hypertension. J Am Coll Cardiol 2016;68(23):2525–36.

25. Ponikowski P, Voors AA, Anker SD, et al. 2016 ESC Guidelines for the diagnosis and treatment of acute and chronic heart failure. Eur Heart J 2016;37(27): 2129–200.

26. Maddox TM, Januzzi JL, Allen LA, et al. 2021 update to the 2017 ACC Expert consensus decision pathway for optimization of heart failure treatment: answers to 10 pivotal issues about heart failure with reduced ejection fraction. J Am Coll Cardiol 2021;77(6):772–810.

27. Armstrong PW, Pieske B, Anstrom KJ, et al. Vericiguat in patients with heart failure and reduced ejection fraction. New Engl J Med 2020;382(20): 1883–93.

28. Jessica Wearden, Augustus Hough, Stephanie Kaiser. Vericiguat in heart failure with reduced ejection fraction. New Engl J Med 2020;383(15):1496–7.

29. McMurray JJV, Solomon SD, Inzucchi SE, et al. Dapagliflozin in patients with heart failure and reduced ejection fraction. New Engl J Med 2019;381(21): 1995–2008.

30. Packer M, Kitzman DW. Obesity-related heart failure with a preserved ejection fraction. JACC: Heart Fail 2018;6(8):633–9.

31. Benza RL, Raina A, Abraham WT, et al. Pulmonary hypertension related to left heart disease: insight from a wireless implantable hemodynamic monitor. The J Heart Lung Transplant 2015;34(3):329–37.

32. Solomon SD, McMurray JJV, Anand IS, et al. Angiotensin–neprilysin inhibition in heart failure with pre-served ejection fraction. New Engl J Med 2019; 381(17):1609–20.

33. Pitt B, Pfeffer MA, Assmann SF, et al. Spironolactone for heart failure with preserved ejection fraction. New Engl J Med 2014 Apr 10;370(15):1383–92.

34. Yancy CW, Jessup M, Bozkurt B, et al. 2017 ACC/AHA/HFSA focused update of the 2013 ACCF/AHA Guideline for the management of heart failure: a Report of the American College of Cardiology/American heart association task force on clinical Practice Guidelines and the heart failure Society of America. Circulation 2017;23(8):628–51.

35. Armstrong PW, Lam CSP, Anstrom KJ, et al. Effect of vericiguat vs placebo on quality of life in patients

with heart failure and preserved ejection fraction. JAMA 2020;324(15):1512–21.

36. Udelson JE, Lewis GD, Shah SJ, et al. Effect of praliciguat on peak rate of oxygen consumption in patients with heart failure with preserved ejection fraction. JAMA 2020;324(15):1522–31.

37. Pieske B, Maggioni AP, Lam CSP, et al. Vericiguat in patients with worsening chronic heart failure and preserved ejection fraction: results of the SOluble guanylate Cyclase stimulatoR in heArT failurE patientS with PRESERVED EF (SOCRATES-PRESERVED) study. Eur Heart J 2017;38(15):1119–27.

38. Kosiborod M, Cavender MA, Fu AZ, et al. Lower risk of heart failure and death in patients initiated on sodium-glucose cotransporter-2 inhibitors versus Other glucose-Lowering drugs. Circulation 2017; 136(3):249–59.

39. Bermejo J, Yotti R, García-Orta R, et al. Sildenafil for improving outcomes in patients with corrected valvular heart disease and persistent pulmonary hypertension: a multicenter, double-blind, randomized clinical trial. Eur Heart J 2018;39(15):1255–64.

40. Koller B, Steringer-Mascherbauer R, Ebner CH, et al. Pilot study of endothelin receptor blockade in heart failure with diastolic dysfunction and pulmonary hypertension (BADDHY-Trial). Heart Lung Circ 2017; 26(5):433–41.

41. Vachiéry J-L, Delcroix M, Al-Hiti H, et al. Macitentan in pulmonary hypertension due to left ventricular dysfunction. Eur Respir J 2018;51(2):1701886.

42. Shah MR, Stinnett SS, McNulty SE, et al. Hemodynamics as surrogate end points for survival in advanced heart failure: an analysis from FIRST. Am Heart J 2001;141(6):908–14.

43. Liu LCY, Hummel YM, van der Meer P, et al. Effects of sildenafil on cardiac structure and function, cardiopulmonary exercise testing and health-related quality of life measures in heart failure patients with preserved ejection fraction and pulmonary hypertension. Eur J Heart Fail 2017;19(1):116–25.

44. Hoendermis ES, Liu LCY, Hummel YM, et al. Effects of sildenafil on invasive haemodynamics and exercise capacity in heart failure patients with preserved ejection fraction and pulmonary hypertension: a randomized controlled trial. Eur Heart J 2015;36(38): 2565–73.

Lung Disease–Related Pulmonary Hypertension

Kareem Ahmad, MD*, Vikramjit Khangoora, MD, Steven D. Nathan, MD

KEYWORDS

- Pulmonary hypertension • Chronic lung disease • WHO group 3 PH • COPD
- Interstitial lung disease • Cor pulmonale

KEY POINTS

- Concomitant pulmonary hypertension worsens the prognosis of patients with both obstructive and restrictive lung diseases.
- Optimizing the underlying lung disease remains the major goal of medical therapy.
- Emerging evidence attests to the benefit of pulmonary vasodilator therapy with recent approval in the United States of inhaled treprostinil for patients with pulmonary hypertension owing to chronic lung disease.
- Lung transplantation may be the best option in select patients and should be sought early in appropriate candidates.

INTRODUCTION
History

Right heart failure in the setting of lung disease
"Cor pulmonale" has been used in the medical literature to denote right heart failure owing to chronic respiratory disease since the 1960s.[1] It represents 6% to 7% of all types of adult heart disease and accounts for 10% to 30% of heart failure admissions in the United States.[2] The role of right ventricular (RV) stiffening, ventriculoarterial uncoupling, and RV dyssynchrony are now noted features in right heart failure from pulmonary vascular disease.[3] It can be difficult to discern group 1 pulmonary hypertension (PH) (pulmonary arterial hypertension [PAH]) from group 3 PH, but what is clear is that any lung disease in those with hemodynamics suggestive of PAH portends a poor prognosis; alternatively, PH owing to chronic lung disease (PH-CLD) of varied etiologies is likewise associated with worse outcomes.[4]

CURRENT UNDERSTANDING OF PATHOPHYSIOLOGY

The mechanisms driving the development of PH-CLD remain incompletely understood but are likely multifactorial. Hypoxic pulmonary vasoconstriction (HPVC), which may be amplified by hypercapnia and acidemia, can certainly play a role.[5] A study of patients with chronic obstructive pulmonary disease (COPD) with isolated hypoxia, isolated hypercapnia, or a combination thereof showed that just hypercapnia without hypoxemia-induced increases in the mean pulmonary artery pressure (mPAP).[6] In contrast with the systemic circulation, which dilates in response to hypoxia, decreased alveolar oxygen tension results in increased pulmonary vascular tone. HPVC is a regulatory physiologic mechanism that functions to limit ventilation/perfusion mismatching by decreasing blood flow to hypoxic alveoli. As a result, systemic oxygen saturation remains near normal as blood flow is shunted away from poorly ventilated areas of the lung, at the cost of increased pulmonary vascular resistance (PVR). Short-term HPVC is reversible with supplemental oxygen; however, chronic HPVC may result in increased pulmonary vascular remodeling, which may not reverse with correction of hypoxia.[7] Furthermore, chronic HPVC may result in an imbalance of pulmonary vasoactive peptides, perpetuating pulmonary vasoconstriction. A decrease in

Transplant Department, Advanced Lung Disease and Lung Transplant, Inova Fairfax Medical Center, 3300 Gallows Road, Falls Church, VA 22042, USA
* Corresponding author.
E-mail address: Kareem.Ahmad@inova.org

Cardiol Clin 40 (2022) 77–88
https://doi.org/10.1016/j.ccl.2021.08.005
0733-8651/22/© 2021 Elsevier Inc. All rights reserved.

endothelial nitric oxide synthase production resulting in decreased bioavailable nitric oxide and an upregulation of endothelin-1 expression have been observed in patients with COPD and idiopathic pulmonary fibrosis (IPF).[8–10] Increases in multiple cytokines and growth factors in CLD further promulgate pulmonary vascular remodeling via medial hypertrophy, abnormal collagen matrix deposition, and intimal hyperplasia[8] (**Fig. 1**). Extrapulmonary effects of hypoxia include polycythemia, which compounds PH by increasing the viscosity of the blood.[11] In those with obstructive sleep apnea or obesity hypoventilation syndrome, vasoreactivity has been shown to diminish over time, leading to permanent remodeling of vessels. The use of positive airway pressure therapy can be effective in mitigating this.[12] Notably, the amount of parenchymal disease does not necessarily correlate with the presence or severity of PH.[7] This finding suggests that other factors, including genetic polymorphisms, might be at play, leading to significant variability in the prevalence of PH-CLD.[13]

CLINICAL FEATURES

Owing to the significant overlap in symptoms with the underlying lung disease, the diagnosis of PH is often delayed. The most common presenting symptoms are increasing dyspnea with exertion and rapid desaturation and fatigue with exercise. As RV function worsens, signs and symptoms of RV failure may develop. As the hemodynamic consequences of PH become more prominent, patients may present with increased hypoxemia,

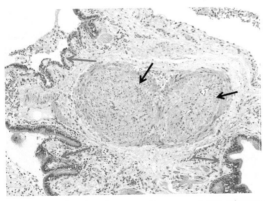

Fig. 1. Vascular changes seen in group 3 PH. Histopathology from a lung biopsy specimen of an interstitial lung disease patient shows presence of neointimal thickening (*arrows*) occurring even in lung tissue with well-preserved parenchymal structure. (*Courtesy of* Haresh Mani, MD; Inova Fairfax Hospital, Falls Church, VA.)

tachypnea, and tachycardia. In cases of mild and well-compensated PH, there may not be additional or unique physical examination findings, apart from an increased P2 heart sound. Overt signs of RV failure in patients with lung disease are uncommon, although patients with more severe PH can develop peripheral edema, increased abdominal girth, and weight gain. Auscultation of the lungs may reveal a variety of sounds related to the primary lung disease, including Velcro-like inspiratory crackles in fibrotic diseases, high-pitched rhonchi in bronchiolitis and bronchiectasis, and wheezing or poor air movement in COPD.

DIAGNOSTIC TESTING FOR PULMONARY HYPERTENSION IN PATIENTS WITH LUNG DISEASE

Commonly available noninvasive modalities that may suggest the presence of group 3 PH include:

- Pulmonary function testing (spirometry, lung volumes, diffusion capacity): the presence of a severely reduced single breath diffusing capacity of the lung for carbon monoxide (DL_{CO} of <30% predicted) is associated with a twofold increase in the likelihood of PH in IPF.[14] Prognostically, patients in group 3 with more severely decreased DL_{CO}s have significantly increased 1- and 5-year mortality compared with those with less severe diffusion defects.[15]
- Six-minute walk test: A decreased 6-minute walk test distance (6MWD), low and progressive desaturation should raise suspicion for the development of group 3 PH. Furthermore, a decreased heart rate recovery 1 minute after exercise cessation (<13 beats per minute) has been shown to predict PH in patients with IPF.[16]
- Chest computed tomography (CT) scan: In patients with IPF, a pulmonary artery to aorta diameter of 1.0 or greater has been shown to correlate with the presence of PH and is an independent predictor of mortality.[17] Additionally, in patients with ILD, an RV to left ventricle ratio of greater than 1 on CT imaging is associated with an increased PVR and mortality[18] (**Fig. 2**).
- Plasma biomarkers: Brain natriuretic peptide or N-terminal pro brain natriuretic peptide are elevated in severe group 3 PH, but their sensitivity and specificity are lower than that for group 1 PH, because it is more likely to be confounded by comorbid left heart abnormalities.[19]

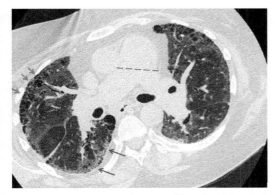

Fig. 2. CT imaging in pulmonary fibrosis with PH. CT imaging shows an enlarged pulmonary artery (PA) segment (*blue dotted line*) in a patient with IPF with severe PAH (mean PA pressure ~60 mm Hg) with characteristic subpleural "honeycombing" (*red arrows*) and fibrosis (*purple line*).

- Echocardiography: Two-dimensional transthoracic echocardiography is the best and most frequently used screening tool for group 3 PH. The RV systolic pressure can be calculated from the maximum tricuspid regurgitant jet velocity. However, the concurrent presence of lung disease may impair the ability to obtain adequate echocardiographic images and subsequently may result in an inaccurate estimation of pulmonary artery pressures.[20] Recent studies have suggested that using alternate echocardiographic measures such as RV outflow tract diameter, fractional area change, and tricuspid annular plane systolic excursion may be more accurate in screening for group 3 PH.[21] In a study of patients with group 3 PH, 3-dimensional echo-derived fractional area change of more than and less than 28% discriminated both risk of mortality and heart failure hospitalization.[22] In a mixed cohort of patients with PH, including those with PH-CLD, the presence of depressed RV strain by speckle tracking also predicted mortality.[23]

Right heart catheterization (RHC) remains the gold standard for the diagnosis of PH, including group 3 PH. An RHC should be performed in patients with CLD with symptoms and/or testing considered to be disproportionately abnormal in relation to the severity of their underlying primary pulmonary process. RHC is mandatory in any patient with lung disease undergoing a transplant evaluation. The Sixth World Symposium on Pulmonary Hypertension suggested adapting the definition for PH in the context of CLD as follows[4]:

1. CLD without PH (mPAP of <21 mm Hg, or mPAP of 21–24 mm Hg with a PVR of <3 Woods units [WU]).
2. CLD with PH (mPAP of 21–24 mm Hg with a PVR of ≥3 WU, or a mPAP of 25–34 mm Hg).
3. CLD with severe PH (mPAP of >35 mm Hg, or mPAP of >25 mm Hg with a low cardiac index [<2.0 L min^{-1} m^2]) (CLD-severe PH).

RHC data in patients with CLD with PH show similar elevation in right atrial pressure and decrease in cardiac index to patients with PAH.[24] PVR elevation has repeatedly been shown to predict mortality, with a PVR of 7 WU or more carrying a 3-fold increased risk of mortality compared with a PVR of less than 7 WU.[24,25] There is currently a limited role for the use of acute pulmonary vasodilator testing in group 3 PH, with low rates of vasoreactivity reported. However, a lack of response is predictive of worse survival.[24] Additionally, in the setting of an increased incidence of left sided heart disease, the use of exercise RHC should be considered and may be useful in unmasking underlying group 2 PH (PH owing to left heart disease).[26]

It can be difficult to distinguish between severe group 3 PH and group 1 PH in the context of comorbid lung disease. A thorough evaluation of pulmonary function tests, high-resolution CT imaging, pulmonary hemodynamic profile, and cardiopulmonary exercise testing (in select cases), may help to clarify whether the PH is attributable to the underlying pulmonary process[4] (**Table 1**). When there is uncertainty as to the best category for a patient with lung disease and PH, the patient should be referred to centers with expertise in both PH and CLD, especially with regard to the institution of a PH therapy. There are no guidelines on when or how often to screen for patients with PH with CLD; however, many of the standard of care longitudinal CLD testing (pulmonary function tests, 6-minute walk test, chest CT scan) do provide screening information. In addition, we recommend a screening transthoracic echocardiography annually or as triggered by a change in symptoms.

TREATMENT OF THE UNDERLYING DISEASE

An essential first step in the treatment of PH-CLD is optimizing therapy of the underlying disease process. In addition, reversible comorbid conditions that might contribute to the development or perpetuation of PH should be sought and addressed (**Fig. 3**).

Obstructive Lung Disease

In patients with COPD, PH is an independent prognostic factor for mortality regardless of degree of

Table 1
Differentiating group 1 from group 3 PH[a]

Criteria Favoring Group 1 (PAH)	Testing	Criteria Favoring Group 3 (PH Owing to Lung Disease)
Extent of lung disease		
Normal or mildly impaired: FEV_1 of >60% predicted (COPD) FVC of >70% predicted (IPF) Low diffusion capacity in relation to obstructive/restrictive changes	Pulmonary function testing	Moderate to very severely impaired: FEV_1 of <60% predicted (COPD) FVC of <70% predicted (IPF) Diffusion capacity corresponds with obstructive/restrictive changes
Absence of or only modest airway or parenchymal abnormalities	High-resolution CT scan[b]	Characteristic airway and/or parenchymal abnormalities
Haemodynamic profile		
Moderate-to-severe PH	RHC Echocardiogram	Mild-to-moderate PH
Ancillary testing		
Present	Further PAH risk factors (eg, HIV, connective tissue disease, *BMPR2* mutations, etc)	Absent
Features of exhausted circulatory reserve: Preserved breathing reserve Reduced oxygen pulse Low CO/V_{O_2} slope Mixed venous oxygen saturation at lower limit No change or decrease in $P_a{CO_2}$ during exercise	Cardiopulmonary exercise test[c] [$Pa{CO_2}$ particularly relevant in COPD]	Features of exhausted ventilatory reserve: Reduced breathing reserve Normal oxygen pulse Normal CO//0, slope Mixed venous oxygen saturation above lower limit Increase in $P_a{CO_2}$ during exercise
Predominant obstructive/restrictive profile		
Predominant hemodynamic profile		

Abbreviations: BMPR2, bone morphogenetic protein receptor type 2; CO, cardiac output; CT, computed tomography; FEV_1, forced expiratory volume in 1 second; FVC, forced vital capacity; $Pa{CO_2}$, arterial carbon dioxide tension; VO_2, oxygen uptake.
[a] Patients in groups 2 and 4 are excluded based on the diagnostic criteria of these groups.
[b] Parenchymal changes linked to pulmonary veno-occlusive disease may be discriminated from those associated with diffuse parenchymal lung diseases.
[c] Features of a limited circulatory reserve may be noted in severe COPD-PH and severe IPF-PH.
From Nathan SD, Barbera JA, Gaine SP, et al. Pulmonary hypertension in chronic lung disease and hypoxia. Eur Respir J. 2019;53(1):1801914.

obstruction.[21] Correction of chronic hypoxia with long-term oxygen therapy (LTOT) has been shown to reverse the progression of PH in some patients, if not at least stabilizing it in others.[27] Unlike more generalized data showing that LTOT has no effect on outcomes of patients with COPD, in those with PH the daily duration of LTOT use is associated directly with improved hemodynamic results.[28] Cigarette smoke can induce PH independently,

with evidence of both direct endothelial cell oxidative damage and downregulation of inducible nitric oxide synthase.[29] Therefore, smoking cessation is integral in limiting direct toxicity. In addition to its impact on function and outcomes, PH in COPD is also associated with an increased risk of acute exacerbations, and hence requirement for emergency room treatment or hospitalization. Although disease-stabilizing inhalers have no direct effect

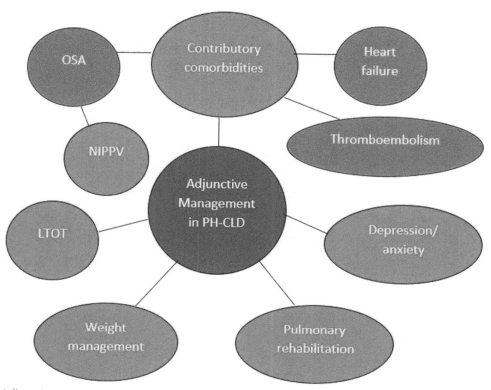

Fig. 3. Adjunctive management in PH-CLD. Long-term oxygen therapy (LTOT) can prevent sequelae of HPVC. Noninvasive positive pressure ventilation (NIPPV) should be used to overcome sleep apnea (OSA) and carbon dioxide retention, which worsens pulmonary vasoconstriction. Concomitant coronary artery disease, arrhythmias, and left heart failure can compound PH. Depression and anxiety are common and can exacerbate dyspnea and overall morbidity. Deconditioning can be combated with the institution of regular exercise, supervised in pulmonary rehabilitation or independently by patients. Pulmonary cachexia can be combated with adequate caloric intake, although obesity leads to pulmonary restriction.

on PH, roflumilast, a phosphodiesterase 4 inhibitor that is approved for the prevention of frequent exacerbations, has some preclinical evidence of attenuating pulmonary vascular remodeling.[30] Lung volume reduction surgery has been shown in a large cohort to immediately decrease the mPAP.[31] However, a subset analysis of the National Emphysema Treatment Trial showed no significant difference in terms of mPAP or PVR 6 months after the surgical intervention.[32] Novel endobronchial valve therapy as an alternative to lung volume reduction surgery has yet to be investigated similarly.

Interstitial Lung Disease

IPF is the most common form of ILD, accounting for nearly 25% of cases, with PH complicating the course in about one-third of these patients.[33] There are 2 approved antifibrotic agents for the treatment of IPF. Nintedanib is a tyrosine kinase inhibitor with known effects on multiple growth

factor receptors. Nintedanib has been assessed in combination with sildenafil, but the study failed to meet its primary end point of improvement in quality of life (QOL) as evaluated by the St. George's Respiratory Questionnaire. However, secondary end points, including the UCSD Shortness of Breath Questionnaire and forced vital capacity, did suggest a potential benefit.[34] Pirfenidone, the other available antifibrotic, has also been studied in combination with sildenafil, but this combination did not show any benefit in reducing disease progression.[35] The second largest group of ILD patients is those with connective tissue diseases (scleroderma lung disease, rheumatoid arthritis-associated ILD, among others). Owing to the independent association of connective tissue diseases with the development of PAH, patients with connective tissue disease are generally classified within 1 group as it may be especially difficult to discern group 1 versus group 3 PH. Other inflammatory and fibrotic lung diseases including non-IPF idiopathic interstitial pneumonias and chronic hypersensitivity pneumonitis also have an increased risk of developing PH.[36,37] Both sarcoidosis and lymphangioleiomyomatosis are diffuse parenchymal processes that can develop PH, with lymphangioleiomyomatosis categorized as group 3 and sarcoidosis categorized as group 5 PH owing its multifactorial pathophysiology.

Pulmonary Vasodilator Therapy

Multiple studies have been conducted in group 3 PH with existing PAH therapies. The results have been mixed and until recently there was no approved therapy for group 3 PH (**Table 2**).

Phosphodiesterase Inhibitors

The widespread use of this class of agents in both obstructive and restrictive lung diseases was owing to their ease in dosing and relative low cost. Sildenafil is the most widely tested of all PAH agents.[38,39] In 1 COPD-PH study, a benefit in functional capacity and reduced symptom burden was demonstrated with a modest decrease in PVR.[40] Interestingly, a previous study in patients with COPD (with and without known PH) failed to show any benefit in terms of maximal exercise capacity or in hemodynamic parameters. In fact, any benefit was only seen in those with documented PH, whereas it was detrimental in those without known PH.[41] A large study of tadalafil in COPD showed no benefit for patients with mild PH by echocardiographic findings.[42] The evidence for benefit in ILD has been suggested in multiple studies, including a large trial of sildenafil in IPF. Although this study failed to meet its primary end point of a 20% improvement in the 6MWD, secondary end points including oxygenation, DL_{CO}, and QOL did suggest some benefit.[43] In addition, a further subgroup analysis did demonstrate that those patients with RV dysfunction on echocardiogram had improved QOL and exercise capacity with sildenafil treatment.[44]

Direct Soluble Guanylate Cyclase Inhibitors

The direct soluble guanylcyclase inhibitor, riociguat, has been studied in PH owing to ILD; unfortunately, it resulted in harm, with increased mortality in a large trial resulting in early study termination.[45] Riociguat also garnered attention for patients with COPD after showing preclinical benefit. A pilot study demonstrated improvement in hemodynamic parameters in 23 patients after single dose testing.[46] A small series showed sustained benefit after up to 7 months of use, although the authors noted that there was a tendency for lower oxygen saturations with exercise.[47]

Endothelin Receptor Antagonists

Preclinical models have suggested that endothelin receptor antagonists might have antifibrotic properties, resulting in all 3 endothelin receptor antagonists being studied in IPF.[48] No benefit was seen with either bosentan or macitentan in their respective IPF clinical trials, but ambrisentan demonstrated harm, with increased rates of hospitalization and increased mortality.[49–51] Bosentan had conflicting results in patients with COPD, with 1 trial noting a significant worsening in hypoxia, providing a cautionary note to the use of endothelin receptor antagonist in these patients.[52,53]

Prostanoids

The most potent group of vasodilators, the prostacyclin analogues, have also been studied in patients with group 3 PH. The first available inhalational form of pulmonary vasodilator therapy, iloprost, was trialed in COPD and severe IPF.[54] Early studies showed promising results, but further prospective investigation in COPD failed to show a benefit.[55] The study of inhaled iloprost in IPF demonstrated a paradoxic worsening in the 6MWD.[56] Recently, inhaled treprostinil was assessed in the largest randomized, placebo-controlled trial of patients with ILD to date. Results showed a significant improvement in 6MWD, decreased rates of clinical worsening, and a decrease in NT-proBNP.[57] This agent was approved for PH-ILD on April 1, 2021, by the US Food and Drug Administration, and is the first and therefore only approved pulmonary vasodilator for group 3 PH. A parallel study of inhaled treprostinil in patients with COPD is currently enrolling, with the results eagerly awaited. There have been no trials of oral treprostinil for PH in ILD and only a small case series of selexipag in COPD suggesting some improvement in functional capacity.[58] The intravenous and subcutaneous administration of prostacyclin therapy is typically reserved for patients with New York Heart Association functional class III or IV and a high risk for mortality. To date, there are no large clinical trials, but reported studies document some success with these parenteral agents in patients with CLD.[59,60] The parenteral prostanoids are often used as salvage therapy in those with the severest hemodynamic impairment and sometimes serve as a bridge to lung transplantation.

Other Forms of Inhaled Therapy

Inhaled nitric oxide is a well-established agent for vasodilator testing during hemodynamic evaluation. Attempts to use it outside the critical care

Table 2
Select randomized control trials of pulmonary vasodilators in PH-CLD

Author (Year)	Disease	Diagnosis of PH	Therapy	Duration	Primary End Point Result	Additional Key Outcomes
Vonbank,[60] 2003	COPD	RHC: mPAP of $\geq$25 mm Hg	Pulsed iNO	3 mo	PVRi and CO improved	No worsened hypoxemia
Stolz,[51] 2008	COPD	Echo	Bosentan	12 wk	No significant effect on 6MWD	Worsened hypoxemia and QOL
Valerio,[50] 2009	COPD	RHC	Bosentan	18 mo	No defined primary	mPAP, PVR, and 6MWD improved.
Rao,[36] 2011	COPD	Echo: sPAP of >40 mm Hg	Sildenafil	12 wk	Increased 6MWD	Decrease in sPAP
Blanco,[37] 2013	COPD	RHC: mPAP of $\geq$25 mm Hg or Echo: sPAP of $\geq$35 mm Hg	Sildenafil	3 mo	No change in cycle endurance	No effect on 6MWD, peak V_{O_2}, QOL or oxygenation
Goudie,[40] 2014	COPD	Echo: PA acceleration time of <120 ms or sPAP of >30 mm Hg	Tadalafil	12 wk	6MWD, no change	Decreased sPAP, no difference in QOL, BNP or oxygenation
Vitulo,[38] 2016	COPD	RHC: mPAP >35 mm Hg (if FEV_1<30%); mPAP of $\geq$30 mm Hg (if FEV_1 of $\geq$30%)	Sildenafil	16 wk	Decrease in PVR	CI and QOL improved
Han,[42] 2013	IPF	Echo: RVSD	Sildenafil	12 wk	Decrease in declining 6MWD	Improvement in QOL
Corte,[48] 2014	ILD	RHC: mPAP of $\geq$25 mm Hg	Bosentan	16 wk	No significant decline in PVRi	No change in FC or symptoms.
Raghu,[47] 2013	IPF	RHC	Ambrisentan	52+ weeks	Unfavorable trend in disease progression, terminated early	Increased hospitalization in treatment
Nathan,[43] 2019	ILD	RHC	Riociguat	26 wk	No difference in 6MWD at study halt	Study stopped early for increased harm to riociguat arm (death and hospitalization)
Nathan,[61] 2020	ILD	Echo	Pulsed iNO	8 wk	Increased MVPA	No change in saturation or 6MWD

(continued on next page)

Table 2
(continued)

Author (Year)	Disease	Diagnosis of PH	Therapy	Duration	Primary End Point Result	Additional Key Outcomes
Behr,[33] 2020	IPF	Echo/RHC	Sildenafil Pirfenidone	52 wk	No difference in disease progression	No significant treatment-emergent adverse events
Waxman,[55] 2021	ILD	RHC	Treprostonil (inhaled)	16 wk	Significantly increased 6MWD	Decreased NT-proBNP and clinical worsening, no difference in QOL

Abbreviations: 6MWD, 6 minute walk distance; BNP, brain natriuretic peptide; FC, functional class; FEV$_1$, forced expiratory volume in 1 s; ILD, interstitial lung diseases; iNO, inhaled nitric oxide; MVPA, moderate to vigorous physical activity; PA, pulmonary artery; PVR(i), pulmonary vascular resistance (indexed); QOL, quality of life; RVSD, right ventricular systolic dysfunction; sPAP, systolic pulmonary artery pressure; V$_{O_2}$, oxygen uptake.

setting have been difficult, but the initial use of nitric oxide for patients with PH-CLD dates back to the late 1990s. Early studies in patents with COPD demonstrated that continuous inhalation during exercise mitigated exertional desaturation, likely through improved ventilation/perfusion matching.[61] Use of pulsed inhalation with oxygen has been shown to be safe and effective in patients with COPD, with a sustained benefit after 3 months.[62] Additionally, pulsed inhaled nitric oxide is currently under investigation, with early data showing safety and efficacy in PH-ILD.[63]

Lung Transplantation

For select patients, lung transplantation can be the best and most viable treatment option. Patients with significant PH-CLD may pose significant challenges in the perioperative period. Higher rates of post-transplant complications and increased 1-year mortality have been reported in patients with PH-CLD than in those without PH.[64–66] This difference may reflect the later stage of the underlying disease or could be explained by early hemodynamic instability, a greater propensity for primary graft dysfunction or other unheralded factors.[67] Patients may benefit from extracorporeal life support to help safely transition into transplant surgery and out to recovery.[68,69] Often, extracorporeal life support will be maintained for up to 1 week postoperatively to "rest" the RV with a new low PVR, enabling a more gradual normalization of ventricular–arterial coupling. Also, transient left ventricle dysfunction has been described in patients with significant PH after transplantation, with subsequent improvement as intraventricular dependence recalibrates.[70] Despite the inherent short-term and long-term risks, lung transplantation is often a life-saving procedure for the sickest patients. Given the progressive and unpredictable nature of CLD and the poorer outcomes in those with PH, early discussion and preparation of patients and caregivers for transplantation remains an integral part of care.

Lung transplantation may not always be an option for patients owing to age, as well as other medical and psychosocial reasons. In these patients, palliative care should be offered for symptom management and end-of-life planning to improve QOL and minimize futile invasive interventions.[71]

SUMMARY

PH-CLD remains a challenge, with poor outcomes for patients facing respiratory failure compounded by RV dysfunction. A high index of clinical suspicion for complicating PH should be maintained in the longitudinal follow-up of these patients, with close monitoring of readily available testing, including DL_{CO} and 6MWD. Echocardiography is the best screening tool, but RHC remains the gold standard for diagnosis. Optimizing therapy of the underlying lung disease and addressing contributory comorbidities should be foremost in the management of PH-CLD. Inhaled vasodilator therapy is now a viable intervention with the recent approval of inhaled treprostinil.

CLINICS CARE POINTS

- A high index of clinical suspicion should prompt evaluation for PH-CLD. Conversely, all patients being evaluated for idiopathic PAH should undergo screening for underlying lung disease.
- RHC remains the gold standard for diagnosing group 3 PH.
- Group 3 PH has limited treatment options, and hence optimization of the underlying lung disease and treating contributory comorbidities are the cornerstones of care.
- The recent approval of inhaled treprostonil heralds a new era in the management of this sick patient population, with more of these patients likely to be referred for RHC.

DISCLOSURE

S.D. Nathan is a consultant for United Therapeutics, Bellerophon, Bayer, Boerhinger-Ingelham, Merck, and Roche. K. Ahmad and V. Khangoora do not have any significant disclosures related to publication of this article.

REFERENCES

1. Dankmeijer J, Herles F, Ibrahim M, et al. Chronic cor pulmonale: report of an expert committee. WHO Technical Report Series No. 213. Circulation 1963; 27:594–615.
2. Han MK, McLaughlin VV, Criner GJ, et al. Pulmonary diseases and the heart. Circulation 2007;116(25): 2992–3005.
3. Rubin LJ. Cor pulmonale revisited. From Ferrer and Harvey to the present. Ann Am Thorac Soc 2018; 15(Suppl 1):S42–4.
4. Nathan SD, Barbera JA, Gaine SP, et al. Pulmonary hypertension in chronic lung disease and hypoxia. Eur Respir J 2019;53(1):1801914.

5. Hawrylkiewicz I, Sliwinski P, Gorecka D, et al. Pulmonary haemodynamics in patients with OSAS or an overlap syndrome. Monaldi Arch Chest Dis 2004; 61(3):148–52.

6. Zuoyou L, Shiota S, Morio Y, et al. Borderline pulmonary hypertension associated with chronic hypercapnia in chronic pulmonary disease. Respir Physiol Neurobiol 2019;262:20–5.

7. Klinger JR. Group III pulmonary hypertension: pulmonary hypertension associated with lung disease—epidemiology, pathophysiology, and treatments. Cardiol Clin 2016;34(3):413–33.

8. Zhao YY, Zhao YD, Mirza MK, et al. Persistent eNOS activation secondary to caveolin-1 deficiency induces pulmonary hypertension in mice and humans through PKG nitration. J Clin Invest 2009;119: 2009–18.

9. Yamakami T, Taguchi O, Gabazza EC, et al. Arterial endothelin-1 level in pulmonary emphysema and interstitial lung disease. Relation with pulmonary hypertension during exercise. Eur Respir J 1997;10(9): 2055–60.

10. Saleh D, Furukawa K, Tsao MS, et al. Elevated expression of endothelin-1 and endothelin converting enzyme-1 in idiopathic pulmonary fibrosis: possible involvement of proinflammatory cytokines. Am J Respir Cell Mol Biol 1997;16(2):187–93.

11. Janssens SP, Thompson BT, Spence CR, et al. Polycythemia and vascular remodeling in chronic hypoxic pulmonary hypertension in Guinea pigs. J Appl Physiol (1985) 1991;71(6):2218–23.

12. Held M, Walthelm J, Baron S, et al. Functional impact of pulmonary hypertension due to hypoventilation and changes under noninvasive ventilation. Eur Respir J 2014;43(1):156–65.

13. Eddahibi S, Chaouat A, Morrell N, et al. Polymorphism of the serotonin transporter gene and pulmonary hypertension in chronic obstructive pulmonary diseases. Circulation 2003;108:1839–44.

14. Nathan SD, Shlobin OA, Ahmad S, et al. Pulmonary hypertension and pulmonary function testing in idiopathic pulmonary fibrosis. Chest 2007;131(3): 657–63.

15. Rose L, Prins KW, Archer SL, et al. Survival in pulmonary hypertension due to chronic lung disease: influence of low diffusion capacity of the lungs for carbon monoxide. J Heart Lung Transpl 2019; 38(2):145–55.

16. Swigris JJ, Olson AL, Shlobin OA, et al. Heart rate recovery after six-minute walk test predicts pulmonary hypertension in patients with idiopathic pulmonary fibrosis. Respirology 2011;16(3):439–45.

17. Yagi M, Taniguchi H, Kondoh Y, et al. CT-determined pulmonary artery to aorta ratio as a predictor of elevated pulmonary artery pressure and survival in idiopathic pulmonary fibrosis. Respirology 2017; 22(7):1393–9.

18. Bax S, Jacob J, Ahmed R, et al. Right ventricular to left ventricular ratio at CT pulmonary angiogram predicts mortality in interstitial lung disease. Chest 2020;157(1):89–98.

19. Leuchte HH, Baumgartner RA, Nounou ME, et al. Brain natriuretic peptide is a prognostic parameter in chronic lung disease. Am J Respir Crit Care Med 2006;173(7):744–50.

20. Arcasoy SM, Christie JD, Ferrari VA, et al. Echocardiographic assessment of pulmonary hypertension in patients with advanced lung disease. Am J Respir Crit Care Med 2003;167(5):735–40.

21. Nowak J, Hudzik B, Jastrzebski D, et al. Pulmonary hypertension in advanced lung diseases: echocardiography as an important part of patient evaluation for lung transplantation. Clin Respir J 2018;12(3): 930–8.

22. Prins KW, Rose L, Archer SL, et al. Clinical determinants and prognostic implications of right ventricular dysfunction in pulmonary hypertension caused by chronic lung disease. J Am Heart Assoc 2019;8: e011464.

23. Fine NM, Chen L, Bastiansen PM, et al. Outcome prediction by quantitative right ventricular function assessment in 575 subjects evaluated for pulmonary hypertension. Circ Cardiovasc Imaging 2013;6(5): 711–21.

24. Awerbach JD, Stackhouse KA, Lee J, et al. Outcomes of lung disease-associated pulmonary hypertension and impact of elevated pulmonary vascular resistance. Respir Med 2019;150:126–30.

25. Wang L, Zhao QH, Pudasaini B, et al. Clinical and hemodynamic characteristics of pulmonary hypertension associated with interstitial lung disease in China. Clin Respir J 2018;12(3):915–21.

26. Jose A, King CS, Shlobin OA, et al. Exercise pulmonary haemodynamic response predicts outcomes in fibrotic lung disease. Eur Respir J 2018;52(3): 1801015.

27. Kim V, Benditt JO, Wise RA, et al. Oxygen therapy in chronic obstructive pulmonary disease. Proc Am Thorac Soc 2008;5:513–8.

28. Xiong W, Zhao Y, Gong S, et al. Prophylactic function of excellent compliance with LTOT in the development of pulmonary hypertension due to COPD with hypoxemia. Pulm Circ 2018;8(2). 2045894018765835.

29. Wright JL, Levy RD, Churg A. Pulmonary hypertension in chronic obstructive pulmonary disease: current theories of pathogenesis and their implications for treatment. Thorax 2005;60:605–9.

30. Izikki M, Raffestin B, Klar J, et al. Effects of roflumilast, a phosphodiesterase-4 inhibitor, on hypoxia- and monocrotaline-induced pulmonary hypertension in rats. J Pharmacol Exp Ther 2009;330(1):54–62.

31. Caviezel C, Aruldas C, Franzen D, et al. Lung volume reduction surgery in selected patients with emphysema and pulmonary hypertension. Eur J

Cardiothorac Surg 2018. https://doi.org/10.1093/ejcts/ezy092.

32. Criner GJ, Scharf SM, Falk JA, et al. Effect of lung volume reduction surgery on resting pulmonary hemodynamics in severe emphysema. Am J Respir Crit Care Med 2007;176:253–60.

33. Nathan SD, Noble PW, Tuder RM. Idiopathic pulmonary fibrosis and pulmonary hypertension: connecting the dots. Am J Respir Crit Care Med 2007;175:875–80.

34. Behr J, Kolb M, Song JW, et al. Nintedanib and sildenafil in patients with idiopathic pulmonary fibrosis and right heart dysfunction. A prespecified subgroup Analysis of a double-blind randomized clinical trial (INSTAGE). Am J Respir Crit Care Med 2019;200(12):1505–12.

35. Behr J, Nathan SD, Wuyts WA, et al. Efficacy and safety of sildenafil added to pirfenidone in patients with advanced idiopathic pulmonary fibrosis and risk of pulmonary hypertension: a double-blind, randomised, placebo-controlled, phase 2b trial. Lancet Respir Med 2021;9(1):85–95.

36. Hallowell RW, Reed RM, Fraig M, et al. Severe pulmonary hypertension in idiopathic nonspecific interstitial pneumonia. Pulm Circ 2012;2(1):101–6.

37. Koschel DS, Cardoso C, Wiedemann B, et al. Pulmonary hypertension in chronic hypersensitivity pneumonitis. Lung 2012;190(3):295–302.

38. Rao RS, Singh S, Sharma BB, et al. Sildenafil improves six-minute walk distance in chronic obstructive pulmonary disease: a randomised, double-blind, placebo-controlled trial. Indian J Chest Dis Allied Sci 2011;53(2):81–5.

39. Blanco I, Santos S, Gea J, et al. Sildenafil to improve respiratory rehabilitation outcomes in COPD: a controlled trial. Eur Respir J 2013;42(4):982–92.

40. Vitulo P, Stanziola A, Confalonieri M, et al. Sildenafil in severe pulmonary hypertension associated with chronic obstructive pulmonary disease: a randomized controlled multicenter clinical trial. J Heart Lung Transpl 2017;36(2):166–74.

41. Lederer DJ, Bartels MN, Schluger NW, et al. Sildenafil for chronic obstructive pulmonary disease: a randomized crossover trial. COPD 2012;9(3):268–75.

42. Goudie AR, Lipworth BJ, Hopkinson PJ, et al. Tadalafil in patients with chronic obstructive pulmonary disease: a randomised, double-blind, parallel-group, placebo-controlled trial. Lancet Respir Med 2014;2(4):293–300.

43. Zisman DA, Schwarz M, Anstrom K, et al. A controlled trial of sildenafil in advanced idiopathic pulmonary fibrosis. N Engl J Med 2010;363(7):620–8.

44. Han MK, Bach DS, Hagan PG, et al. Sildenafil preserves exercise capacity in patients with idiopathic pulmonary fibrosis and right-sided ventricular dysfunction. Chest 2013;143(6):1699–708.

45. Nathan SD, Behr J, Collard HR, et al. Riociguat for idiopathic interstitial pneumonia-associated pulmonary hypertension (RISE-IIP): a randomised, placebo-controlled phase 2b study. Lancet Respir Med 2019;7(9):780–90.

46. Ghofrani HA, Staehler G, Grünig E, et al. Acute effects of riociguat in borderline or manifest pulmonary hypertension associated with chronic obstructive pulmonary disease. Pulm Circ 2015;5(2):296–304.

47. Pichl A, Sommer N, Bednorz M, et al. Riociguat for treatment of pulmonary hypertension in COPD: a translational study. Eur Respir J 2019;53(6):1802445.

48. Clozel M, Salloukh H. Role of endothelin in fibrosis and anti-fibrotic potential of bosentan. Ann Med 2005;37(1):2–12.

49. Raghu G, Behr J, Brown KK, et al. Treatment of idiopathic pulmonary fibrosis with ambrisentan: a parallel, randomized trial. Ann Intern Med 2013;158(9):641–9.

50. Corte TJ, Keir GJ, Dimopoulos K, et al. Bosentan in pulmonary hypertension associated with fibrotic idiopathic interstitial pneumonia. Am J Respir Crit Care Med 2014;190(2):208–17.

51. Bellaye PS, Yanagihara T, Granton E, et al. Macitentan reduces progression of TGF-β1-induced pulmonary fibrosis and pulmonary hypertension. Eur Respir J 2018;52(2):1701857.

52. Valerio G, Bracciale P, Grazia D'Agostino A. Effect of bosentan upon pulmonary hypertension in chronic obstructive pulmonary disease. Ther Adv Respir Dis 2009;3(1):15–21, 72.

53. Stolz D, Rasch H, Linka A, et al. A randomised, controlled trial of bosentan in severe COPD. Eur Respir J 2008;32(3):619–28.

54. Wang L, Jin YZ, Zhao QH, et al. Hemodynamic and gas exchange effects of inhaled iloprost in patients with COPD and pulmonary hypertension. Int J Chron Obstruct Pulmon Dis 2017;12:3353–60.

55. Lammi MR, Ghonim MA, Johnson J, et al. Acute effect of inhaled iloprost on exercise dynamic hyperinflation in COPD patients: a randomized crossover study. Respir Med 2021;180:106354.

56. Krowka MJ, Ahmad S, Andrade J, et al. A randomized, double-blind, placebo-controlled study to evaluate the safety and efficacy of iloprost inhalation in adults with abnormal pulmonary arterial pressure and exercise limitation associated with idiopathic pulmonary fibrosis. Chest 2007;132:633S.

57. Waxman A, Restrepo-Jaramillo R, Thenappan T, et al. Inhaled treprostinil in pulmonary hypertension due to interstitial lung disease. N Engl J Med 2021;384(4):325–34.

58. Abuserewa S, Selim AMA, Lowes BD, et al. Role of selexipag in COPD patients with out of proportion pulmonary hypertension. J Card Fail 2019;25(8):S45.

59. Olschewski H, Ghofrani HA, Walmrath D, et al. Inhaled prostacyclin and iloprost in severe

pulmonary hypertension secondary to lung fibrosis. Am J Respir Crit Care Med 1999;160(2):600–7.

60. Shimizu M, Imanishi J, Takano T, et al. Disproportionate pulmonary hypertension in a patient with early-onset pulmonary emphysema treated with specific drugs for pulmonary arterial hypertension. Intern Med 2011;50(20):2341–6.

61. Roger N, Barberà JA, Roca J, et al. Nitric oxide inhalation during exercise in chronic obstructive pulmonary disease. Am J Respir Crit Care Med 1997; 156(3 Pt 1):800–6.

62. Vonbank K, Ziesche R, Higenbottam TW, et al. Controlled prospective randomised trial on the effects on pulmonary haemodynamics of the ambulatory long term use of nitric oxide and oxygen in patients with severe COPD. Thorax 2003;58(4): 289–93.

63. Nathan SD, Flaherty KR, Glassberg MK, et al. A randomized, double-blind, placebo-controlled study of pulsed, inhaled nitric oxide in subjects at risk of pulmonary hypertension associated with pulmonary fibrosis. Chest 2020;158(2):637–45.

64. Hayes D Jr, Tumin D, Budev MM, et al. Adverse outcomes associated with pulmonary hypertension in chronic obstructive pulmonary disease after bilateral lung transplantation. Respir Med 2017;128:102–8.

65. Andersen KH, Schultz HH, Nyholm B, et al. Pulmonary hypertension as a risk factor of mortality after lung transplantation. Clin Transpl 2016;30(4): 357–64.

66. Kim CY, Park JE, Leem AY, et al. Prognostic value of pre-transplant mean pulmonary arterial pressure in lung transplant recipients: a single-institution experience. J Thorac Dis 2018;10(3):1578–87.

67. Porteous MK, Lee JC, Lederer DJ, et al, Lung Transplant Outcomes Group. Clinical risk factors and prognostic model for primary graft dysfunction after lung transplantation in patients with pulmonary hypertension. Ann Am Thorac Soc 2017;14(10): 1514–22.

68. Chicotka S, Pedroso FE, Agerstrand CL, et al. Increasing opportunity for lung transplant in interstitial lung disease with pulmonary hypertension. Ann Thorac Surg 2018;106(6):1812–9.

69. Hayanga JWA, Chan EG, Musgrove K, et al. Extracorporeal membrane oxygenation in the perioperative care of the lung transplant patient. Semin Cardiothorac Vasc Anesth 2020;24(1):45–53.

70. Verbelen T, Van De Bruaene A, Cools B, et al. Postoperative left ventricular function in different types of pulmonary hypertension: a comparative study. Interact Cardiovasc Thorac Surg 2018;26:813–9.

71. Boland J, Martin J, Wells AU, et al. Palliative care for people with non-malignant lung disease: summary of current evidence and future direction. Palliat Med 2013;27(9):811–6.

Surgical Management of Chronic Thromboembolic Pulmonary Hypertension

Andrew M. Vekstein, MD[a],*, Joseph R. Nellis, MD, MBA[a],
Sharon L. McCartney, MD[b], John C. Haney, MD[a]

KEYWORDS

- Pulmonary thromboendarterectomy • Pulmonary embolism • Circulatory arrest
- Pulmonary hypertension • Reperfusion

KEY POINTS

- Pulmonary thromboendarterectomy (PTE) is the standard of care for management of chronic thromboembolic pulmonary hypertension.
- Although right ventricular dysfunction, distal disease, and pulmonary vascular resistance (PVR) greater than 1000 dyn·s/cm^5 are known risk factors for morbidity and mortality, patients with severely elevated PVR also have the greatest potential for symptomatic and hemodynamic improvement after PTE.
- In order to achieve a complete thromboendarterectomy without impaired visualization from bronchial arterial back-bleeding, periods of deep hypothermic circulatory arrest are necessary.
- Complete resection of obstructing disease is the most important predictor of hemodynamic and functional outcomes after PTE.
- Reperfusion pulmonary edema is the most complicating factor after successful PTE, and postoperative care should be tailored to degree of edema and right ventricular function.

INTRODUCTION

Chronic thromboembolic pulmonary hypertension (CTEPH) is a condition characterized by the incomplete resolution of thromboembolic material within the pulmonary vasculature, endothelial dysfunction, vascular remodeling, and ultimately, pulmonary hypertension.[1,2] After the recommended 6 months of therapeutic anticoagulation for acute pulmonary embolism (PE), 30% to 50% of patients continue to experience a perfusion defect.[3] Although a majority go on to develop some degree of chronic thromboembolic disease or chronic thromboembolic pulmonary vascular disease, only 0.4% to 6.2% develop evidence of right heart failure and CTEPH.[4–7] Risk factors for progression to CTEPH after acute PE include inflammatory disorders (eg, inflammatory bowel disease), history of splenectomy, and known hypercoagulable states (eg, factor V Leiden).[8] Left unaddressed, the 3-year mortality for CTEPH is more than 50%.[9,10] Medical therapies have helped extend life expectancy to a median survival of 6 to 7 years, although surgery continues to be the standard of care.[11,12] Surgical management of CTEPH with pulmonary thromboendarterectomy (PTE) has evolved significantly over the past 30 years and now represents the standard of care to improve survival, functional status, and quality of life for patients with CTEPH.[13–17] The

Funding: This work was supported by the National Institutes of Health (5T32HL069749-17 to Dr Vekstein).
[a] Division of Cardiovascular and Thoracic Surgery, Department of Surgery, Duke University Medical Center, DUMC Box 3483, 8665A HAFS, Durham, NC 27710, USA; [b] Division of Cardiothoracic Anesthesia, Department of Anesthesiology, Duke University Medical Center, DUMC Box 3094, Durham, NC 27710, USA
* Corresponding author. DCRI, 300 W. Morgan Street, Desk 8108, Durham, NC 27701.
E-mail address: andrew.vekstein@duke.edu
Twitter: @AndrewVekstein (A.M.V.)

Cardiol Clin 40 (2022) 89–101
https://doi.org/10.1016/j.ccl.2021.08.008
0733-8651/22/© 2021 Elsevier Inc. All rights reserved.

following review summarizes the current literature on CTEPH from a surgeon's perspective, including the operative evaluation, treatment selection, preoperative patient optimization, operative best practices, complications, expected outcomes, and postoperative surveillance.

MAKING THE OPERATIVE DIAGNOSIS

Outcomes following PTE rest on patient selection and technical insight. Patients presenting with fatigue, dyspnea, and exercise intolerance can generate a broad differential diagnosis, and most have undergone an extensive diagnostic workup before referral to surgery. Ventilation/perfusion (V/Q) scintigraphy is a standard of care for initial screening for CTEPH. This imaging modality is noninvasive and relatively inexpensive and has sensitivity of 90% to 100% and specificity of 93% to 100% for chronic thromboembolic disease.[18,19]

Abnormal or positive V/Q scans with suspicion for CTEPH should prompt anatomic imaging in order to confirm anatomic disease and correlate with hemodynamics, allowing for targeted risk stratification and operative planning.[20] Although chest computed tomography angiography (CTA) classically underdiagnoses chronic thromboembolism, recent improvements in this technique have led to similar sensitivity (94%–100%) and specificity (93%–100%) compared with V/Q.[21,22] Pulmonary angiography continues to be the gold standard for describing segmental and subsegmental pulmonary artery (PA) filling defects, but ongoing advancements in noninvasive imaging continue to challenge this position. In a study of 24 patients with CTEPH, CTA was more sensitive than angiography at the main and lobar levels (66%–76% vs 100%, respectively), whereas angiography had higher sensitivity at the subsegmental level (97% vs 80%).[21] Short breath-holds (<5 seconds), thin collimation, and less than 1-mm slices reconstructed in 3 dimensions can improve the subsegmental sensitivity of CTA. Gated acquisition, although not common, can also improve CTA resolution.

Preoperative right heart catheterization (RHC) helps to confirm the diagnosis and risk-stratify patients.[23] Although there is no specified degree of right ventricular (RV) dysfunction that precludes PTE in the appropriate setting, known risk factors for worse outcomes following surgery include preexisting RV failure, chronic obstructive or restrictive lung disease, lack of disease in the lower lobes, preoperative pulmonary vascular resistance (PVR) greater than 1000 dyn·s/cm^5, and predominately distal disease.[24–26]

Although preoperative risk calculators have not yet been developed for PTE, the Jamieson classification system is commonly used to reference preoperative and intraoperative disease location.[27] Type I disease (fresh thrombus within the main or lobar arteries) and type II disease (intimal thickening and fibrosis proximal to the segmental arteries) are considered proximal disease and amenable to PTE. Type III disease (thromboembolic material within the distal segmental arteries only) and type IV disease (distal arteriolar vasculopathy without visible thromboembolic material) are considered distal and classically less amenable to PTE. A 2002 study by Thistlethwaite and colleagues[28] showed significant decreases in PA systolic pressures (35–36 mm Hg) and PVR (660–560 dyn·s/cm^5) following PTE for type I and II disease. PTE for type III and IV disease had little to no effect. Surgery may still be offered for type III disease by experienced operators, however, as the hemodynamic outcomes are directly related to the completeness of endarterectomy.

For patients with mixed disease involving both proximal and distal lesions, or concern for a component of primary pulmonary hypertension, examination of the pulmonary arterial waveform on RHC may allow better characterization of disease burden and candidacy for PTE. Patients with predominantly distal thromboembolic disease with or without concurrent primary pulmonary hypertension have a significantly lower pulse pressure compared with those with more proximal and resectable disease (**Fig. 1**).[29] Furthermore, the PA occlusion waveform can help predict patients' operative response to PTE. In a small series of 26 patients, patients with poor outcomes following PTE were found to have a gradual pressure decline toward the PA occlusion pressure, indicating high resistive indices distally in the small vessels and capillary beds.[30] By contrast, patients with proximal disease had a more rapid decline in PA pressures toward occlusion (**Fig. 2**). Mapping out the rate of decline toward wedge pressures, the group showed a near linear relationship between increasing distal disease, higher post-PTE PVR, mean PA pressures, and mortality.

Multidisciplinary teams consisting of pulmonologists, radiologists, and surgeons should discuss and evaluate each patient individually.[11] In addition to patients' radiographic and hemodynamic data, functional status and existing comorbidities also play a role in selecting the proper patients for PTE. Severe obstructive or restrictive pulmonary disease is a contraindication to PTE given the concern for reperfusion injury and minimal expected benefit for restoring perfusion to poorly ventilated parenchyma.[13] Hepatic or renal

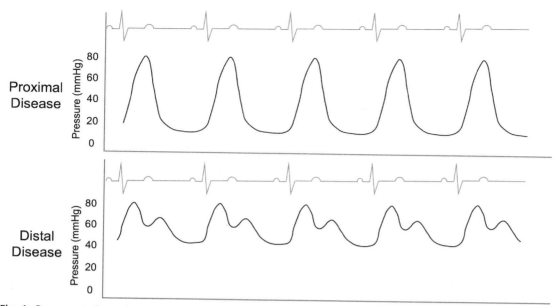

Fig. 1. Representative pulmonary arterial tracings in patients with predominantly proximal versus distal thromboembolic disease burden. Despite similar systolic pulmonary arterial pressures, there is notably lower pulse pressure in patients with distal disease.

insufficiency secondary to right heart failure and malignancy is another controversial condition, although not absolutely contraindicated if the expectation is resolution with improvement in the venous congestion. Centers of excellence have demonstrated the safe repair of concurrent cardiac lesions, although experience remains limited.[31]

OPERATIVE CANDIDATES

Operative candidates are patients with type I and II, as well as appropriate type III, disease with visible thromboembolic material that correlates with their hemodynamic compromise.[32,33] Bilateral disease located in the lower lobes with a rapid deterioration in the pulmonary wedge pressure is a good prognostic feature.[23] Preoperative PVR greater than 1000 dyn·s/cm^5, although a risk factor, also identifies patients with the most to gain from operative intervention.[12,16] Elevated PVR is not a contraindication to PTE on its own and should be further characterized using pulmonary wedge tracings to identify the predominant distribution of underlying disease.[23] Historically, 50% to 70% of patients are operative candidates at the time of initial consultation.[30]

INOPERABLE PATIENTS

Patients ineligible for surgery are classically those with type IV disease, hemodynamic compromise that is out of proportion to the degree of visible thromboembolic material, or markedly elevated PVR that is associated with a distal disease pattern on PA and occlusion RHC tracings. The usual comorbidities and overall debilitation should also be considered before offering surgery. Approximately 37% of patients at their initial consultation is inoperable. Distal disease is the most common reason for patients to be declined for surgery (48%), followed by patient comorbidities (13%), and elevated PVR (10%).[30]

MEDICAL AND INTERVENTIONAL MANAGEMENT

Several different pulmonary vascular agents have been applied to the CTEPH population. The AIR and CTREPH trials demonstrated benefits of inhaled (iloprost) or subcutaneous (treprostinil) prostacyclin analogues in terms of functional classification, 6-minute walk distance, brain natriuretic peptide (BNP) levels, cardiac indices, pulmonary vascular indices in an overall pulmonary arterial hypertension, and CTEPH-specific populations.[34,35] Although endothelin agonists (eg, bosentan and macitentan) have shown improvements in PVR and cardiac indices, the BENEFiT and MERIT-1 trials failed to demonstrate benefits in terms of functional status or 6-minute walk distances.[36,37] More recently, the CHEST-1 and CHEST-2 trials found that riociguat, a guanylate cyclase agonist, significantly improved the 6-minute walk, functional classification, PVR, and BNP in patients with inoperable CTEPH.[38] Riociguat is

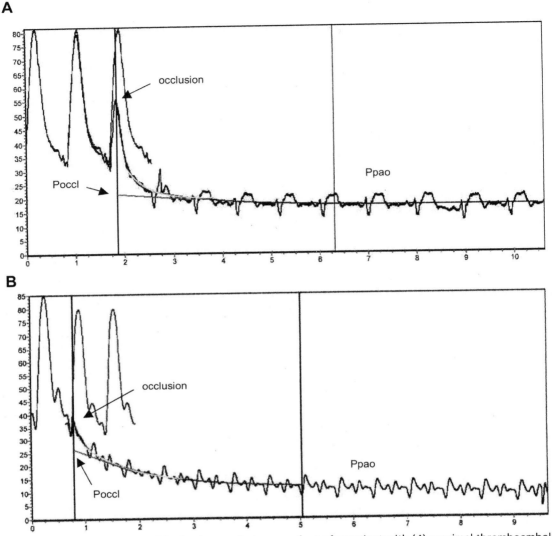

Fig. 2. Pulmonary arterial transitioning into occlusion waveforms for patient with (*A*) proximal thromboembolic disease and (*B*) distal thromboembolic disease. Proximal disease was associated with a more rapid drop in pressure to the occlusion pressure (Poccl). Ppao, pulmonary artery occluded pressure. (*From* Kim NHS, Fesler P, Channick RN, et al. Preoperative partitioning of pulmonary vascular resistance correlates with early outcome after thromboendarterectomy for chronic thromboembolic pulmonary hypertension. Circulation 2004;109:18-22.)

the only approved drug for the medical management of CTEPH and is now considered a standard of therapy for distal disease.[39] Medical management has significantly improved outcomes for inoperable patients with CTEPH from a median survival of 3 years to 6 to 7 years today.[8,9,32] In patients being evaluated for PTE, medical management of pulmonary hypertension may be beneficial in those with decompensated RV failure, but has not been shown to significantly improve the chance of becoming an operative candidate.[40]

In addition to medical management, inoperable patients may also be candidates for balloon pulmonary angioplasty (BPA), an approach that has evolved significantly since it was introduced in the 1990s. Procedural techniques and outcomes of BPA are discussed more extensively in a separate article in this issue of *Cardiology Clinics*. After a multidisciplinary evaluation, BPA may represent an excellent adjunct to medical therapy, particularly in patients with more distal disease. Furthermore, BPA used as part of a hybrid approach after PTE for mixed proximal and distal disease has been reported, although the evidence remains limited.[41] At the authors' institution, a hybrid technique of unilateral PTE through a minimally invasive thoracotomy with staged contralateral BPA has been used for patients with differential proximal and distal disease burdens on each side.

OPERATIVE APPROACH

A standard approach to PTE has evolved primarily over the 30 years of experience at the University of California San Diego (UCSD) under the leadership of Drs Jamieson and Madani.[42–44] There has been significant evolution in this approach, and the authors' institution has developed several adaptations, which are described here.

Anesthesia Considerations

An experienced cardiothoracic anesthesia team is essential to safely manage perioperative care during PTE. Intubation with standard single-lumen endotracheal tube is typically performed, with the largest size for the patient's anatomy (typically 8.0 mm) preferred to allow bronchoscopic examination during the perioperative period as needed. Cardiovascular collapse on induction is a concern in all CTEPH patients, but particularly those with PVR greater than 1000 $dyn \cdot s/cm^5$, severe tricuspid insufficiency, and RV end-diastolic pressure greater than 14 mm Hg. A 9F high-flow triple-lumen central line is placed in either the internal jugular or the subclavian vein position, through which a Swan-Ganz pulmonary arterial catheter is floated and positioned in the main PA before incision. In this disease process, the thromboembolic disease is chronic and fixed, so embolization of acute thrombus is typically not encountered, and thus, PA catheter insertion is not contraindicated. Radial, and at some centers, femoral arterial monitoring lines should be inserted. Because antegrade cerebral perfusion is not typically used, arterial catheters may be placed in either extremity. Temperature monitoring with nasopharyngeal and bladder probes is crucial for the confirmation of profound hypothermia before circulatory arrest. A comprehensive transesophageal echocardiogram (TEE) is performed before and after the procedure. In addition to overall cardiac function, there should also be careful examination for interatrial flow because of atrial septal defect (ASD) or patent foramen ovale (PFO), typically including a bubble study, and for evaluation of aortic insufficiency, if aortic cross-clamp is not going to be used during cardiopulmonary bypass. The presence of interatrial shunting, especially if large, is typically addressed surgically

because of the elevated right-sided pressures and the contribution to hypoxemia that this may pose. In addition, if significant aortic insufficiency is present (> moderate), an aortic cross-clamp should be used. Finally, Bispectral Index or formal electroencephalography (EEG) electrodes are placed to confirm electrocerebral inactivity before circulatory arrest.

Incision

- Standard sternotomy is the most commonly performed incision, allowing excellent exposure of bilateral branch pulmonary arteries.
- Unilateral or bilateral anterior thoracotomy is used at some institutions, often as part of "hybrid" operation with BPA performed for contralateral disease.

Cannulation and Venting

- Arterial cannulation is performed in the distal ascending aorta or proximal aortic arch. In a thoracotomy approach, direct aortic, right axillary, or femoral arterial cannulation may be used.
- Bicaval venous cannulation is used to allow complete decompression of the right heart and achieve a bloodless field. Cannulation of the superior vena cava (SVC) should be performed in the most superior aspect of the pericardial space to prevent the cannula from interfering with exposure of the right pulmonary artery (RPA). In a thoracotomy approach, percutaneous bicaval drainage is used.
- A direct PA vent is placed, with plans to remove and subsequently replace after left-sided thromboendarterectomy.
- Left ventricular venting is typically performed through the right superior pulmonary vein.

Cooling and Myocardial Protection

- After initiation of cardiopulmonary bypass, the patient is systematically cooled in coordination with the perfusion team with a 10°C differential between arterial inflow and venous outflow. External cooling pads are often used to expedite this process.
- Many institutions performing this operation use aortic cross-clamp and cardioplegic myocardial arrest once the temperature reaches 20°C and EEG confirms electrical inactivity.
- At the authors' institution, they favor avoiding aortic cross-clamping, allowing a slow ventricular fibrillation rhythm with excellent left ventricular venting confirmed multiple times

throughout the operation. This approach is discussed in more detail later in the article.

Exposure of the Bilateral Branch Pulmonary Arteries

- Dissection is typically performed within the pericardium. Extension into the pleural space on either side is not necessary. Some institutions intentionally open the right pleural space widely in order to "dislocate" the apex of the left ventricle rightward, facilitating exposure of the left pulmonary artery (LPA).[45] At the authors' institution, they favor the use of a Heart-Net (DMC Medical, County Clare, Ireland) to achieve similar retraction without entering the right pleural space.
- RPA: The SVC is circumferentially dissected from the RPA. A self-retaining (Henly or cerebellar) retractor is then placed between the SVC and ascending aorta, nicely exposing the RPA from the main to lobar branches. Longitudinal pulmonary arteriotomy is then performed from the bifurcation to the first branching (**Fig. 3**).
- LPA: The apex of the heart is retracted to the right with the HeartNet, which is secured to the sternal retractor. A curvilinear pulmonary arteriotomy is then performed from the main PA extending down the LPA toward the pericardial reflection (**Fig. 4**).

Thromboendarterectomy

- Back-bleeding from bronchial arterial collaterals impairs visualization, which necessitates circulatory arrest for any more distal thromboendarterectomy.
- Circulatory arrest intervals: Circulatory arrest intervals typically last 20 minutes. Although many institutions limit to 1 interval for each side, the authors' institution uses repeated circulatory arrest intervals, with intervening reperfusion times of around 5 minutes, in order to optimize time to perform complete endarterectomy.
- Instruments: Specialized instruments developed by the UCSD group, including short and long double-action forceps, microsuction, and micro-endarterectomy spatula, are essential for any institution performing this operation.
- Any acute thrombotic material is easily extracted to allow unobstructed exposure of mature thromboembolic disease.
- The critical aspect of the operation is the appropriate development and maturation of the endarterectomy plane (**Fig. 5**). This plane

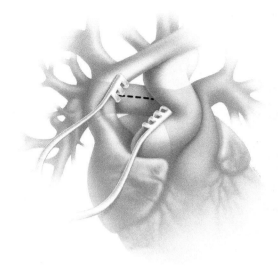

Fig. 3. Exposure of the right main PA and planned arteriotomy. (Illustrated by Megan Llewellyn, MSMI, CMI; copyright Duke University; with permission under a CC BY-ND 4.0 license.)

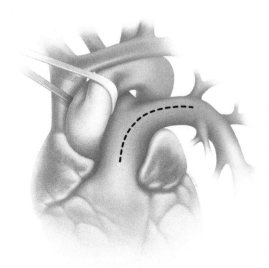

Fig. 4. Exposure of the left main PA and planned arteriotomy. (Illustrated by Megan Llewellyn, MSMI, CMI; copyright Duke University; with permission under a CC BY-ND 4.0 license.)

is initially developed with the scalpel and spatula within the main PA and then extended with microsuction, balancing adequate depth to achieve complete endarterectomy with the potential risk of vessel perforation. Appropriate depth yields a pearly white layer, and any yellow atheromatous material within the wall should lift up with the endarterectomy specimen. Excessive depth can result in a striated, "sticky" dissection or reveal a purplish discoloration consistent with exposed adventitia. This finding may be tolerated within the main PA; if extended distally, however, this may result in endobronchial hemorrhage.

- Once a proper plane has been developed, double-action forceps are used to grasp and withdraw the specimen hand over hand as the endarterectomy plane is extended into the lobar and segmental vessels. The native vessel should be gently teased away from the specimen with a sweeping motion.
- The surgical assistant should aid in maintaining gentle grasp of the endarterectomy specimen, as avulsing the central specimen may cause subsegmental disease to retract into the vessel.
- Pulmonary arteriotomy is closed with 5-0 or 6-0 polypropylene suture in a continuous

fashion. Pledgeted reinforcement sutures or patch augmentation is rarely needed.

Rewarming and Weaning from Cardiopulmonary Bypass

- Following completion of bilateral PTE, rewarming should be performed at the same rate as the cooling process with 10°C differential between bypass inflow and outflow, in addition to external warming devices.
- Any concomitant procedures, such as coronary artery bypass, may be performed during this period. If prebypass TEE revealed any interatrial communication, this should be repaired through a right atriotomy during the rewarming period. Some institutions perform right atriotomy to visually examine the atrial septum, regardless of TEE findings, given the importance of closing an ASD/PFO in this population.
- Once temperature is greater than 32°C, the heart is defibrillated if normal sinus rhythm has not resumed spontaneously.
- Some institutions regularly administer methylprednisolone and mannitol during the rewarming period.[46]
- Low fractional inspired oxygen (<30%) ventilation is used after separation from cardiopulmonary bypass to minimize ischemia-reperfusion injury, as pulmonary flow has drastically improved compared with preoperatively. Inhaled pulmonary vasodilators may be added with ventilation.
- Typical hemodynamics include significant vasoplegia requiring vasopressors while weaning from CPB. Depending on findings on TEE, inotropes may be necessary to support primarily the right ventricle during weaning. Although RV hypertrophy and some degree of dilation may still be present, both the echocardiographic appearance and the hemodynamic profile will typically be improved.

Indications for Extracorporeal Membrane Oxygenation

Delayed cardiopulmonary recovery may prompt the need for mechanical support with veno-arterial (VA) or veno-venous (VV) extracorporeal membrane oxygenation (ECMO) during the process of weaning from cardiopulmonary bypass or in the early postoperative period. Although the overall indications for these advanced forms of mechanical support are similar to other causes for cardiovascular or respiratory failure, there are specific considerations in the context of PTE.

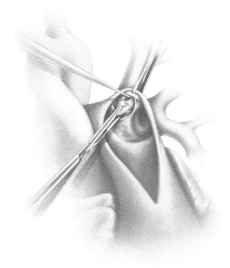

Fig. 5. Establishing proper endarterectomy plane with micro-endarterectomy spatula and double-action forceps. (Illustrated by Megan Llewellyn, MSMI, CMI; copyright Duke University; with permission under a CC BY-ND 4.0 license.)

The most common indication for VV-ECMO after PTE is severe reperfusion pulmonary edema. In the San Diego experience, patients with a Pao_2-to-Fio_2 ratio less than 0.6, $Paco_2$ greater than 60, impaired lung compliance of 30 mL/cm H_2O with tidal volume of 10 mL/kg, or elevated peak inspiratory pressures greater than 30 mm Hg with pneumothorax were considered candidates for VV-ECMO.[47] Successful decannulation and survival to discharge were 40% and 30%, respectively, in this series.

VA-ECMO is most commonly indicated in patients with severe RV dysfunction on intraoperative TEE, with escalating inotrope requirement. In the authors' experience, aggressive support is necessary when complete thromboendarterectomy could not be achieved owing to distal unresectable disease. In these cases, PVR remains elevated and is exacerbated by hypoxic vasoconstriction. VA-ECMO allows for RV decompression to promote recovery, whereas the residual pulmonary hypertension is managed medically. VA-ECMO may also be applied in cases of endobronchial hemorrhage, in which decompressing the PA and gently reversing anticoagulation may resolve bleeding. In a series of 7 patients requiring VA-ECMO after PTE by Berman and colleagues,[48] 5 patients were decannulated, and 4 patients survived to discharge.

Pulmonary Thromboendarterectomy Without Aortic Cross-Clamp

Many institutions perform PTE under cardioplegic myocardial arrest with aortic cross-clamping. This approach, paired with periods of circulatory arrest, achieves the bloodless field necessary for endarterectomy. However, at the authors' institution, they have found that resecting a complete endarterectomy specimen often requires multiple 20-minute periods of circulatory arrest, particularly when patients present with bilateral and distal disease. As such, the authors favor performing the operation without aortic cross-clamp, allowing the adequately vented heart to fibrillate throughout the operation. This technique eases the pressure on the surgeon to minimize cross-clamping time and allows a focus on complete endarterectomy tailored to patients with significant segmental and subsegmental disease (**Table 1**). Furthermore, the cross-clamp can mechanically impair exposure of the branch pulmonary arteries.

In the authors' experience, they have not seen a significant increase in stroke or other neurologic complications with prolonged total circulatory arrest times, nor have they observed increased myocardial dysfunction in the early

Table 1 Comparison of pulmonary thromboendarterectomy with versus without aortic cross-clamp		
	With Cross-Clamp	Without Cross-Clamp
Heart temperature	4–8°C	17°C
Electrical activity	None	Slow VF
Myocardial ischemic time	Entire operative period Single	20-min intervals Repeated

postoperative period, as they think the most important predictor of RV dysfunction is inadequate resection of the obstructing thromboembolic disease.

POSTOPERATIVE CARE
Respiratory

Reperfusion pulmonary edema is a ubiquitous challenge, and, in fact, represents technical success of PTE. The authors' institution favors maintaining mechanical ventilation for at least 12 to 24 hours after surgery with positive end-expiratory pressure of 5 to 8 cm H_2O to help reduce the edema. Patients may require higher than expected Fio_2 and minute ventilation in the early postoperative period, which is generally tolerated, as edema typically improves within days.[49] Aggressive diuresis may not be feasible in the immediate postoperative period because of peripheral vasodilation after deep hypothermia and/or acute kidney injury. The authors typically initiate intravenous diuretics postoperative day 1 as the hemodynamics allow. In patients with more severe reperfusion injury, prolonged intubation is sometimes necessary. At the authors' institution, they advocate for early tracheostomy (postoperative day 5–7) in such patients to promote earlier mobilization and slow weaning from mechanical ventilatory support. VV-ECMO is rarely needed, but may provide appropriate bridging to recovery when needed.

Cardiovascular

Postoperative hemodynamics are highly dependent on the reduction in pulmonary artery pressure (PAP) at the completion of the operation.[50] In patients with a significant reduction in PAP, cardiac output is usually adequate or overly robust in the context of reduced RV afterload, which may exacerbate pulmonary edema. Any systemic hypotension is usually due to vasoplegia after deep hypothermia and should be managed with vasopressors rather than aggressive fluid resuscitation. In patients with persistent PAP elevation, RV dysfunction is common postoperatively, particularly when moderate to severe RV dysfunction was present before the operation. Inotropic support with epinephrine and/or dopamine is typically favored in the postoperative period, with the latter preferred because of the potential to promote autodiuresis. Patients are frequently managed with inhaled pulmonary vasodilators (inhaled nitric oxide, epoprostenol, iloprost, or treprostinil) for at least 24 hours postoperatively, as there may be dynamic vasoconstriction of the pulmonary arterial bed despite relief of the mechanical obstruction.[34,51,52]

Anticoagulation

Although postoperative coagulopathy is rare after PTE, chest tube output and laboratory values must be monitored in the standard fashion as after any cardiac surgery. Once deemed safe, anticoagulation should be resumed according to institutional preference. Most patients are initiated on unfractionated heparin infusion or subcutaneous enoxaparin, and subsequently transitioned to their preoperative regimen, whether with warfarin or with direct oral anticoagulant (DOAC). Importantly, DOACs should be avoided in patients with known or highly suspected hypercoagulable states, such as antiphospholipid syndrome.

OUTCOMES
Operative Outcomes

Modern 30-day mortality after PTE has been reported as low as 1% to 2%, but more commonly between 5% and 8%, depending on institutional and surgeon experience.[40,51,53] Disease categorization and preoperative versus postoperative hemodynamics have important implications for operative mortality. Postoperative PVR greater than 500 dyn·s/cm^5 is associated with a 10% to 30% operative mortality, whereas patients with PVR less than 500 dyn·s/cm^5 experience an operative mortality of 0% to 1%.[54] Severe reperfusion pulmonary injury leading to prolonged respiratory failure, as discussed previously, is the most common cause of morbidity, with an incidence as high as 40%.[55] Endobronchial hemorrhage owing to transmural dissection during endarterectomy is a feared complication, with associated mortality approaching 70%. Multiple approaches to manage this complication have been proposed,

including endobronchial balloon occlusion, various hemostatic agents, or bridging with ECMO.[56,57] Six percent to 9% of patients require tracheostomy for prolonged respiratory failure after PTE.[58] Acute kidney injury is another common complication, with an incidence between 25% and 45% depending on definition and rates of new dialysis between 3% and 5%, similar to published rates after hypothermic circulatory arrest during aortic arch surgery.[59,60]

In terms of hemodynamic improvement, the goal of PTE is usually to achieve a 50% reduction in PVR and mean PAP. The largest single-institution series has presented a 65% reduction in PVR and 45% reduction in mean PAP, with a trend toward greater reduction in both hemodynamic parameters in patients undergoing PTE in the most recent era of experience.[12] As expected, hemodynamic improvements are most significant for patients undergoing PTE for type I or II disease.[27] Registry data have shown that about one-third of patients experience persistent pulmonary hypertension after PTE.[27]

Long-Term Outcomes

The long-term survival and quality-of-life benefits from PTE have continued to improve in the modern era.[61] Overall patient survival at 1, 3, 5, and 10 years has been reported as 86% to 93%, 84% to 91%, 79% to 89%, and 72% to 82%, respectively.[15,32,62,63] Specifically, the UCSD group cites 6-year survival of 75% based on recent survey-assessed follow-up.[64] Postoperative improvement in pulmonary pressure has classically been cited as the most important predictor of long-term survival.[15,65] Reduction in pulmonary pressure correlates well with improvement in exercise tolerance and heart failure symptoms. A study linked to national survival data in the United Kingdom examined the subset of patients surviving at least 3 months after PTE. When divided into 2 groups, based on follow-up mean PAP less than or greater than 30 mm Hg (mean 20 ± 5 vs 38 ± 8 mm Hg), there was no significant difference in 5-year survival. However, patients with follow-up mean PAP less than 30 mm Hg had longer 6-minute walk distance (386 ± 106 vs 337 ± 97 m, $P<.001$) and improved New York Heart Association (NYHA) functional class (88.1 vs 68.9% NYHA I/II; $P<.001$).[61] Despite these differences in outcomes, this institution observed improvements in functional status and quality of life even if PAP remained high after surgery, with overall 45% increase in 6-minute walk distance, indicating that even an incomplete result may generate substantial symptomatic improvements.[14]

The optimal assessment of hemodynamic outcome of PTE is somewhat controversial. In patients progressing well after surgery with subjective improvement, invasive catheterization to measure resultant right heart pressures may be unnecessary. Blanchard and colleagues[66] have proposed the Tei Index as a noninvasive assessment of preoperative and postoperative CTEPH. A measure of myocardial performance during transthoracic echocardiography, the Tei Index uses Doppler measure of ventricular inflow and outflow. When applied to the right ventricle, the Tei Index has been demonstrated to correlate well with PVR and mean PAP before and after PTE when compared with RHC parameters.

SUMMARY

CTEPH is a progressive and debilitating disease with limited options for medical management. V/Q scanning followed by anatomic imaging (CTA or pulmonary angiography) allows for diagnosis and anatomic characterization of disease burden. Although RV dysfunction, distal disease, and PVR greater than 1000 dyn·s/cm^5 are known risk factors, patients with severely elevated PVR have the greatest potential for symptomatic and hemodynamic improvement after PTE. Operative technique has evolved significantly over the past 30 years, with corresponding improvement in outcomes. Deep hypothermic circulatory arrest is used to perform complete endarterectomy into segmental and subsegmental arterial branches. The authors' institution has adapted to perform the procedure without aortic cross-clamp, allowing more time to perform complete distal resection of disease, which is the most important step to optimize functional and hemodynamic outcome.

CLINICS CARE POINTS

- All patients with chronic thromboembolic pulmonary hypertension should be evaluated by a multidisciplinary team of pulmonary vascular physicians, cardiac surgeons, interventional cardiologists, and radiologists.
- Initial screening with ventilation/perfusion scanning should be followed with anatomic assessment with computed tomography angiography and/or pulmonary angiography to determine potential for technical success with pulmonary thromboendarterectomy and to risk-stratify patients for this operation.

- Pulmonary thromboendarterectomy is most successful in patients with proximal disease (Jamieson type I or II), predominantly lower lobar vessels affected, no or mild right ventricular dysfunction, and without severely debilitating comorbidities.
- Achieving a complete thromboendarterectomy is the highest operative priority and has the most significant implications for operative and long-term outcomes.

DISCLOSURES

The authors have nothing to disclose.

REFERENCES

1. Simonneau G, Montani D, Celermajer DS, et al. Haemodynamic definitions and updated clinical classification of pulmonary hypertension. Eur Respir J 2019;53(1):1801913.
2. Simonneau G, Gatzoulis MA, Adatia I, et al. Updated clinical classification of pulmonary hypertension. J Am Coll Cardiol 2013;62(25_Supplement):D34–41.
3. Wartski M, Collignon MA. Incomplete recovery of lung perfusion after 3 months in patients with acute pulmonary embolism treated with antithrombotic agents. THESEE Study Group. Tinzaparin ou Heparin Standard: evaluation dans l'Embolie Pulmonaire Study. J Nucl Med 2000;41:1043–8.
4. Poli D, Grifoni E, Antonucci E, et al. Incidence of recurrent venous thromboembolism and of chronic thromboembolic pulmonary hypertension in patients after a first episode of pulmonary embolism. J Thromb Thrombolysis 2010;30:294–9.
5. Pengo V, Lensing AW, Prins MH, et al. Incidence of chronic thromboembolic pulmonary hypertension after pulmonary embolism. N Engl J Med 2004;350:2257–64.
6. Held M, Hesse A, Gött F, et al. A symptom-related monitoring program following pulmonary embolism for the early detection of CTEPH: a prospective observational registry study. BMC Pulm Med 2014;14:141.
7. Klok FA, van Kralingen KW, van Dijk AP, et al. Prospective cardiopulmonary screening program to detect chronic thromboembolic pulmonary hypertension in patients after acute pulmonary embolism. Haematologica 2010;95:970–5.
8. Bonderman D, Jakowitsch J, Adlbrcht C, et al. Medical conditions increasing the risk of chronic thromboembolic pulmonary hypertension. Thromb Haemost 2005;93:512–6.
9. Kunieda T, Nakanishi N, Satoh T, et al. Prognoses of primary pulmonary hypertension and chronic major

vessel thromboembolic pulmonary hypertension determined from cumulative survival curves. Intern Med 1999;38:543–6.

10. Riedel M, Stanek V, Widimsky J, et al. Longterm follow-up of patients with pulmonary thromboembolism. Late prognosis and evolution of hemodynamic and respiratory data. Chest 1982;81:151–8.

11. Taniguchi Y, Jaïs X, Jevnikar M, et al. Predictors of survival in patients with not-operated chronic thromboembolic pulmonary hypertension. J Heart Lung Transpl 2019;38:833–42.

12. Galiè N, Hoeper MM, Humbert M, et al. Guidelines for the diagnosis and treatment of pulmonary hypertension. Eur Respir J 2009;34:1219–63.

13. Madani MM, Auger WR, Pretorius V, et al. Pulmonary endarterectomy: recent changes in a single institution's experience of more than 2,700 patients. Ann Thorac Surg 2012;94(1):97–103.

14. Banks DA, Pretorius GV, Kerr KM, et al. Pulmonary endarterectomy: part I. Pathophysiology, clinical manifestations, and diagnostic evaluation of chronic thromboembolic pulmonary hypertension. Semin Cardiothorac Vasc Anesth 2014;18:319–30.

15. Freed DH, Thomson BM, Tsui SSL, et al. Functional and haemodynamic outcome 1 year after pulmonary thromboendarterectomy. Eur J Cardiothorac Surg 2008;34(3):525–30.

16. Ishida K, Masuda M, Tanabe N, et al. Long-term outcome after pulmonary endarterectomy for chronic thromboembolic pulmonary hypertension. J Thorac Cardiovasc Surg 2012;144:321–6.

17. Mayer E, Jenkins D, Lindner J, et al. Surgical management and outcome of patients with chronic thromboembolic pulmonary hypertension: results from an international prospective registry. J Thorac Cardiovasc Surg 2011;141:702–10.

18. Galiè N, Humbert M, Vachiery JL, et al. 2015 ESC/ERS Guidelines for the diagnosis and treatment of pulmonary hypertension: the Joint Task Force for the Diagnosis and Treatment of Pulmonary Hypertension of the European Society of Cardiology (ESC) and the European Respiratory Society (ERS). Eur Respir J 2015;46:903–75.

19. Tunariu N, Gibbs SJR, Win Z, et al. Ventilation-perfusion scintigraphy is more sensitive than multidetector CTPA in detecting chronic thromboembolic pulmonary disease as a treatable cause of pulmonary hypertension. J Nucl Med 2007;48:680–4.

20. Ley S, Ley-Zaporozhan J, Pitton MB, et al. Diagnostic performance of state-of-the-art imaging techniques for morphological assessment of vascular abnormalities in patients with chronic thromboembolic pulmonary hypertension (CTEPH). Eur Radiol 2012;22:607–16.

21. McLaughlin VV, Langer A, Tan M, et al. Contemporary trends in the diagnosis and management of pulmonary arterial hypertension: an initiative to close the care gap. Chest 2013;143:324–32.

22. Reichelt A, Hoeper MM, Galanski M, et al. Chronic thromboembolic pulmonary hypertension: evaluation with 64-detector row CT versus digital subtraction angiography. Eur Radiol 2009;71:49–54.

23. Jenkins D, Mayer E, Screaton N, et al. State-of-the-art chronic thromboembolic pulmonary hypertension diagnosis and management. Eur Respir Rev 2012;21:32–9.

24. Kim NH, Delcroix M, Jais X, et al. Chronic thromboembolic pulmonary hypertension. Eur Respir J 2019;53:1801915.

25. Dartevelle P, Fadel E, Mussot S, et al. Chronic thromboembolic pulmonary hypertension. Eur Respir J 2004;23:637–48.

26. Tscholl D, Langer F, Wendler O, et al. Pulmonary thromboendarterectomy – risk factors for early survival and hemodynamic improvement. Eur J Cardiothorac Surg 2001;19(6):771–6.

27. Jamieson SW, Kapelanski DP. Pulmonary endarterectomy. Curr Probl Surg 2000;37:165–252.

28. Thistlethwaite PA, Mo M, Madani MM, et al. Operative classification of thromboembolic disease determines outcome after pulmonary endarterectomy. J Thorac Cardiovasc Surg 2002;124:1203–11.

29. Nakayama Y, Nakanishi N, Sugimachi M, et al. Characteristics of pulmonary artery pressure waveform for differential diagnosis of chronic pulmonary thromboembolism and primary pulmonary hypertension. J Am Coll Cardiol 1997;29(6):1311–6.

30. Kim NHS, Fesler P, Channick RN, et al. Preoperative partitioning of pulmonary vascular resistance correlates with early outcome after thromboendarterectomy for chronic thromboembolic pulmonary hypertension. Circulation 2004;109:18–22.

31. Thistlethwaite PA, Auger WR, Madani MM, et al. Pulmonary thromboendarterectomy combined with other cardiac operations: indications, surgical approach, and outcome. Ann Thorac Surg 2001;72:13–7.

32. Pepke-Zaba J, Delcroix M, Lang I, et al. Chronic thromboembolic pulmonary hypertension (CTEPH): results from an international prospective registry. Circulation 2011;124:1973–81.

33. Fedullo P, Kerr KM, Kim NH, et al. Chronic thromboembolic pulmonary hypertension. Am J Respir Crit Care Med 2011;183:1605–13.

34. Sadushi-Kolici R, Pavel J, Kopec G, et al. Subcutaneous treprostinil for the treatment of severe non-operable chronic thromboembolic pulmonary hypertension (CTREPH): a randomised phase 3 trial. Lancet Respir Med 2019;7:239–48.

35. Olschewski H, Simonneau G, Galiè N, et al. Inhaled iloprost for severe pulmonary hypertension. N Engl J Med 2002;347(5):322–9.

36. Ghofrani H-A, Simonneau G, D'Armini AM, et al. Macitentan for the treatment of inoperable chronic

thromboembolic pulmonary hypertension (MERIT-1): results from the multicentre, phase 2, randomised, double-blind, placebo-controlled study. Lancet Respir Med 2017;5(10):785–94.

37. Jaïs X, D'Armini AM, Jansa P, et al. Bosentan for treatment of inoperable chronic thromboembolic pulmonary hypertension: BENEFiT (Bosentan Effects in iNopErable Forms of chronIc Thromboembolic pulmonary hypertension), a randomized, placebo-controlled trial. J Am Coll Cardiol 2008; 52(25):2127–34.

38. Ghofrani H-A, D'Armini AM, Grimminger F, et al. Riociguat for the treatment of chronic thromboembolic pulmonary hypertension. N Engl J Med 2013; 369(4):319–29.

39. Hoeper MM. Pharmacological therapy for patients with chronic thromboembolic pulmonary hypertension. Eur Respir Rev 2015;24:272–82.

40. Delcroix M, Lang I, Pepke-zaba J, et al. Long-term outcome of patients with chronic thromboembolic pulmonary hypertension. Results from an international prospective registry. Circulation 2016;133: 859–71.

41. Yanaka K, Nakayama K, Shinke T, et al. Sequential hybrid therapy with pulmonary endarterectomy and additional balloon pulmonary angioplasty for chronic thromboembolic pulmonary hypertension. J Am Heart Assoc 2018;7:e008838.

42. Madani MM, Jamieson SW. Technical advances of pulmonary endarterectomy for chronic thromboembolic pulmonary hypertension. Semin Thorac Cardiovasc Surg 2006;18(3):243–9.

43. Madani MM. Surgical treatment of chronic thromboembolic pulmonary hypertension: pulmonary thromboendarterectomy. Methodist Debakey Cardiovasc J 2016;12(4):213–8.

44. Daily PO, Dembitsky WP, Jamieson SW. The evolution and the current state of the art of pulmonary thromboendarterectomy. Semin Thorac Cardiovasc Surg 1999;11(2):152–63.

45. Biancosino C, Tudorache I, Iablonskii P, et al. Facilitated pulmonary thromboendarterectomy on the left side through cardiac dislocation. Oper Tech Thorac Cardiovasc Surg 2015;20(4):355–69.

46. Kerr KM, Auger WR, Marsh JJ, et al. Efficacy of methylprednisolone in preventing lung injury following pulmonary thromboendarterectomy. Chest 2012;141(1):27–35.

47. Thistlethwaite PA, Madani MM, Kemp AD, et al. Venovenous extracorporeal life support after pulmonary endarterectomy: indications, techniques, and outcomes. Ann Thorac Surg 2006;82(6): 2139–45.

48. Berman M, Tsui S, Vuylsteke A, et al. Successful extracorporeal membrane oxygenation support after pulmonary thromboendarterectomy. Ann Thorac Surg 2008;86(4):1261–7.

49. Fedullo PF, Auger WR, Dembitsky WP. Postoperative management of the patient undergoing pulmonary thromboendarterectomy. Semin Thorac Cardiovasc Surg 1999;11(2):172–8.

50. Mayer E. Surgical and post-operative treatment of chronic thromboembolic pulmonary hypertension. Eur Respir Rev 2010;19(115):64–7.

51. Kramm T, Eberle B, Krummenauer F, et al. Inhaled iloprost in patients with chronic thromboembolic pulmonary hypertension: effects before and after pulmonary thromboendarterectomy. Ann Thorac Surg 2003;76(3):711–8.

52. Gårdebäck M, Larsen FF, Rådegran K. Nitric oxide improves hypoxaemia following reperfusion oedema after pulmonary thromboendarterectomy. Br J Anaesth 1995;75(6):798–800.

53. Archibald CJ, Auger WR, Fedullo PF. Outcome after pulmonary thromboendarterectomy. Semin Thorac Cardiovasc Surg 1999;11(2):164–71.

54. Jamieson SW, Kapelanski DP, Sakakibara N, et al. Pulmonary endarterectomy: experience and lessons learned in 1,500 cases. Ann Thorac Surg 2003; 76(5):1457–64.

55. Bates DM, Fernandes TM, Duwe BV, et al. Efficacy of a low–tidal volume ventilation strategy to prevent reperfusion lung injury after pulmonary thromboendarterectomy. Ann Am Thorac Soc 2015;12(10): 1520–7.

56. Shetty DP, Nair HC, Shetty V, et al. A novel treatment for pulmonary hemorrhage during thromboendarterectomy surgery. Ann Thorac Surg 2015;99(3):e77–8.

57. Dalia AA, Streckenbach S, Andrawes M, et al. Management of pulmonary hemorrhage complicating pulmonary thromboendarterectomy. Front Med 2018;5:326.

58. D'Armini AM, Morsolini M, Mattiucci G, et al. Pulmonary endarterectomy for distal chronic thromboembolic pulmonary hypertension. J Thorac Cardiovasc Surg 2014;148(3):1005–12.e2.

59. Zhang C, Wang G, Zhou H, et al. Preoperative platelet count, preoperative hemoglobin concentration and deep hypothermic circulatory arrest duration are risk factors for acute kidney injury after pulmonary endarterectomy: a retrospective cohort study. J Cardiovasc Surg 2019;14(1):220.

60. Vekstein AM, Yerokun BA, Jawitz OK, et al. Does deeper hypothermia reduce the risk of acute kidney injury after circulatory arrest for aortic arch surgery? Eur J Cardiothorac Surg 2021;60(2):314–21.

61. Freed DH, Thomson BM, Berman M, et al. Survival after pulmonary thromboendarterectomy: effect of residual pulmonary hypertension. J Thorac Cardiovasc Surg 2011;141(2):383–7.

62. Cannon John E, Su Li, Kiely David G, et al. Dynamic risk stratification of patient long-term outcome after pulmonary endarterectomy. Circulation 2016; 133(18):1761–71.

63. Saouti N, Morshuis WJ, Heijmen RH, et al. Long-term outcome after pulmonary endarterectomy for chronic thromboembolic pulmonary hypertension: a single institution experience. Eur J Cardiothorac Surg 2009;35:947–52.

64. Madani M, Mayer E, Fadel E, et al. Pulmonary endarterectomy. Patient selection, technical challenges, and outcomes. Ann Am Thorac Soc 2016; 13(Supplement_3):S240–7.

65. Hartz RS, Byrne JG, Levitsky S, et al. Predictors of mortality in pulmonary thromboendarterectomy. Ann Thorac Surg 1996;62:1255–9.

66. Blanchard DG, Malouf PJ, Gurudevan SV, et al. Utility of right ventricular tei index in the noninvasive evaluation of chronic thromboembolic pulmonary hypertension before and after pulmonary thromboendarterectomy. JACC Cardiovasc Imaging 2009;2(2):143–9.

Interventional Management of Chronic Thromboembolic Pulmonary Hypertension

J.D. Serfas, MD, Richard A. Krasuski, MD*

KEYWORDS

- Chronic thromboembolic pulmonary hypertension • Balloon pulmonary angioplasty
- Pulmonary endarterectomy • Interventional cardiology

KEY POINTS

- Balloon pulmonary angioplasty (BPA) is an emerging and effective therapy for inoperable chronic thromboembolic pulmonary hypertension that should be performed in expert centers after multidisciplinary discussion.
- Refinements in procedural technique have reduced complication rates and improved BPA efficacy.
- Further research, including randomized clinical trials, is needed to establish the efficacy of BPA and determine appropriate therapeutic end points.

INTRODUCTION

Chronic thromboembolic pulmonary hypertension (CTEPH) is a well-defined class of pulmonary hypertension and represents about 19% of all pulmonary hypertension.[1] Its pathophysiology, diagnosis, and management are all distinct from other forms of pulmonary hypertension, and it is unique in that it is potentially reversible with pulmonary thromboendarterectomy (PTE), an operation associated with major clinical and hemodynamic improvement and low operative mortality in experienced centers.[2] However, many patients are not ideal candidates for PTE, or have residual or recurrent pulmonary hypertension after PTE; for these patients, medical and interventional therapy may play a pivotal role. Balloon pulmonary angioplasty (BPA) is a rapidly developing catheter-based therapy that is increasingly used in such patients. This article summarizes the pathophysiology, diagnosis, and management of CTEPH, with a particular focus on BPA.

CHRONIC THROMBOEMBOLIC PULMONARY HYPERTENSION PATHOPHYSIOLOGY

CTEPH is characterized by the deposition of chronic thrombotic material in the pulmonary arterial tree, leading to obstruction to flow, as well as remodeling of the microvasculature.[3,4] Most cases occur in patients with known prior pulmonary embolism (PE), but a substantial minority of patients (up to 38%) have no such history.[1] However, only ~3% of patients with an acute PE go on to develop CTEPH, and the factors that lead to the development of chronic thrombus and eventual CTEPH are not fully understood, although thrombophilic disorders, cancer, splenectomy, inflammatory and infectious disorders, non-O blood

Disclosures: Dr R.A. Krasuski has received honoraria from Actelion Pharmaceuticals and research grants from Actelion Pharmaceuticals, Edwards Lifesciences, Corvia, CryoLife, and the Adult Congenital Heart Association. Dr J.D. Serfas has nothing to disclose.
Section of Adult Congenital Heart Disease, Division of Cardiology, Duke University Medical Center, 2301 Erwin Road, Durham, NC 27710, USA
* Corresponding author. Duke University Medical Center, Box 3012, Durham, NC 27710.
E-mail address: richard.krasuski@duke.edu

Cardiol Clin 40 (2022) 103–114
https://doi.org/10.1016/j.ccl.2021.08.009
0733-8651/22/© 2021 Elsevier Inc. All rights reserved.

group, abnormalities in platelet function and fibrinolytic activity, and genetic factors are all thought to play a role.[4]

DIAGNOSIS AND EVALUATION

Because the presenting symptoms of CTEPH are nonspecific and it is an important form of pulmonary hypertension with unique treatment algorithms, a high index of suspicion is mandatory in patients presenting with shortness of breath or functional limitation and in patients with evidence of pulmonary hypertension on prior testing. According to the 2015 ESC/European Respiratory Society (ERS) Pulmonary Hypertension Guidelines, any patient with suspicion for pulmonary hypertension that is not easily explained by left heart disease or parenchymal lung disease after clinical evaluation and echocardiography should undergo ventilation/perfusion (V/Q) scintigraphy to evaluate for the presence of CTEPH.[5] V/Q scintigraphy is more sensitive for distal thrombotic disease than computed tomography pulmonary angiography (CTPA); therefore, CTPA should not be used as the sole screening modality for CTEPH.[6] The diagnosis of CTEPH is confirmed when evidence of chronic thrombus on V/Q scintigraphy or CTPA is present together with invasive demonstration of precapillary pulmonary hypertension, defined by the 6th World Symposium on Pulmonary Hypertension as a mean pulmonary artery pressure (mPAP) greater than 20 mm Hg, a pulmonary capillary wedge pressure (PCWP) less than or equal to 15 mm Hg, and a pulmonary vascular resistance (PVR) greater than or equal to 3 Wood units (WU).[7]

CTPA nonetheless plays an important role in the evaluation of CTEPH, because it provides excellent visualization of the proximal pulmonary arteries, as well as the heart and pulmonary parenchyma, which can allow for risk stratification and uncovering of alternate diagnoses.[8] CTPA also informs treatment decisions and procedural planning for both PTE and BPA. Recent advances in computed tomography (CT) technology have improved the utility of CTPA in the evaluation of CTEPH, and specifically include the development of dual energy CT (DECT) and cone-beam CT. DECT may be used to generate an iodine perfusion map of the pulmonary parenchyma (**Fig. 1**), and can be used to help differentiate acute PE from CTEPH as well as CTEPH from World Health Organization (WHO) group 1 pulmonary arterial hypertension (PAH).[2] Flat-panel cone-beam CT can be used on a C-arm to provide better visualization of distal arteries and lesions than most other available imaging technologies, and can be useful for the planning of BPA procedures.[9] The limited availability and cost of both of these imaging modalities limit their widespread use.

In most centers, invasive pulmonary angiography, typically paired with right heart catheterization, remains the gold standard assessment of the pulmonary vasculature for determination of anatomic candidacy for PTE and/or BPA.[10] Although protocols differ from center to center, this typically includes the use of digital subtraction angiography (DSA) with frontal and lateral angiograms of each lung, and allows the identification and characterization of CTEPH lesions out to the subsegmental level. Selective segmental or subsegmental injections are often required for complete characterization of more distal lesions and are typically performed at the time of BPA. Lesions are grouped into 1 of 5 types: ringlike stenoses, web lesions, subtotal occlusion, total occlusions or pouch defects, and tortuous lesions, with the first 4 types typically being found in the segmental and subsegmental arteries, and tortuous lesions occurring distal to the subsegmental arteries. Understanding of the differing types of lesions is critical, because it can inform target lesion selection; lesion-specific success rates are highest with ringlike and web lesions, whereas total occlusions and tortuous lesions have much lower success rates and are at higher risk for complications.[11]

MANAGEMENT

The cornerstone of therapy for CTEPH is PTE, which should be considered for all patients with CTEPH as soon as the diagnosis is identified. However, some patients are poor candidates for PTE, because of comorbidities, acuity of illness, or surgical inaccessibility of the disease (in general, more proximal disease [ie, in the main, lobar, and segmental arteries] is surgically accessible, whereas more distal disease is not). For the latter patients, BPA is an appealing treatment strategy. Medical therapy should be offered alongside surgical and/or interventional therapy and includes chronic anticoagulation with a vitamin K antagonist or direct oral anticoagulant and advanced medical therapies developed for PAH, as well as supportive measures such as diuretics and oxygen as needed. The soluble guanylate cyclase stimulator riociguat is the preferred advanced medical therapy for CTEPH. It was approved by the US Food and Drug Administration (FDA) based on the double-blind placebo-controlled Chronic Thromboembolic Pulmonary Hypertension Soluble Guanylate Cyclase Stimulator Trial-1 (CHEST-1),[12] which showed significant improvements in 6minute walk distance (6MWD) and PVR with riociguat. Although additional therapies

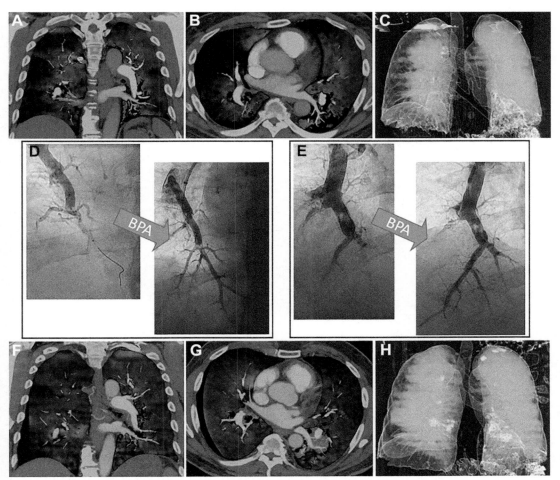

Fig. 1. Dual energy CTPA before and after a first session of BPA. Iodine density map imaging in coronal (*A*) and axial (*B*) views show multifocal wedge-shaped areas of decreased perfusion in the periphery of the right lung, which is also seen on total pulmonary blood volume imaging (*C*). BPA was performed on multiple complex web and subtotal lesions in the right lung (*D, E*). Post-BPA dual energy CTPA shows increased areas of peripheral perfusion in iodine mapping (*F, G*) and total pulmonary blood volume imaging (*H*).

are often used to treat inoperable and recurrent CTEPH based on the results of combination therapy trials in PAH, no other medications are currently FDA approved. The endothelin receptor antagonist macitentan showed statistically significant reductions in PVR and improvement in 6MWD in the double-blind placebo-controlled Macitentan for the Treatment of Inoperable Chronic Thromboembolic Pulmonary Hypertension Trial (MERIT-1).[13] High-dose open-label subcutaneous treprostinil showed improvement in 6MWD compared with low-dose subcutaneous treprostinil in advanced functional class (III or IV) patients in the Subcutaneous Treprostinil for the Treatment of Severe Non-operable Chronic Thromboembolic Pulmonary Hypertension (CTREPH) trial.[14] Bosentan showed improvement in PVR but not 6MWD in

the Bosentan Effects in Inoperable Forms of Chronic Thromboembolic Pulmonary Hypertension (BENEFiT) Study.[15] The ultimate treatment strategy should be determined at an expert center after multidisciplinary discussion.

BALLOON PULMONARY ANGIOPLASTY
History

Balloon angioplasty in the pulmonary arteries has long been performed in congenital heart disease, beginning in the 1980s,[16–18] and was first reported for CTEPH in a 1988 case report.[19] In 2001, Feinstein and colleagues[20] presented a series of 18 patients with CTEPH who underwent BPA with improvements in New York Heart Association (NYHA) functional class, 6MWD, and mPAP.

However, the complication rate was high, with most patients developing pulmonary edema, 3 requiring mechanical ventilation, and 1 dying a week after the procedure related to right ventricular failure. As a result, the procedure was largely abandoned in the United States and Europe for many years. However, refinements continued in Japan, with progressive changes in procedural technique and splitting of the procedure into multiple sessions, which helped reduce complication rates; several publications have since shown acceptable safety profiles and promising efficacy, starting in the 2010s.[21–27] Since that time, the procedure has been rapidly adopted and further refined at several European and, eventually, American centers, with generally favorable results.[10,28–35] It is now offered at select expert centers for appropriate patients with CTEPH across the globe.

Patient Selection

In general, patients should be considered for BPA when they are deemed inoperable candidates for PTE, whether because of surgically inaccessible distal disease, patient comorbidities, frailty, or patient preference.[36] It may also be used for patients with residual pulmonary hypertension and distal obstructive disease after PTE, and occasionally as a stabilizing procedure in critically ill patients,[37] or as a rescue option after failed PTE.[38] Large, central clots and unilateral total occlusion of a branch pulmonary artery are not technically amenable to BPA (**Fig. 2**), and BPA should not be attempted for such lesions. Certain patients have severe microvascular disease that is out of proportion to their vascular occlusions; these patients may be less likely to benefit from BPA.[1]

Outcomes

There is a growing evidence base supporting the use of BPA in nonoperative candidates, with demonstrated benefits in several clinical factors. The bulk of the evidence is composed of small and single-center studies,[11,28–31,33,35,39–52] which have consistently shown improved hemodynamics with reductions in mPAP and PVR and increases in cardiac index, and typically improvements in WHO functional class (most patients achieving WHO I or II status) and increase in 6MWD by 50 to 100 m. Most studies have also measured brain natriuretic peptide levels and shown improvements post-BPA, and selected studies have shown improvements in imaging parameters, with smaller right ventricular and larger left ventricular volumes and reduction in ventricular dyssynchrony post-BPA,[39] improvements in

pulmonary artery energetics by MRI,[43] and improved echo parameters of right ventricular systolic and diastolic function.[45,47] These findings have been corroborated in larger, multicenter studies as well,[32,34,53–56] with the largest study to date[57] being a 7-center registry including 308 patients who underwent 1408 BPA procedures in Japan. Results in this study were impressive, with reductions in mPAP from 43 mm Hg to 23 mm Hg, PVR from 10.7 WU to 3.6 WU, brain natriuretic peptide (BNP) level from 240 pg/mL to 39 pg/mL, and improvements in WHO class and increase in 6MWD by 111 m, with reductions in oxygen use and need for advanced medical therapy for pulmonary hypertension. There have additionally been signals in some studies of improved survival with BPA; in a comparison of 160 patients in Poland who underwent PTE (n = 31), BPA and medical therapy (58), or medical therapy alone (69), BPA patients had the highest 2-year survival at 92% (compared with 79% for PTE or medical therapy alone), and use of BPA was found to be a significant predictor of survival in multivariable regression (hazard ratio [HR] for death 0.35; confidence interval [CI], 0.13–0.94; P = .037).[31] In an analysis of the French experience with patients with nonoperable CTEPH from 2006 to 2016, BPA was independently associated with survival (HR for mortality 0.31; CI, 0.10–0.96; P = .042), and there was a clear improvement in survival between the pre-BPA era (2006–2012) and the BPA era (2013–2016).[58] A meta-analysis of 17 of the studies mentioned earlier including 670 patients with CTEPH showed decreases in mPAP of 14.2 mm Hg, PVR of 3.8 WU, and mean right atrial pressure of 2.7 mm Hg, as well as increases in 6MWD of 67.3 m and cardiac output of 0.2 L/min,[59] and a separate systematic review and meta-analysis suggested a benefit of BPA compared with riociguat therapy for CTEPH, with greater improvements in right atrial pressure, mPAP, PVR, NYHA class, and 6MWD.[60] The Riociguat Versus BPA in Nonoperable CTEPH (RACE) trial, which has yet to be published as of this writing, was presented at the ERS meeting in 2019, and randomized 124 patients with CTEPH to BPA or riociguat therapy. BPA was associated with greater reductions in PVR, mPAP, mean right atrial pressure, and N-terminal pro–BNP level, and a greater improvement in functional class. Complications were unsurprisingly more common in the BPA group.[61]

The hemodynamic improvements seen after BPA are generally not immediate but are often seen in later follow-up.[62] This finding is thought to be caused by ongoing flow-mediated vascular remodeling that takes place over the days and

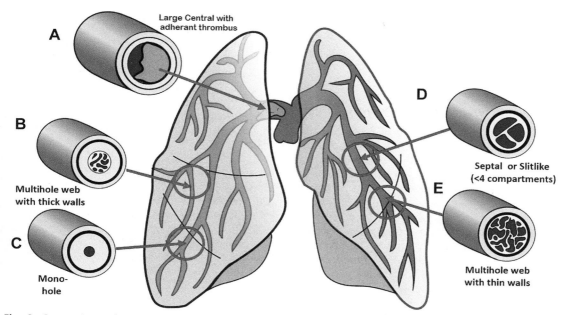

Fig. 2. Comparison of a proximal lesion (A) that is most amenable to pulmonary thromboendarterectomy compared with the optical coherence tomography–described lesions in vessels 2 to 5 mm in diameter, which are most amenable to BPA. The latter include multihole web lesions with thick walls (B), monohole lesions with thick walls (C), slitlike lesions with thin walls and less than 4 compartments (D), and multihole webs with thin walls (E).

weeks after BPA. The exact timing of the hemodynamic improvements remains to be elucidated. Thankfully, these hemodynamic improvements seem to be durable, with sustained hemodynamic improvements out to 4 years in 1 study.[63]

The complication rate of BPA, which was initially the reason for its disuse in the early 2000s, has improved dramatically with refinements in technique, but complications are still common.[49,51] At the 6th World Symposium on Pulmonary Hypertension, the complications of BPA were classified into several categories that are recommended for use in BPA centers for tracking and reporting purposes.[64] The most common complication is vascular injury, whether caused by wire perforation, balloon overdilation, or high-pressure contrast injection, and can result in a variety of manifestations, ranging from asymptomatic infiltrate on postprocedural chest imaging to massive intrathoracic hemorrhage and death. Other common manifestations are extravasation of contrast on angiography, cough, hemoptysis, hypoxemia, tachycardia, and increased pulmonary artery pressures. Although many of these manifestations were previously thought to be caused by reperfusion pulmonary edema, as has been observed with PTE, they are now more accurately recognized as complications of vascular injury. Other complications include vascular dissection, allergic

or adverse reactions to contrast media and/or sedation, renal dysfunction, and access site complications. Minor complications are common, with 36% of patients in the largest registry experiencing at least 1 complication,[57] but more serious complications are thankfully rare. Importantly, complication rates vary depending on the type of lesion treated, with web and ringlike lesions having the lowest complication rates and total occlusions and tortuous lesions having the highest rates[11]; this relationship has been corroborated on subsequent imaging studies, with web and bandlike lesions having low rates (~8%–10%) of angiogram- or CT-detected pulmonary hemorrhage and much higher rates (~37%) seen after interventions to occlusive lesions.[41] Higher preprocedural pulmonary artery pressure has also been considered a risk factor for the development of complications; in Feinstein and colleagues'[20] original article in 2001, mPAP greater than 35 mm Hg correlated with the development of pulmonary edema, and Kataoka and colleagues[21] found mPAP to be higher in patients who developed pulmonary edema. Pulmonary edema is more common after initial BPA procedures than after subsequent sessions. Inami and colleagues[25] proposed the Pulmonary Edema Predictive Scoring Index (PEPSI), which is a composite score of baseline PVR and change in Pulmonary Flow

Grade score, which is an angiographic assessment of pulmonary artery and vein flow, as a predictor of pulmonary edema post-BPA. In that study, PEPSI was the strongest predictor of pulmonary edema on multivariable analysis.

Balloon Pulmonary Angioplasty Procedural Details

Typically, BPA is performed over the course of several sessions; this is done to limit radiation and contrast exposure and reduce the risk of severe complications arising in multiple lung fields. End points for each session vary significantly from center to center, although they typically involve limits on contrast, radiation dose, fluoroscopy time, and number of segments treated. The University of California in San Diego reports limits of 400 mL of contrast, 2-Gy radiation exposure, and 3 to 5 diseased segments treated.[10] Typically, 4 to 6 sessions per patient are required. The procedure is performed under conscious or moderate sedation, without use of general anesthesia or endotracheal intubation. Heparin is given to maintain an activated clotting time of 200 to 250 seconds. Femoral or internal jugular venous access is used, and a long (~90 cm) 6-French, 7-French, or 8-French sheath is advanced into the target pulmonary artery; a 6-French or 7-French preshaped guide catheter is advanced through the sheath and positioned in the target segment. The long sheath serves to stabilize the guide catheter, buttressing it against the movements of the right ventricle. A 0.36-mm or 0.46-mm (0.014″ or 0.018″) guidewire is advanced across the target lesion, and an appropriately sized balloon is inflated within the lesion. Appropriate guidewire positioning is crucial, as straight as possible within the distal vessel, ideally with the distal tip knuckled in a J conformation to mitigate the risk of guidewire perforation.[65] First-line guidewires should generally be soft and atraumatic, and polymer-jacketed guidewires should be avoided, because they have been anecdotally associated with higher risk for vascular injury.[10] Microcatheters, guide extensions, and balloon catheters may be used to support workhorse wires, and judicious guidewire escalation may be used with caution for the most difficult lesions. Balloons are typically semicompliant or noncompliant and are initially undersized to minimize the risk of vascular injury and reperfusion edema. Balloons with 2.0-mm diameter are often the initial size, especially for more distal lesions, although smaller diameters are sometimes used. Larger diameters are often necessary in more proximal lesions,[66] and, rarely, use of sculpting or cutting balloons has been reported, although

these should be used only with extreme caution and in experienced hands.[10] Guide catheter selection should be tailored to the target segment and lesions, but, generally, Judkins right and multipurpose catheters are often useful in the right lung, whereas Amplatz left-shaped catheters are often helpful for accessing lesions in the left lung.[1] Inspiratory breath holds can be helpful for crossing and dilating difficult lesions, especially in the lower lung fields.

Lesion selection

Most patients with CTEPH have diffuse disease, with several potential target lesions. Selection of initial targets depends primarily on 3 factors: (1) location and severity of perfusion defects identified on perfusion scintigraphy, DECT, and/or nonselective DSA; (2) probability of complications based on lesion morphology; and (3) likelihood of benefit based on lung zone (ie, the lower lung zones typically receive greater perfusion under physiologic conditions, and thus patients are likely to derive greater benefit from reperfusion of these areas). Complex webs and slitlike lesions that cause significant perfusion defects may be difficult to appreciate on nonselective angiography, and so perfusion defects should guide selection of segments to interrogate with selective angiography, even if specific lesions are not clearly seen on the initial imaging.[66] Thus, the most ideal lesions for BPA are webs and ringlike lesions in the distal lower lung zones in areas with significant perfusion defects, whereas tortuous lesions and complete occlusions in the upper lung zones are generally treated only if hemodynamic and symptomatic goals have not been met and there are no remaining untreated lower-risk lesions.

Mechanism of improvement

In contrast with the soft, lipid-rich plaques and acute obstructing thrombus that is encountered in the coronary arteries, the obstructive lesions in CTEPH are composed of a network of fibrotic, collagen-rich, partially recanalized organized thrombus that is adherent to the vessel wall.[2] The fibrotic material can be clearly visualized with optical coherence tomography (OCT), and lesions have been categorized into 4 categories according to their OCT appearance: (1) septum, in which the fibrotic material partitions the arterial lumen into 4 or fewer compartments; (2) multihole with thin walls, in which there are 5 or more lumens divided by thin fibrous partitions; (3) multihole with thick walls; and (4) monohole, in which there is 1 central small lumen through the organized thrombus (see **Fig. 2**).[67] Histologic and intravascular imaging evaluation of CTEPH lesions after

BPA have shown that the fibrotic material is displaced to the side of the vessel,[68,69] but that most of the luminal increase is associated with stretch of the native artery rather than compression of the fibrotic material, at least in more proximal vessels.[69] In smaller, more distal vessels, in which the vessel walls become more muscular and less distensible, there is a smaller degree of vessel expansion and the luminal increase depends more on compression of the organized thrombus.[70] However, in addition to vessel stretch, dissection of the arterial media may occur, causing a pseudovascular space to form that then becomes a new lumen, as has been shown histologically.[71] This dissection plane can resemble what is done with PTE, and may not be appreciable by angiography at the time of BPA.

The precise mechanism of improvement in BPA is not fully settled; interestingly, the total pulmonary artery compliance improves shortly after completion of the BPA procedure, but intravascular ultrasonography (IVUS)–based estimations of local pulmonary artery distensibility and compliance at the area of the BPA do not change.[72] Furthermore, microvascular disease often coexists to varying degrees with the larger fibrotic occlusions, and can be present even in patients whose hemodynamics normalize, in both BPA-treated and BPA-untreated segments of lung.[68] Determining the presence and extent of this microvascular disease preprocedurally could potentially help identify patients who are most and least likely to benefit from either BPA or advanced medical therapy.

Procedural safety

Although post-BPA CT scans detect evidence of pulmonary hemorrhage in a large proportion of patients (47%), most of these have no or limited clinical manifestations and are often not readily appreciable on angiography; in contrast, angiographically detected vascular injury at the time of BPA is a potent predictor of the need for mechanical ventilation.[73] Such vascular injury is the most common cause of adverse events after BPA, and is related to vessel trauma from wire manipulation or balloon overdistension; therefore, great care should be taken to avoid both. Techniques to minimize procedural risks are summarized in **Box 1**.

A thorough understanding of the pathobiology discussed earlier informs techniques to minimize the risk of adverse outcomes. For example, the distensibility of the native pulmonary artery with its accompanying propensity for dissection underscores the importance of undersizing balloons, especially in lesions with the highest burden of minimally compressible fibrous thrombus (ie, subtotal and total occlusions).

As mentioned previously, meticulous attention to wire positioning is critical, and the most atraumatic wires and catheters should be used with only very rare and cautious escalation to more aggressive equipment. Balloons should be undersized, especially in initial sessions, high-risk lesions, and in patients with severely increased pulmonary pressures. Low-risk lesions, such as webs and ringlike lesions, should be treated preferentially to subtotal and total occlusions and tortuous lesions.

Based on the observation that BPA-treated lesions continue to improve with time beyond what is achieved at the time of the initial ballooning both angiographically[74] and by pressure wire gradient,[75] and out of concern for exposing the distal microvasculature to high pressure, some groups have advocated an approach that involves treating as many lesions as possible with small (~2 mm) balloons in initial sessions, and only dilating lesions up to more appropriate sizes in subsequent sessions. An alternative approach is predicated on the observation that mPAP greater than or equal to 35 mm Hg has been consistently shown to be a risk factor for poor outcomes, and consists of limiting the number of segments treated in each session until mPAP decreases to less than 35 mm Hg, after which more aggressive ballooning is likely safer.[66]

Many interventionalists have used pressure wires to guide therapy and ensure safety; balloon dilation is performed until distal to proximal pressure ratio (Pd/Pa) is greater than 0.8, or until Pd exceeds 35 mm Hg, whichever comes first.[56] Increased postprocedure Pd has been associated with the incidence of lung injury.[40] Optimizing medical therapy for pulmonary hypertension before first BPA has also been proposed.[76]

IVUS and OCT have both been described to guide lesion and balloon selection,[67,77] but have been acknowledged as impractical, because they can add significant time and complexity to the procedure, and many lesions are not able to be reliably imaged.[69]

In addition, operators must be prepared to manage complications swiftly as they arise. Vascular injury must be recognized and treated promptly; methods for doing so include prolonged balloon sealing, heparin reversal, covered stent placement, and vessel occlusion with coils or preferably resorbable gel.[78,79] BPA should not be attempted without the necessary expertise and equipment to manage said complications, and the ready availability of traditional life support measures is mandatory, including intubation and mechanical ventilation, bronchoscopy, and surgical and intensive care expertise.

Box 1
Techniques to minimize balloon pulmonary angioplasty risk

- Optimize medical pulmonary hypertension therapy before first BPA session
- Use atraumatic workhorse wires without polymer jacketing
- Knuckle the distal tip of the guidewire in the distal pulmonary vasculature
- Undersize balloons, especially if mPAP is greater than or equal to 35 mm Hg
- Prioritize web and ring lesions; approach subtotal and total occlusions with caution
- If using a flow wire, stop if distal to proximal pressure ratio reaches 0.8 or distal pressure reaches 35 mm Hg
- Do not treat more than 3 to 5 segments in a single BPA session
- Stock equipment to quickly address complications (covered stents, coils, Gelfoam, and so forth)

Therapeutic targets

There is no agreement currently on final end points for BPA. Although individual sessions are typically limited by safety concerns, the markers of completion of therapy are poorly defined. Early targets were typically hemodynamic, with therapy continuing until mPAP was below a certain threshold, often 25 mm Hg.[50,57] However, alternative targets, such as perfusion measured by scintigraphy, completeness of angiographic revascularization, right ventricular size and function, functional class, or other clinical parameters, could all be considered. Ultimately, the decision must be individualized to the patient's goals and clinical status.

SUMMARY

BPA is an emerging and promising therapy for the treatment of inoperable CTEPH, and its role in comprehensive CTEPH management is expected to continue to grow. Complications are becoming less common with refinements in procedural technique; careful planning and meticulous attention to optimal technique are critical for procedural success. Further research, including adequately powered randomized controlled trials, is needed to determine efficacy and to refine the approach to patient selection, preprocedure and postprocedure noninvasive evaluation, and procedural techniques for efficacy and safety.

CLINICS CARE POINTS

- CTEPH is a unique form of pulmonary hypertension that is potentially reversible with PTE
- Management decisions for patients with CTEPH should be made in multidisciplinary discussion at an expert CTEPH center
- BPA results in several clinical improvements and should be considered for all patients with inoperable CTEPH
- Mitigating risk of complications with BPA is of paramount importance and meticulous care must be paid to procedural techniques

ACKNOWLEDGMENTS

The authors would like to acknowledge Thomas M. Bashore, MD, for his fantastic artwork and inspirational mentorship, and Dr Joseph G. Mammarappallil, MD, PhD, for his expertise and assistance regarding dual-energy CT imaging.

REFERENCES

1. Rotzinger DC, Rezaei-Kalantari K, Aubert J-D, et al. Pulmonary angioplasty: a step further in the continuously changing landscape of chronic thromboembolic pulmonary hypertension management. Eur J Radiol 2021;136:109562.
2. Delcroix M, Torbicki A, Gopalan D, et al. ERS statement on chronic thromboembolic pulmonary hypertension. Eur Respir J 2020. https://doi.org/10.1183/13993003.02828-2020.
3. Dorfmüller P, Günther S, Ghigna M-R, et al. Microvascular disease in chronic thromboembolic pulmonary hypertension: a role for pulmonary veins and systemic vasculature. Eur Respir J 2014;44(5):1275–88.
4. Simonneau G, Torbicki A, Dorfmüller P, et al. The pathophysiology of chronic thromboembolic pulmonary hypertension. Eur Respir Rev 2017;26(143). https://doi.org/10.1183/16000617.0112-2016.
5. Galiè N, Humbert M, Vachiery J-L, et al. 2015 ESC/ERS Guidelines for the diagnosis and treatment of pulmonary hypertension: the Joint Task Force for the Diagnosis and Treatment of Pulmonary Hypertension of the European Society of Cardiology (ESC) and the European Respiratory Society (ERS): Endorsed by: Association for European Paediatric and Congenital Cardiology (AEPC),

International Society for Heart and Lung Transplantation (ISHLT). Eur Heart J 2016;37(1):67–119.

6. Rogberg AN, Gopalan D, Westerlund E, et al. Do radiologists detect chronic thromboembolic disease on computed tomography? Acta Radiol 2019; 60(11):1576–83.

7. Simonneau G, Montani D, Celermajer DS, et al. Haemodynamic definitions and updated clinical classification of pulmonary hypertension. Eur Respir J 2019;53(1). https://doi.org/10.1183/13993003.01913-2018.

8. Narechania S, Renapurkar R, Heresi GA. Mimickers of chronic thromboembolic pulmonary hypertension on imaging tests: a review. Pulm Circ 2020;10(1). 2045894019882620.

9. Hinrichs JB, Renne J, Hoeper MM, et al. Balloon pulmonary angioplasty: applicability of C-Arm CT for procedure guidance. Eur Radiol 2016;26(11): 4064–71.

10. Mahmud E, Madani MM, Kim NH, et al. Chronic thromboembolic pulmonary hypertension: evolving therapeutic approaches for operable and inoperable disease. J Am Coll Cardiol 2018;71(21): 2468–86.

11. Kawakami T, Ogawa A, Miyaji K, et al. Novel angiographic classification of each vascular lesion in chronic thromboembolic pulmonary hypertension based on selective angiogram and results of balloon pulmonary angioplasty. Circ Cardiovasc Interv 2016; 9(10). https://doi.org/10.1161/CIRCINTERVENTIONS.115.003318.

12. Ghofrani H-A, D'Armini AM, Grimminger F, et al. Riociguat for the treatment of chronic thromboembolic pulmonary hypertension. N Engl J Med 2013; 369(4):319–29.

13. Ghofrani H-A, Simonneau G, D'Armini AM, et al. Macitentan for the treatment of inoperable chronic thromboembolic pulmonary hypertension (MERIT-1): results from the multicentre, phase 2, randomised, double-blind, placebo-controlled study. Lancet Respir Med 2017. https://doi.org/10.1016/S2213-2600(17)30305-3.

14. Sadushi-Kolici R, Jansa P, Kopec G, et al. Subcutaneous treprostinil for the treatment of severe non-operable chronic thromboembolic pulmonary hypertension (CTREPH): a double-blind, phase 3, randomised controlled trial. Lancet Respir Med 2019; 7(3):239–48.

15. Jaïs X, D'Armini AM, Jansa P, et al. Bosentan for treatment of inoperable chronic thromboembolic pulmonary hypertension: BENEFiT (Bosentan Effects in iNopErable Forms of chronIc Thromboembolic pulmonary hypertension), a randomized, placebo-controlled trial. J Am Coll Cardiol 2008; 52(25):2127–34.

16. Lock JE, Castaneda-Zuniga WR, Fuhrman BP, et al. Balloon dilation angioplasty of hypoplastic and stenotic pulmonary arteries. Circulation 1983;67(5): 962–7.

17. Kreutzer J, Landzberg MJ, Preminger TJ, et al. Isolated peripheral pulmonary artery stenoses in the adult. Circulation 1996;93(7):1417–23.

18. Martin EC, Diamond NG, Casarella WJ. Percutaneous transluminal angioplasty in nonatherosclerotic disease. Radiology 1980;135(1): 27–33.

19. Voorburg JA, Cats VM, Buis B, et al. Balloon angioplasty in the treatment of pulmonary hypertension caused by pulmonary embolism. Chest 1988;94(6): 1249–53.

20. Feinstein JA, Goldhaber SZ, Lock JE, et al. Balloon pulmonary angioplasty for treatment of chronic thromboembolic pulmonary hypertension. Circulation 2001;103(1):10–3.

21. Kataoka M, Inami T, Hayashida K, et al. Percutaneous transluminal pulmonary angioplasty for the treatment of chronic thromboembolic pulmonary hypertension. Circ Cardiovasc Interv 2012;5(6): 756–62.

22. Sugimura K, Fukumoto Y, Satoh K, et al. Percutaneous transluminal pulmonary angioplasty markedly improves pulmonary hemodynamics and long-term prognosis in patients with chronic thromboembolic pulmonary hypertension. Circ J 2012;76(2):485–8.

23. Taniguchi Y, Miyagawa K, Nakayama K, et al. Balloon pulmonary angioplasty: an additional treatment option to improve the prognosis of patients with chronic thromboembolic pulmonary hypertension. EuroIntervention 2014;10(4):518–25.

24. Fukui S, Ogo T, Morita Y, et al. Right ventricular reverse remodelling after balloon pulmonary angioplasty. Eur Respir J 2014;43(5):1394–402.

25. Inami T, Kataoka M, Shimura N, et al. Pulmonary edema predictive scoring index (PEPSI), a new index to predict risk of reperfusion pulmonary edema and improvement of hemodynamics in percutaneous transluminal pulmonary angioplasty. JACC Cardiovasc Interv 2013;6(7):725–36.

26. Yanagisawa R, Kataoka M, Inami T, et al. Safety and efficacy of percutaneous transluminal pulmonary angioplasty in elderly patients. Int J Cardiol 2014; 175(2):285–9.

27. Sato H, Ota H, Sugimura K, et al. Balloon pulmonary angioplasty improves biventricular functions and pulmonary flow in chronic thromboembolic pulmonary hypertension. Circ J 2016;80(6):1470–7.

28. Kriechbaum SD, Wiedenroth CB, Wolter JS, et al. N-terminal pro-B-type natriuretic peptide for monitoring after balloon pulmonary angioplasty for chronic thromboembolic pulmonary hypertension. J Heart Lung Transpl 2018;37(5):639–46.

29. Velázquez M, Albarrán A, Hernández I, et al. Balloon pulmonary angioplasty for inoperable patients with chronic thromboembolic pulmonary hypertension.

observational study in a referral unit. Rev Esp Cardiol (Engl Ed) 2019;72(3):224–32.

30. Brenot P, Jaïs X, Taniguchi Y, et al. French experience of balloon pulmonary angioplasty for chronic thromboembolic pulmonary hypertension. Eur Respir J 2019;53(5). https://doi.org/10.1183/13993003.02095-2018.

31. Siennicka A, Darocha S, Banaszkiewicz M, et al. Treatment of chronic thromboembolic pulmonary hypertension in a multidisciplinary team. Ther Adv Respir Dis 2019;13. 1753466619891529.

32. Maschke SK, Hinrichs JB, Renne J, et al. C-Arm computed tomography (CACT)-guided balloon pulmonary angioplasty (BPA): evaluation of patient safety and peri- and post-procedural complications. Eur Radiol 2019;29(3):1276–84.

33. Godinas L, Bonne L, Budts W, et al. Balloon pulmonary angioplasty for the treatment of nonoperable chronic thromboembolic pulmonary hypertension: single-center experience with low initial complication rate. J Vasc Interv Radiol 2019;30(8):1265–72.

34. van Thor MCJ, Lely RJ, Braams NJ, et al. Safety and efficacy of balloon pulmonary angioplasty in chronic thromboembolic pulmonary hypertension in the Netherlands. Neth Heart J 2020;28(2):81–8.

35. Hoole SP, Coghlan JG, Cannon JE, et al. Balloon pulmonary angioplasty for inoperable chronic thromboembolic pulmonary hypertension: the UK experience. Open Heart 2020;7(1):e001144.

36. Lang I, Meyer BC, Ogo T, et al. Balloon pulmonary angioplasty in chronic thromboembolic pulmonary hypertension. Eur Respir Rev 2017;26(143). https://doi.org/10.1183/16000617.0119-2016.

37. Tsuji A, Ogo T, Demachi J, et al. Rescue balloon pulmonary angioplasty in a rapidly deteriorating chronic thromboembolic pulmonary hypertension patient with liver failure and refractory infection. Pulm Circ 2014;4(1):142–7.

38. Collaud S, Brenot P, Mercier O, et al. Rescue balloon pulmonary angioplasty for early failure of pulmonary endarterectomy: the earlier the better? Int J Cardiol 2016;222:39–40.

39. Yamasaki Y, Nagao M, Abe K, et al. Balloon pulmonary angioplasty improves interventricular dyssynchrony in patients with inoperable chronic thromboembolic pulmonary hypertension: a cardiac MR imaging study. Int J Cardiovasc Imaging 2017;33(2):229–39.

40. Kinutani H, Shinke T, Nakayama K, et al. High perfusion pressure as a predictor of reperfusion pulmonary injury after balloon pulmonary angioplasty for chronic thromboembolic pulmonary hypertension. Int J Cardiol Heart Vasc 2016;11:1–6.

41. Ikeda N, Kubota S, Okazaki T, et al. The predictors of complications in balloon pulmonary angioplasty for chronic thromboembolic pulmonary

hypertension. Catheter Cardiovasc Interv 2019; 93(6):E349–56.

42. Kimura M, Kohno T, Kawakami T, et al. Shortening hospital stay is feasible and safe in patients with chronic thromboembolic pulmonary hypertension treated with balloon pulmonary angioplasty. Can J Cardiol 2019;35(2):193–8.

43. Nagao M, Yamasaki Y, Abe K, et al. Energy efficiency and pulmonary artery flow after balloon pulmonary angioplasty for inoperable, chronic thromboembolic pulmonary hypertension: analysis by phase-contrast MRI. Eur J Radiol 2017;87: 99–104.

44. Yokokawa T, Sugimoto K, Nakazato K, et al. Electrocardiographic criteria of right ventricular hypertrophy in patients with chronic thromboembolic pulmonary hypertension after balloon pulmonary angioplasty. Intern Med 2019;58(15):2139–44.

45. Broch K, Murbraech K, Ragnarsson A, et al. Echocardiographic evidence of right ventricular functional improvement after balloon pulmonary angioplasty in chronic thromboembolic pulmonary hypertension. J Heart Lung Transpl 2016;35(1): 80–6.

46. Tatebe S, Sugimura K, Aoki T, et al. Multiple beneficial effects of balloon pulmonary angioplasty in patients with chronic thromboembolic pulmonary hypertension. Circ J 2016;80(4):980–8.

47. Moriyama H, Murata M, Tsugu T, et al. The clinical value of assessing right ventricular diastolic function after balloon pulmonary angioplasty in patients with chronic thromboembolic pulmonary hypertension. Int J Cardiovasc Imaging 2018;34(6):875–82.

48. Kimura M, Kohno T, Kawakami T, et al. Midterm effect of balloon pulmonary angioplasty on hemodynamics and subclinical myocardial damage in chronic thromboembolic pulmonary hypertension. Can J Cardiol 2017;33(4):463–70.

49. Kurzyna M, Darocha S, Pietura R, et al. Changing the strategy of balloon pulmonary angioplasty resulted in a reduced complication rate in patients with chronic thromboembolic pulmonary hypertension. A single-centre European experience. Kardiol Pol 2017;75(7):645–54.

50. Ogo T, Fukuda T, Tsuji A, et al. Efficacy and safety of balloon pulmonary angioplasty for chronic thromboembolic pulmonary hypertension guided by cone-beam computed tomography and electrocardiogram-gated area detector computed tomography. Eur J Radiol 2017;89:270–6.

51. Mizoguchi H, Ogawa A, Munemasa M, et al. Refined balloon pulmonary angioplasty for inoperable patients with chronic thromboembolic pulmonary hypertension. Circ Cardiovasc Interv 2012;5(6): 748–55.

52. Aoki T, Sugimura K, Tatebe S, et al. Comprehensive evaluation of the effectiveness and safety of balloon

pulmonary angioplasty for inoperable chronic thrombo-embolic pulmonary hypertension: long-term effects and procedure-related complications. Eur Heart J 2017;38(42):3152–9.

53. Shimura N, Kataoka M, Inami T, et al. Additional percutaneous transluminal pulmonary angioplasty for residual or recurrent pulmonary hypertension after pulmonary endarterectomy. Int J Cardiol 2015; 183:138–42.

54. Olsson KM, Wiedenroth CB, Kamp J-C, et al. Balloon pulmonary angioplasty for inoperable patients with chronic thromboembolic pulmonary hypertension: the initial German experience. Eur Respir J 2017;49(6). https://doi.org/10.1183/13993003.02409-2016.

55. Inami T, Kataoka M, Ando M, et al. A new era of therapeutic strategies for chronic thromboembolic pulmonary hypertension by two different interventional therapies; pulmonary endarterectomy and percutaneous transluminal pulmonary angioplasty. PLoS One 2014;9(4):e94587.

56. Inami T, Kataoka M, Shimura N, et al. Pressure-wire-guided percutaneous transluminal pulmonary angioplasty: a breakthrough in catheter-interventional therapy for chronic thromboembolic pulmonary hypertension. JACC Cardiovasc Interv 2014;7(11): 1297–306.

57. Ogawa A, Satoh T, Fukuda T, et al. Balloon pulmonary angioplasty for chronic thromboembolic pulmonary hypertension: results of a multicenter registry. Circ Cardiovasc Qual Outcomes 2017;10(11). https://doi.org/10.1161/CIRCOUTCOMES.117.004029.

58. Taniguchi Y, Jaïs X, Jevnikar M, et al. Predictors of survival in patients with not-operated chronic thromboembolic pulmonary hypertension. J Heart Lung Transpl 2019;38(8):833–42.

59. Khan MS, Amin E, Memon MM, et al. Meta-analysis of use of balloon pulmonary angioplasty in patients with inoperable chronic thromboembolic pulmonary hypertension. Int J Cardiol 2019;291:134–9.

60. Wang W, Wen L, Song Z, et al. Balloon pulmonary angioplasty vs riociguat in patients with inoperable chronic thromboembolic pulmonary hypertension: a systematic review and meta-analysis. Clin Cardiol 2019;42(8):741–52.

61. Jais X, Brenot P, Bouvaist H, et al. Late breaking abstract - balloon pulmonary angioplasty versus riociguat for the treatment of inoperable chronic thromboembolic pulmonary hypertension: results from the randomised controlled RACE study. Eur Respir J 2019;54(Suppl 63):RCT1885.

62. Hosokawa K, Abe K, Oi K, et al. Negative acute hemodynamic response to balloon pulmonary angioplasty does not predicate the long-term outcome in patients with chronic thromboembolic pulmonary hypertension. Int J Cardiol 2015;188:81–3.

63. Inami T, Kataoka M, Yanagisawa R, et al. Long-term outcomes after percutaneous transluminal pulmonary angioplasty for chronic thromboembolic pulmonary hypertension. Circulation 2016;134(24):2030–2.

64. Kim NH, Delcroix M, Jais X, et al. Chronic thromboembolic pulmonary hypertension. Eur Respir J 2019; 53(1).

65. Ogo T. Balloon pulmonary angioplasty for inoperable chronic thromboembolic pulmonary hypertension. Curr Opin Pulm Med 2015;21(5):425–31.

66. Coghlan JG, Rothman AM, Hoole SP. Balloon pulmonary angioplasty: state of the art. Interv Cardiol 2020;16:e02.

67. Inohara T, Kawakami T, Kataoka M, et al. Lesion morphological classification by OCT to predict therapeutic efficacy after balloon pulmonary angioplasty in CTEPH. Int J Cardiol 2015;197:23–5.

68. Ogawa A, Kitani M, Mizoguchi H, et al. Pulmonary microvascular remodeling after balloon pulmonary angioplasty in a patient with chronic thromboembolic pulmonary hypertension. Intern Med 2014; 53(7):729–33.

69. Shimokawahara H, Ogawa A, Mizoguchi H, et al. Vessel stretching is a cause of lumen enlargement immediately after balloon pulmonary angioplasty: intravascular ultrasound analysis in patients with chronic thromboembolic pulmonary hypertension. Circ Cardiovasc Interv 2018;11(4):e006010.

70. Magoń W, Stępniewski J, Waligóra M, et al. Virtual histology to evaluate mechanisms of pulmonary artery lumen enlargement in response to balloon pulmonary angioplasty in chronic thromboembolic pulmonary hypertension. J Clin Med 2020;9(6).

71. Kitani M, Ogawa A, Sarashina T, et al. Histological changes of pulmonary arteries treated by balloon pulmonary angioplasty in a patient with chronic thromboembolic pulmonary hypertension. Circ Cardiovasc Interv 2014;7(6):857–9.

72. Magoń W, Stępniewski J, Waligóra M, et al. Pulmonary artery elastic properties after balloon pulmonary angioplasty in patients with inoperable chronic thromboembolic pulmonary hypertension. Can J Cardiol 2019;35(4):422–9.

73. Ejiri K, Ogawa A, Fujii S, et al. Vascular injury is a major cause of lung injury after balloon pulmonary angioplasty in patients with chronic thromboembolic pulmonary hypertension. Circ Cardiovasc Interv 2018;11(12):e005884.

74. Nagayoshi S, Ogawa A, Matsubara H. Spontaneous enlargement of pulmonary artery after successful balloon pulmonary angioplasty in a patient with chronic thromboembolic pulmonary hypertension. EuroIntervention 2016;12(11):e1435.

75. Shimokawahara H, Nagayoshi S, Ogawa A, et al. Continual improvement in pressure gradient at the lesion after balloon pulmonary angioplasty for chronic thromboembolic pulmonary hypertension.

Can J Cardiol 2021. https://doi.org/10.1016/j.cjca.2021.03.009.

76. Wiedenroth CB, Ghofrani HA, Adameit MSD, et al. Sequential treatment with riociguat and balloon pulmonary angioplasty for patients with inoperable chronic thromboembolic pulmonary hypertension. Pulm Circ 2018;8(3). 2045894018783996.

77. Nagayoshi S, Fujii S, Nakajima T, et al. Intravenous ultrasound-guided balloon pulmonary angioplasty in the treatment of totally occluded chronic thromboembolic pulmonary hypertension. EuroIntervention 2018;14(2):234–5.

78. Hosokawa K, Abe K, Oi K, et al. Balloon pulmonary angioplasty-related complications and therapeutic strategy in patients with chronic thromboembolic pulmonary hypertension. Int J Cardiol 2015;197:224–6.

79. Ejiri K, Ogawa A, Matsubara H. Bail-out technique for pulmonary artery rupture with a covered stent in balloon pulmonary angioplasty for chronic thromboembolic pulmonary hypertension. JACC Cardiovasc Interv 2015;8(5):752–3.

Management of Pulmonary Hypertension in the Pediatric Patient

Rebecca Epstein, MD, Usha S. Krishnan, MD, DM (Card)*

KEYWORDS

- Pulmonary hypertension • Pediatric • Diagnosis and management principles

KEY POINTS

- Pediatric pulmonary hypertension (PH), although similar to adult PH, is a unique entity with its own particular pathogeneses, presentation, and management.
- Targeted PH therapies have significantly improved survival in the pediatric PH population in the past 20 years.
- New PH treatments and interventional procedures have shown potential to continue to improve outcomes of children with PH.

INTRODUCTION

Pediatric pulmonary hypertension (PH) is a rare disease with high morbidity and mortality if not diagnosed and treated early. The rarity of sustained pediatric PH has been demonstrated in multiple studies, with an estimated prevalence of 20 to 40 cases per million in Europe. Pulmonary arterial hypertension (PAH), a subset of PH in which the disease is primarily in the precapillary pulmonary arterioles, has a prevalence of 3.0 to 3.7 cases per million children.[1–4]

In the past 20 years, there has been a growing recognition that pediatric PH, although having some similarities to adult PH, is a unique entity with its own particular pathogeneses, presentation, and management.[5,6] Importantly, pediatric PH especially in preterm infants is often a direct sequela of inappropriate lung growth and development and is directly impacted by pulmonary adaptations to fetal and postnatal life. Additional differences between pediatric and adult PH includes their genetic basis, natural history, and responsiveness to PAH-directed therapies.

As experience with adult PAH has grown, targeted PAH therapies have been developed that are increasingly used in younger patients, with sildenafil now approved in children in Europe and bosentan approved for children older than 3 years in the United States. Most of the other medications used in adults including parenteral prostanoids are used in combination therapies for children with significant PAH. Furthermore, interventional strategies like atrial septostomy and reversed Potts shunt in specific patients with severe disease have improved morbidity and mortality.[7,8] Owing to these recent advances, survival of children with PH has significantly improved, with 1-, 5-, and 10-year survivals at 97%, 97%, and 78%.[9] Therapeutic advances have not only increased survival rates but also significantly improved quality of life in children with PAH.[10]

This article reviews the various forms of PH in childhood, with a focus on both established and investigational therapies that are currently available.

DEFINITION AND CLASSIFICATIONS OF PEDIATRIC PULMONARY HYPERTENSION

Pediatric PH is defined as a mean pulmonary artery pressure (mPAP) greater than 20 mm Hg in

Pediatric Cardiology, Columbia University Irving Medical Center, New York Presbyterian Hospital, CHN 2N, #255, 3959 Broadway, New York, NY 10032, USA
* Corresponding author.
E-mail address: usk1@mail.cumc.columbia.edu

Cardiol Clin 40 (2022) 115–127
https://doi.org/10.1016/j.ccl.2021.08.010
0733-8651/22/© 2021 Elsevier Inc. All rights reserved.

cardiology.theclinics.com

children who are at least 3 months of age.[5] PAH, a subset of PH driven by abnormalities in the precapillary arterioles, is defined as an elevated mPAP greater than 20 mm Hg and pulmonary vascular resistance index (PVRi) (>3 Wood units (WU) × m^2) with normal left heart pressures.[11] These definitions, which were published by the 6th World Symposium on Pulmonary Hypertension (WSPH) in 2018,[12] use the cutoff for a normal mPAP of 20 instead of the previously used 25 mm Hg, because mildly increased mPAP (20–24 mm Hg) has been found to independently predict poor survival in adult patients with PH.[13]

The 6th WSPH also refined its universal PH classification system (**Box 2**). This system groups PH into 5 distinct categories, with PAH being group I. As the understanding of the pathobiology of PH has increased, the 6th WSPH made some important changes by expanding the congenital heart disease (CHD) categories, moving hematologic conditions to group V, and also incorporating complex CHD into WSPH Group V PH, which includes PH with unclear and/or multifactorial mechanisms.[12]

The Pulmonary Vascular Research Institute (PVRI) Pediatric Task Force recognizing the multifactorial cause of childhood PH updated the definition and classification system for pediatric PH.[14] The PVRI Task Force also noted that patients with single ventricle physiology and passive pulmonary blood flow can have pulmonary vascular disease even without an elevated mPAP and benefit from further lowering the pulmonary arterial pressures (PAP). Children with cavopulmonary anastomoses are therefore considered to have pulmonary hypertensive vascular disease if the PVRi is greater than 3 WU × m^2 or the transpulmonary gradient is greater than 6 mm Hg, even with normal PAPs by conventional definition.[14]

EPIDEMIOLOGY AND CAUSE

Epidemiologic data regarding pediatric PH are largely derived from PH registries. Although there are multiple adult PAH registries, including the REVEAL [Registry to Evaluate Early and Long-term PAH Disease Management][15] and COMPERA [Prospective Registry of Newly Initiated Therapies for Pulmonary Hypertension][16] registries, such robust data collection systems did not initially exist for children. Nonetheless, in the past several years new pediatric PH databases have been developed including the TOPP [Tracking Outcomes and Practice in Pediatric Pulmonary Hypertension] registry, which includes 31 centers from 19 countries[17]; the PPHNet [National Pediatric Pulmonary Hypertension Network], composed of 14 pediatric PH

centers in North America and Canada; the Pediatric & Congenital Heart Disease Taskforce of the Pulmonary Vascular Research Institute; and the Spanish Registry of Pediatric Pulmonary Hypertension (REHIPED).

A critical difference between pediatric and adult PH noted in a large comprehensive Netherlands study was the high incidence of "transient" PH in children (87%), which is due to either a repairable cardiac shunt or persistent PH of the newborn.[2] Although the incidence of all types of pediatric PH, including "transient" PH is 63.7 cases/million children/year, the prevalence of sustained PH is about 20 to 40 cases per million in Europe, and the prevalence of PAH is 3.0 to 3.7 cases/million children.[1–4]

In the TOPP registry, the vast majority (88%) of children with PH had PAH (group I), whereas the remaining patients (12%) had PH from respiratory disease such as bronchopulmonary dysplasia (group III). Of the children with PAH, 57% had PAH that was idiopathic (IPAH) or familial (FPAH) and 43% had associated PAH (APAH) in the presence of other disorders like CHD or rheumatologic conditions.

The median age of pediatric PH diagnosis is 7 years, and registries have reported a gender distribution of about 1:1 females:males,[3,4] suggesting a more equal gender distribution in pediatric PH than in adult PH wherein the ratio is closer to 4:1.[18]

Although the cause of pediatric PH is often multifactorial, the genes encoding the transforming growth factor beta/bone morphogenetic protein (TGF-β/BMP) signaling pathway have been linked to the development of PH. This pathway plays an important role in embryonic heart development and systemic vasculogenesis, and mutations in this pathway have been identified in about 80% of children with FPAH and 20% of children with IPAH.[19–21] The genetics of pediatric PH also differs from that of adult PH in the higher incidence of TBX4 mutations and other novel genes in up to 19% of childhood PH.[22,23]

PATHOGENESIS AND PATHOBIOLOGY OF PEDIATRIC PULMONARY HYPERTENSION

The pathogenesis of pediatric PH is complex and heterogeneous. Nevertheless, there are several mechanisms that are fundamental to the development of PH, such as pulmonary vasoconstriction, endothelial dysfunction, cell proliferation with growth dysregulation, inflammation, and in situ thrombosis. These mechanisms must be intimately understood, because they form the basis for targeted therapy in this population.

Vasoconstriction

Pulmonary vasoconstriction and an imbalance in tissue vasoactive mediators has long been recognized as a critical component of PH. In neonates with pediatric PH, the pulmonary vasculature fails to relax as it normally does in transitioning from fetal to neonatal life, and this elevated pulmonary vascular resistance can become fixed as the vasculature itself thickens. In addition, there is a reduction in arteriolar number and vascular surface area. In contrast, older children with IPAH tend to have smooth muscle cell (SMC) hypertrophy that causes vasoconstriction and usually have less of the plexiform lesions and intimal fibrosis that are typically seen in adult PH. Of note, molecular pathways that are crucial in development of all forms of vasoconstriction are the nitric oxide (NO) pathway, prostacyclin pathway, and endothelin pathway.

- NO pathway: NO is produced in the endothelium by endothelial NO synthetase (eNOS) and stimulates production of cyclic GMP (cGMP), which is a potent vasodilator and has antiproliferative properties.[24,25] The bioavailability of endothelial NO is decreased in many forms of PAH, and there is often increased production of the phosphodiesterase 5 (PDE 5) enzyme, which degrades cGMP. Asymmetric dimethyl arginine, which is elevated in many forms of PAH, acts by the inhibition of eNOS and via direct effects on gene expression.
- Prostacyclin (PGI2) pathway: PGI2 induces smooth muscle relaxation and prevents platelet aggregation via cyclic AMP production. In patients with PAH, there is a disruption between the balance of PGI2 and vasoactive hormones, which leads to vasoconstriction.
- Endothelin pathway: Endothelin-1 (ET-1) leads to vasoconstriction, fibrogenesis, and cell proliferation and acts via ETA and ETB receptors in the SMC. ET-1 levels are increased in lung tissue and circulation in IPAH, in APAH secondary to lung disease and thromboembolism, as well as in patients with congenital diaphragmatic hernia. ET-1 has been shown to act on SMCs to cause vasoconstriction, cell proliferation, and fibrogenesis.[26]

Endothelial Dysfunction

The endothelium of the pulmonary vasculature helps to produce growth factors and cell signals and is critical in maintaining homeostasis and vascular tone.[27] The triggers of endothelial dysfunction in the patient with PH are not fully understood, but there is often abnormal endothelial activation that causes release of vasoproliferative agents (which promote vascular hyperplasia), as well as vasoconstrictive substances (which lead to worsening vascular obstruction).

Cell Proliferation and Apoptosis

In PH, the smooth muscle and endothelial cells of the pulmonary vasculature are more susceptible to apoptosis, migration, and inappropriate proliferation. There are various growth factors that are abnormally elevated in patients with PAH and play a role in this improper balance, such as vascular endothelial growth factor, tumor necrosis factor-α, and platelet-derived growth factor. Mutations in BMPR2, ALK-1, and endoglin lead to vascular remodeling and are potential pathways for therapeutic intervention.

Inflammation

Inflammation is a known trigger in PAH as evidenced by an increase in cytokines, interleukins, and chemokines[28]; this is most often seen in rheumatological diseases where a rheumatic flare can trigger a PH crisis as well and only subsides with appropriate therapy for the underlying condition. Likewise in childhood PH, especially in preterm infants, lung or systemic infection and inflammation trigger worsening PH and improve with resolution of the inflammatory trigger.

PRESENTATION

Children with PH typically present with exertional dyspnea, fatigue, and failure to thrive. Symptoms are often nonspecific and may be attributed to more common childhood disorders before PH is diagnosed. Syncope especially immediately after exercising or early in the morning just after waking is more common in childhood- (25%) versus adult-onset PH (12%)[17] and may be due to children's increased sensitivity to vasoconstrictive triggers and may actually indicate a vasoresponsive phenotype in selected patients. Patients with unrepaired CHD are less likely to present with syncope but do become more cyanotic with activity or even at rest, because they use cardiac shunts as a "pop-off" for right-to-left blood flow during PH crises. In advanced PH, children may develop right ventricular (RV) failure and subsequent fluid congestion and retention with symptoms of hepatomegaly, peripheral edema, ascites, and even malabsorption due to intestinal wall edema.

PATIENT EVALUATION AND DIAGNOSIS

The diagnostic workup for pediatric PH is similar to that of adults (Fig. 1) and begins with a thorough

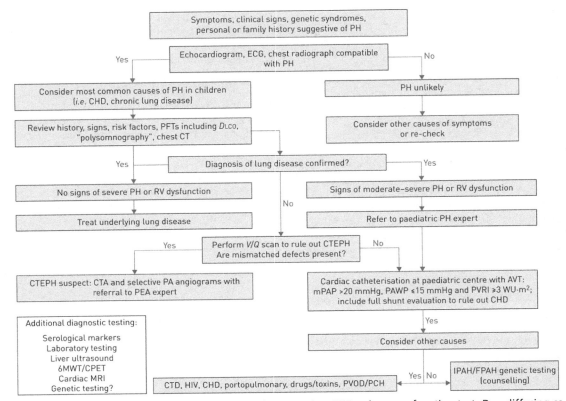

Fig. 1. Diagnostic workup for pediatric pulmonary hypertension. PFT, pulmonary function test; D_{LCO}, diffusing capacity of the lung for carbon monoxide; CT, computed tomography; V/Q, ventilation/perfusion; CTEPH, chronic thromboembolic PH; CTA, CT angiography; PA, pulmonary artery; PEA, pulmonary endarterectomy; AVT, acute vasodilator testing; PAWP, pulmonary arterial wedge pressure; PVRi, pulmonary vascular resistance index; WU, Wood units; 6MWT, 6-minute walk test; CPET, cardiopulmonary exercise test; CTD, connective tissue disease; PVOD, pulmonary veno-occlusive disease; PCH, pulmonary capillary hemangiomatosis. *Reproduced with* permission of the © ERS 2021: European Respiratory Journal 53 (1) 1801916; DOI: 10.1183/13993003.01916- 2018, published January 24, 2019.

individual and family history, physical examination, laboratory tests, genetic evaluation, echocardiography, and ultimately invasive hemodynamic studies. In the initial evaluation of a child with PH, it is also critical to assess for other treatable disorders that may cause PAH and to check for any systemic end-organ injury from PAH such as renal and liver dysfunction.

History and Physical Examination

In addition to obtaining a comprehensive review of systems and complete family history, physicians must pay close attention to a child's growth curve, because failure to thrive and growth retardation can be important signs of chronic disease and right heart failure. A pediatric functional classification system proposed by the PVRI Pediatric Task Force in 2011 takes into account age-related

activity and exercise capacity and can be used as part of the clinical evaluation.[29] Vital signs on examination will often show tachypnea and tachycardia, and patients may have decreased oxygen saturation if an intracardiac "pop-off" shunt is present.

On cardiac examination, palpation may reveal a RV heave (from elevated RV pressure), a RV S3 gallop, and a widened second heart sound with a loud pulmonary component and an early systolic click from the dilated pulmonary artery (PA) may be auscultated. Multiple different murmurs may be heard, including a systolic ejection murmur over the dilated PAs, an early diastolic murmur from pulmonary insufficiency at the right upper sternal border, or a systolic murmur at the right lower sternal border if tricuspid regurgitation (TR) is present. If there is severe PH, intracardiac shunts will not generate a murmur because there is no significant pressure gradient between the right and left ventricles. If there is RV failure, hepatomegaly, ascites, and edema can be present.

Echocardiography

Echocardiography plays a critical role in the diagnosis and monitoring of PH and can be used to check for associated structural heart disease, evaluate cardiac function, risk stratification, and to monitor PAP.

As the RV pressure increases, echocardiography will show ventricular septal flattening and posterior systolic bowing into the left ventricle with systemic or suprasystemic RV pressures (**Fig. 2**). The RV systolic function is difficult to assess because of its complex geometry, but various measures are used to assess for RV dysfunction including tricuspid annular plane systolic excursion, Tei index (which includes both systolic and diastolic time intervals to assess the global cardiac dysfunction), RV fractional area change, and RV ejection fraction.[30] The left ventricular systolic function is typically preserved, although it too can show signs of diastolic dysfunction especially when there is posterior systolic bowing of the ventricular septum. Diastolic dysfunction of the ventricles can be quantified by mitral and tricuspid diastolic inflow velocities, pulmonary and systemic venous flow patterns, RV myocardial performance index, and tissue Doppler imaging of the mitral and tricuspid annulus and at the septum.

RV systolic pressure can be determined by measuring the peak systolic pressure gradient from the RV to the right atrium and is calculated by using the Bernoulli equation $P = 4 \, v^2$, where v is the maximum velocity of the TR jet measured by continuous wave Doppler. Assuming there is no obstruction between the RV to the PA, the TR jet can also be used to estimate the PA pressure and severity of PH (see **Fig. 2**). Clinicians, however, will often rely on additional echocardiographic findings that are suggestive of PH, such as ventricular septal position and motion, systemic to pulmonary shunt gradients at the ventricular or great artery levels, and pulmonary regurgitation Doppler gradients, because there may not be an adequate TR Doppler envelope to estimate pressures and TR jet velocity can overestimate or underestimate the PA pressure especially with nonsedated echocardiograms.[31,32] Of note, echocardiography protocols are available for the pediatric patient with PH (**Box 1**)[33] and should be used for both diagnosis and long-term monitoring of children with PH.

Cardiac Catheterization

Right heart catheterization is considered the gold standard for diagnosing PH and allows for direct measurement of PA pressure and PVR. In 2019, the 6th WSPH modified their criteria for adult PH to include a mean PA pressure greater than 20 mm Hg and a PVR 3 WU[12] or more, and the pediatric task force adopted these criteria as well.[5] Inclusion of PVR in the definition of pediatric PH is particularly useful because, as discussed previously, many children with single ventricle physiology can have normal PA pressures but even mildly elevated pulmonary vascular resistances can lead to severe physiologic consequences and Fontan failure.

During cardiac catheterization, acute vasodilator testing (AVT) (usually with inhaled NO [iNO]) should also be performed. Other medications including inhaled prostanoids have also been used for AVT but are not standardized. AVT responsiveness in adults is defined as a decrease

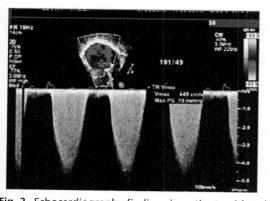
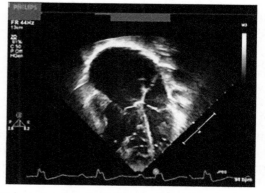

Fig. 2. Echocardiography findings in patients with pulmonary hypertension. (*Left*) Echocardiography continuous wave Doppler imaging across the tricuspid valve showing measurements of the tricuspid valve regurgitation jet using the Bernoulli principle. (*Right*) Apical 4-chamber imaging showing a dilated right atrium and right ventricle, with bowing of the atrial and ventricular septum to the left.

Box 1
Transthoracic echocardiography protocol in pediatric patients with pulmonary hypertension

Variables to be assessed
Estimation of the systolic PAP through the TR jet velocity by CW Doppler
Estimation of mean PAP and end diastolic PAP through CW Doppler of the PR jet
PAAT
RV longitudinal systolic function (eg, TAPSE)
RV fractional area change
RV strain and strain rate measurements
RV systolic to diastolic duration ratio by CW Doppler of the TR jet
Tissue Doppler velocities (eg, E', A' and S')
RV myocardial performance (Tei) index
RV/LV diameter ratio
LV EI (Eccentricity Index)

RV and RA enlargement.
   CW, continuous wave; LV, left ventricle; PR, pulmonary regurgita; RA, right atrium; S', peak systolic velocity; TAPSE, tricuspid annular plane systolic excursion; TR, tricuspid regurgitation; TTE, transthoracic echocardiography; PAAT, pulmonary artery acceleration time; LV EI, left ventricular eccentricity index.
   Note: TTE alone is not sufficient to initiate a targeted therapy.

Koestenberger M, Friedberg MK, Nestaas E, et al. Transthoracic echocardiography in the evaluation of pediatric pulmonary hypertension and ventricular dysfunction. Pulm Circ. 2016;6(1):15–29. https://doi.org/10.1086/68505. © Sage Publications Ltd. 2021. Reprinted by permission of SAGE publications.

Box 2
Updated clinical classification of pulmonary hypertension

1 PAH
1.1 Idiopathic PAH
1.2 Heritable PAH
1.3 Drug- and toxin-induced PAH
1.4 PAH associated with
1.4.1 Connective tissue disease
1.4.2 HIV infection
1.4.3 Portal hypertension
1.4.4 Congenital heart disease
1.4.5 Schistosomiasis
1.5 PAH long-term responders to calcium channel blockers
1.6 PAH with overt features of venous/capillaries (PVOD/PCH) involvement
1.7 Persistent PH of the newborn syndrome
2 PH due to left heart disease
2.1 PH due to heart failure with preserved LVEF
2.2 PH due to heart failure with reduced LVEF
2.3 Valvular heart disease
2.4 Congenital/acquired cardiovascular conditions leading to postcapillary PH
3 PH due to lung diseases and/or hypoxia
3.1 Obstructive lung disease
3.2 Restrictive lung disease
3.3 Other lung disease with mixed restrictive/obstructive pattern
3.4 Hypoxia without lung disease
3.5 Developmental lung disorders
4 PH due to pulmonary artery obstructions
4.1 Chronic thromboembolic PH
4.2 Other pulmonary artery obstructions
5 PH with unclear and/or multifactorial mechanisms
5.1 Hematological disorders
5.2 Systemic and metabolic disorders
5.3 Others
5.4 Complex congenital heart disease

LVEF, left ventricular ejection fraction; PCH, pulmonary capillary hemangiomatosis; PVOD, pulmonary veno-occlusive disease.

Reproduced with permission of the © ERS 2021: European Respiratory Journal 53(1) 180193; DOI 10. 1183/13993003.01913-2018, published January 24, 2019.

---

in mPAP by at least 10 mm Hg to a value of less than 40 mm Hg with sustained cardiac output, or in subjects with baseline mPAP less than 40 mm Hg as a drop of at least 10 mm Hg without a decrease in cardiac output.[5] This definition has been shown to successfully identify patients who will have sustained benefit from calcium channel blocker (CCB) therapy with much better long-term outcomes and should therefore be used in pediatric population as well.[34] In fact, the 6th WSPH have included these patients as a separate category WSPH, group 1.5 (see **Box 2**).

The 6-Minute Walk Test and Cardiopulmonary Exercise Testing

The 6-minute walk test is useful to assess functional capacity, monitor response to therapy, and predict outcomes. Using an actigraph, or a noninvasive monitor of patients' activity levels, provides a continuous real-time monitoring tool and is an attractive option for evaluating activity in patients with PH.[35] Cardiopulmonary exercise testing is another testing modality that has been shown to provide cardiorespiratory parameters that correlate with the degree of pulmonary vascular resistance and disease severity in children[36,37] and can reliably be performed in patients who are at least 7 years old. These tests are performed at 3- to 6-month intervals to guide response to therapy and indicate further interventions or escalation.

Risk Assessment

Risk assessment scores have been available for adult PH; however, it is only recently that the

European Society of Cardiology/European Respiratory Society guidelines and the 6th WSPH proceedings recommended risk scoring for pediatric PAH using the REVEAL registry and the European registries. Pediatric patients with PH had lower median risk scores when compared with adults, but 1-year survival for each risk group was similar to adults, although they separated at 5 years.[38]

TREATMENT

Although there is no uniform therapeutic approach for all children with PH, various treatments have been developed that can improve the survival of pediatric patients with PH.[39,40] As most children with PH have some degree of precapillary PAH, targeted therapies discussed later are geared toward the pediatric patient with PAH. A synopsis of the guidelines specifically for pediatric IPAH/FPAH management is outlined in **Fig. 3** and is reviewed in further depth in the following sections (along with general PAH treatment).

GENERAL MEASURES AND THE PRIMARY CARE PHYSICIAN

Managing children with PH is a team effort with the pediatrician playing an important role. Any fevers should be treated early with antipyretics, to decrease the metabolic demands on an already tenuous cardiorespiratory system. Respiratory infections, which are quite common in children, can

trigger hypoxemia and a PH crisis if not treated aggressively. Some children may require iNO during an acute respiratory illness if they are hospitalized with severe PH. Decongestants containing pseudoephedrine are contraindicated because they can worsen PH symptoms, but antitussives are sometimes used especially if there is a risk of coughing-induced hemoptysis. Annual influenza and pneumococcal vaccines should be provided for primary prevention of respiratory illnesses. Coronavirus disease 2019 vaccination is recommended in children with PH older than 16 years, and currently clinical trials are underway in younger children.

It is also important that pediatricians provide dietary recommendations and even medical therapy to prevent constipation, because straining with bowel movements can decrease venous return to the right side of the heart and can cause a syncopal event. A thorough psychosocial evaluation and close follow-up is highly recommended to identify and manage issues that may impact the quality of life of these fragile patients.

Several goals of targeted therapy for PAH are as follows:

1. Improvement of symptoms and quality of life
2. Improvement of hemodynamics
3. Halting progression of disease
4. Reversal of established pulmonary vascular disease and cardiac hypertrophy (if possible)
5. Reduction of morbidity
6. Increasing life expectancy with the disease

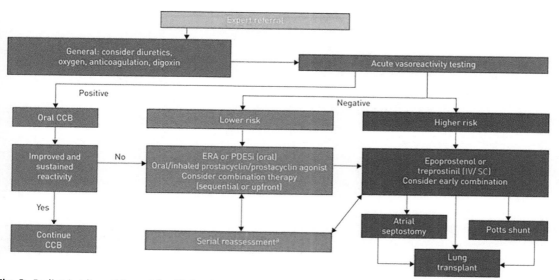

Fig. 3. Pediatric idiopathic and familial pulmonary arterial hypertension treatment algorithm. ERA, endothelin receptor antagonist; PDE5i, phosphodiesterase type 5 inhibitor; IV, intravenous; SC, subcutaneous. [a]Deterioration or not meeting treatment goals. Reproduced with permission of the © ERS 2021: European Respiratory Journal 53 (1) 1801916; DOI: 10.1183/13993003.01916- 2018, published January 24, 2019.

Medical Therapy

Calcium channel blockade

CCBs, which prevent calcium influx into smooth and cardiac muscles, have been shown to be potent pulmonary vasodilators for patients who are "responders" to AVT. Only 5% to 10% of adults with PAH are considered AVT "responders,"[41] whereas some studies have suggested that the response rate in children may be as high as 40%,[9] although other research has not shown such a difference in vasoreactivity.[42] Of note, children with CHD are significantly less likely be AVT responsive, and therefore CCBs often do not help improve PAH in this subgroup.[42] CCBs are only used in children older than 1 year and are contraindicated in AVT nonresponders.

The optimal dosing of CCBs in children has not been established. Studies typically report using relatively high doses of CCBs, such as amlodipine 20 to 40 mg daily and long-acting nifedipine 120 to 240 mg daily, but the optimal dosing of drugs in pediatric PAH is still unknown.

Nitric oxide

inhaled Nitric Oxide (iNO) causes smooth muscle relaxation of the pulmonary vasculature by activating guanylate cyclase and increasing cGMP.[24] iNO may also prevent platelet adhesion to arterial walls via its antiproliferative effect on smooth muscle. iNO in doses of 1 to 20 ppm is used in a multitude of scenarios including treatment of an acute PAH crisis, following cardiac surgery, during right heart catheterization for AVT, and for treatment of persistent PH in the newborn.[43] Weaning iNO has to be done carefully in a carefully monitored intensive care unit setting and often may need to be weaned in fractions of 1 ppm to prevent rebound PH. Sildenafil has been used especially in the postoperative setting as a cGMP donor while weaning off iNO.[44]

Phosphodiesterase inhibitors

Like NO, phosphodiesterase 5 (PDE5) inhibitors cause pulmonary vasodilation by increasing cGMP levels in smooth muscle. PDE5 inhibitors were initially used in patients being weaned off iNO postoperatively,[44] but now they are often first-line therapy along with other medications in treatment of PAH. PDE5 inhibitors have been shown to improve symptoms in pediatric patients with PH, both when used alone and when they are administered as part of combination therapy with prostacyclins.[45,46]

The STARTS-1 trial, a double-blind, multicenter, placebo-controlled study, showed that the PDE5 inhibitor sildenafil improved the functional class and maximal aerobic capacity of pediatric patients with PAH patients.[47] Although its extension study,

the STARTS-2 trial, found that children randomized to higher doses of sildenafil had increased mortality, all sildenafil groups (including the high-dose sildenafil group) had increased survival compared with placebo.[48] Because increased sildenafil dosing was associated with increased mortality, the US Food and Drug Administration (FDA) in 2012 initially advised that chronic sildenafil use was "not recommended in children," but later revised their recommendations to state that there "may be situations in which the risk-benefit profile" of sildenafil "may be acceptable in individual children but should only be administered under expert guidance."[49] Based on the STARTS trial data, sildenafil was approved for use in Europe by the European Medicines Agency.

Sildenafil is typically administered 3 times a day and is enterally dosed as 1 mg/kg per dose in infants, 10 mg for children weighing 10 to 20 kg, and 20 mg per dose for children weighing greater than 20 kg. The intravenous dose is half of the enteral dose. Sildenafil is usually slowly uptitrated to reach the final dose to prevent hypotension and monitor for other side effects. Tadalafil, a newer PDE5 inhibitor, is an attractive alternative to sildenafil, because it is dosed once a day with a similar side effect profile.[50]

Endothelin receptor antagonists

Endothelin-1 (ET-1) is a potent pulmonary vasoconstrictor that is elevated in many patients with PAH, and its level inversely correlates with prognosis. Bosentan, an oral endothelin receptor antagonist (ERA), is now FDA approved in children older than 3 years in the United States. An open-label study in children with group I PAH showed bosentan to be well tolerated and improve hemodynamics at 12-week follow-up.[51,52] Side effects of bosentan include hepatotoxicity and teratogenicity. Bosentan is given at 1 mg/kg per dose twice a day and increased to 2 mg/kg per dose after 2 to 4 weeks, while monitoring liver enzymes. Patients on stable bosentan doses require monthly liver function testing, and postmenarchal girls require monthly pregnancy testing and dual contraception, to prevent teratogenicity of the medication. Ambrisentan is a selective ERA that has been associated with less hepatoxicity and can be administered once daily.[53] Macitentan, a tissue-specific ERA, is now undergoing trials in the pediatric age group.[54] All ERAs are known to be teratogenic in animal studies and hence have the same pregnancy testing and dual contraception instructions.

Prostacyclins

The discovery of prostacyclin's pulmonary vasodilatory effects in the early 1990s revolutionized the medical management of PAH, because its use significantly improved survival and quality of life. Importantly, prostacyclins show a survival benefit even in patients who are unresponsive to AVT, implying that prostacyclin is not only a pulmonary vasodilator but possibly promotes pulmonary vascular remodeling as well.

Epoprostenol, an intravenous prostacyclin, can be chronically administered and has been shown to prolong survival, improve cardiac output, increase exercise capacity, positively alter hemodynamics, and prolong survival in children with PAH.[55,56] Epoprostenol dosing (ng/kg/min) is slowly uptitrated starting at 1 to 2 ng/kg/min to over 100 ng/kg/min.

Because epoprostenol has a very short half-life of 1 to 2 minutes and is chemically unstable at room temperature, it must be delivered using a continuous infusion system with cold packs and a central venous line is typically needed. This form of drug administration is associated with its own challenges including clots and line occlusion, catheter and systemic infection, and pump malfunction, which can either lead to an inadvertent bolus (causing systemic hypotension) or interruption (causing rebound PAH) of epoprostenol. These difficulties have led to a search for alternative forms of prostacyclin that would allow for oral, inhaled, subcutaneous, or long-acting intravenous delivery.

Prostacyclin analogues

Treprostinil sodium can be administered both subcutaneously and intravenously, and in its subcutaneous form the complications of having a central venous line can be avoided. Recent research has described the successful use of subcutaneous treprostinil in young children.[57] Discomfort at the infusion site has been reported, although no other serious side effects related to subcutaneous treprostinil have been noted.[58] Infusion site pain has been noted to be lower in infants when compared with older patients.[57]

Oral prostacyclin analogues Oral treprostinil was approved by the US FDA in 2013 for use in adults with PAH. Although treprostinil has been shown to improve exercise capacity in PAH,[59] it has a significant side effect profile including headaches and gastrointestinal symptoms, and a recent pediatric study found that half of children who were initiated on the drug had stopped it within 2 years mostly because of its side effects.[60]

Other oral prostacyclin analogues include beraprost sodium, which has been approved for PAH in Japan but not in the Europe and the United States, and oral selexipag, a prostacyclin receptor agonist

that has also been shown to decrease the risk of PAH complications and death.[61,62]

Inhaled prostacyclin analogues Inhaled prostacyclins are an attractive choice for prostacyclin administration, because their selective delivery to the lungs avoids more systemic side effects. Direct airway delivery is also thought to cause less V-Q mismatch. Inhaled iloprost has a short half-life of 20 to 25 minutes and must be given every 1 to 4 hours,[43] whereas inhaled treprostinil with its longer half-life can be administered every 6 hours and has been shown to improve exercise capacity and is safe and well tolerated in the pediatric population.[63]

Combination therapy

Similar to cancer therapy experience, combination therapy to target multiple pathways simultaneously has shown benefit in PH therapy. The AMBITION trial demonstrated that the risk of clinical failure was 50% lower in adults on a combination of ambrisentan and tadalafil when compared with monotherapy using either drug.[45] A recent pediatric study including patients with PAH from two US and one European center demonstrated that treatment with combination therapy was strongly associated with improved survival when compared with monotherapy.[39]

Anticoagulation

The role of chronic anticoagulation in pediatric patients with PAH is based on recent adult IPAH studies, which have demonstrated that many adults with IPAH have small PA thromboses on lung pathology. Although the adult COMPERA registry suggested that anticoagulation in adult patients with IPAH is associated with improved survival,[64] the REVEAL registry concluded that anticoagulation is not advantageous and can in certain scenarios even worsen survival.[65] As there is no research to support use of anticoagulation in pediatric PAH, it is currently only used in children with coagulation disorders, significant ventricular systolic dysfunction, thromboembolic PH, and those patients with indwelling lines or minipumps to prevent line occlusion via clot formation.

Novel therapies, ongoing clinical trials, and investigational drugs

Antiproliferative drugs Early PAH management had focused on medications that would cause pulmonary vasodilation. In the last 10 years, however, we have learned that additional pathobiologic mechanisms are involved in PH, including unbridled cell proliferation in the smooth muscle and adventitia of PAs. Some newer PH medications, which were borrowed from the oncology world, target this mechanism. Imatinib, a tyrosine kinase inhibitor that is used to treat chronic myeloid leukemia, inhibits a growth factor receptor on SMCs and has shown early signs of improving symptoms in adults with advanced PAH.[66] Everolimus is another antineoplastic drug, which is an mTOR inhibitor, and in pilot studies has improved PVR and exercise tolerance in children with PAH.[67] Sirolimus has been studied in children with pulmonary vein stenosis in an attempt to halt the progression of disease.[68]

Rho-Kinase inhibitors The RhoA-/Rho-kinase signaling pathway effects vasorelaxation, and when activated can cause sustained SMC contraction. Studies show that drugs that block the rho-kinase pathway, like fasudil, can decrease PAPs in animals with PAH that is refractory to prostanoids and iNO, although this has not been reproduced in humans.[69,70]

Gene therapy With new understanding of the genetic basis of PAH, research has also turned to gene replacement as possible therapy for PAH. Advances in genetic therapy may ultimately hold the key to early detection and perhaps even cure for specific children with known genetic mutations, such as the 2q33 (TGF-β receptor) mutation associated with HPAH and IPAH.[71]

Interventional Therapy

Atrial septostomy
In children with severe PH, an atrial communication allows cardiac output to be maintained via right to left shunting even during a PH crisis. Thus, patients who have PAH with right heart failure or recurrent syncope, but do not have a patent foramen ovale, can benefit clinically and hemodynamically from an atrial septostomy.[8,72] This procedure has been shown to increase survival (1- and 2-year survival is 87% and 76%, respectively, compared with 64% and 42% using conventional therapy alone).

This invasive procedure is associated with significant risks and is usually only performed in patients with syncope or right heart failure despite maximal medical therapy, and potentially as a bridge to transplantation.

Potts shunt
A reverse Potts shunt, which allows for right to left flow from the left PA to the descending aorta, can also help to decompress the RV in the setting of significant PH and can improve hemodynamics and outcomes in the severely ill child.[7,73–77] Unidirectional valved Potts shunts can be used to minimize left to right flow across the shunt when pulmonary pressures drop.[76] A transcatheter approach for placement of the Potts shunt has been suggested as a possible option as well.[77] Use of Potts shunt may improve quality of life as well as survival to transplant.

Lung transplantation
A small number of centers perform pediatric lung transplantation for patients with PAH. Survival rates for patients with PAH who have undergone lung transplantation are quite low: the 1-year, 5-year, and 10-year survivals are 64%, 44%, and 20%, respectively.[78,79] Transplantation should therefore be considered for children who are World Health Organization functional class IV despite maximal medical therapy, and ideally children should be listed when their probability of 2-year survival is less than 50%. Extracorporeal membrane oxygenation, either as a bridge to recovery or to transplant, can also be a feasible option in certain patients.

SUMMARY

Owing to recent advances in PH therapy, children with PH have significantly improved survival, hemodynamics, and quality of life. Patients who are responsive to AVT benefit from CCBs, whereas nonresponsive patients can be assisted with prostanoids and ERAs. Multiple new treatments are on the horizon and have shown promise in adult PAH populations. As our understanding of the genetic basis and pathobiologic mechanisms of PH continue to evolve, we hope that in the future we will be able to better treat, and potentially cure, this disease.

DISCLOSURE

The authors have nothing to disclose.

REFERENCES

1. Fraisse A, Jais X, Schleich JM, et al. Characteristics and prospective 2-year follow-up of children with pulmonary arterial hypertension in France. Arch Cardiovasc Dis 2010;103(2):66–74.
2. Van Loon L, Roofthooft M, Hillege HL, et al. Pediatric Pulmonary Hypertension in the Netherlands Epidemiology and Characterization During the Period 1991 to 2005. 2011. doi:10.1161/CIRCULATIONAHA.
3. Li L, Jick S, Breitenstein S, et al. Pulmonary arterial hypertension in the USA: an epidemiological study in a large insured pediatric population. Pulm Circ 2017;7(1):126–36.
4. Marín MJDC, Rotés AS, Ogando AR, et al. Assessing pulmonary hypertensive vascular disease in

childhood data from the Spanish registry. Am J Respir Crit Care Med 2014;190(12):1421–9.

5. Rosenzweig EB, Abman SH, Adatia I, et al. Paediatric pulmonary arterial hypertension: updates on definition, classification, diagnostics and management. Eur Respir J 2019;53(1). https://doi.org/10.1183/13993003.01916-2018.

6. Simonneau G, Montani D, Celermajer DS, et al. Haemodynamic definitions and updated clinical classification of pulmonary hypertension. Eur Respir J 2019;53(1). https://doi.org/10.1183/13993003.01913-2018.

7. Baruteau AE, Serraf A, Lévy M, et al. Potts shunt in children with idiopathic pulmonary arterial hypertension: long-term results. Ann Thorac Surg 2012;94(3):817–24.

8. Micheletti A, Hislop AA, Lammers A, et al. Role of atrial septostomy in the treatment of children with pulmonary arterial hypertension. Heart 2006;92(7):969–72.

9. Yung D, Widlitz AC, Rosenzweig EB, et al. Outcomes in children with idiopathic pulmonary arterial hypertension. Circulation 2004;110(6):660–5.

10. Mullen MP, Andrus J, Labella MH, et al. Quality of life and parental Adjustment in pediatric pulmonary hypertension. Chest 2014;145(2). https://doi.org/10.1378/chest.13-0636.

11. Hansmann G, Koestenberger M, Alastalo TP, et al. 2019 Updated consensus statement on the diagnosis and treatment of pediatric pulmonary hypertension: the European Pediatric Pulmonary Vascular Disease Network (EPPVDN), endorsed by AEPC, ESPR and ISHLT. J Hear Lung Transpl 2019;38(9):879–901.

12. Galiè N, McLaughlin VV, Rubin LJ, et al. An overview of the 6th World Symposium on pulmonary hypertension. Eur Respir J 2019;53(1). https://doi.org/10.1183/13993003.02148-2018.

13. Douschan P, Kovacs G, Avian A, et al. Mild elevation of pulmonary arterial pressure as a predictor of mortality. Am J Respir Crit Care Med 2018;197(4):509–16.

14. Del Cerro MJ, Abman S, Diaz G, et al. A consensus approach to the classification of pediatric pulmonary hypertensive vascular disease: report from the PVRI pediatric taskforce, Panama 2011. Pulm Circ 2011;1(2):286–98.

15. Benza RL, Miller DP, Gomberg-Maitland M, et al. Predicting survival in pulmonary arterial hypertension: Insights from the registry to evaluate early and long-term pulmonary arterial hypertension disease management (REVEAL). Circulation 2010;122(2):164–72.

16. Hoeper MM, Pausch C, Grünig E, et al. Idiopathic pulmonary arterial hypertension phenotypes determined by cluster analysis from the COMPERA registry. J Hear Lung Transpl 2020;39(12):1435–44.

17. Berger RMF, Beghetti M, Humpl T, et al. Clinical features of paediatric pulmonary hypertension: a registry study. Lancet 2012;379(9815):537–46.

18. Badesch DB, Raskob GE, Elliott CG, et al. Pulmonary arterial hypertension: baseline Characteristics from the REVEAL registry. Chest 2010;137(2). https://doi.org/10.1378/chest.09-1140.

19. Zhu N, Welch CL, Wang J, et al. Rare variants in SOX17 are associated with pulmonary arterial hypertension with congenital heart disease. Genome Med 2018;10(1). https://doi.org/10.1186/s13073-018-0566-x.

20. Levy M, Eyries M, Szezepanski I, et al. Genetic analyses in a cohort of children with pulmonary hypertension. Eur Respir J 2016;48(4):1118–26.

21. Pfarr N, Fischer C, Ehlken N, et al. Hemodynamic and genetic Analysis in children with idiopathic, Heritable, and congenital heart disease associated pulmonary arterial hypertension. Respir Res 2013;14(1):3. https://doi.org/10.1186/1465-9921-14-3.

22. Zhu N, Gonzaga-Jauregui C, Welch CL, et al. Exome Sequencing in children with pulmonary arterial hypertension Demonstrates differences compared with adults. Circ Genomic Precis Med 2018;11(4):e001887.

23. Kerstjens-Frederikse WS, Bongers EMHF, Roofthooft MTR, et al. TBX4 mutations (small patella syndrome) are associated with childhood-onset pulmonary arterial hypertension. J Med Genet 2013;50(8):500–6.

24. Rosenzweig EB, Barst RJ. Congenital heart disease and pulmonary hypertension: Pharmacology and feasibility of late surgery. Prog Cardiovasc Dis 2012;55(2):128–33.

25. Bradley EA, Chakinala M, Billadello JJ. Usefulness of medical therapy for pulmonary hypertension and delayed atrial septal defect closure. Am J Cardiol 2013;112(9):1471–6.

26. Sauvageau S, Thorin E, Caron A, et al. Endothelin-1-Induced pulmonary Vasoreactivity is Regulated by ETA and ETB receptor Interactions. J Vasc Res 2007;44(5). https://doi.org/10.1159/000102534.

27. Veyssier-Belot C, Cacoub P. Role of endothelial and smooth muscle cells in the physiopathology and treatment management of pulmonary hypertension. Cardiovasc Res 1999;44:274–82.

28. Hassoun PM, Mouthon L, Barberà JA, et al. Inflammation, growth factors, and pulmonary vascular remodeling. J Am Coll Cardiol 2009;54(1 Suppl):S10–9. https://doi.org/10.1016/j.jacc.2009.04.006.

29. Lammers AE, Adatia I, Del Cerro MJ, et al. Functional classification of pulmonary hypertension in children: report from the PVRI pediatric taskforce, Panama 2011. Pulm Circ 2011;1(2):280–5.

30. Grünig E, Peacock AJ. Imaging the heart in pulmonary hypertension: an update. Eur Respir Rev 2015;24(138):653–64.

31. Fisher MR, Forfia PR, Chamera E, et al. Accuracy of Doppler echocardiography in the hemodynamic

assessment of pulmonary hypertension. Am J Respir Crit Care Med 2009;179(7):615–21.

32. Greiner S, Jud A, Aurich M, et al. Reliability of noninvasive assessment of systolic pulmonary artery pressure by Doppler echocardiography compared to right heart catheterization: analysis in a large patient population. J Am Heart Assoc 2014;3(4). https://doi.org/10.1161/JAHA.114.001103.

33. Koestenberger M, Friedberg MK, Nestaas E, et al. Transthoracic echocardiography in the evaluation of pediatric pulmonary hypertension and ventricular dysfunction. Pulm Circ 2016;6(1):15–29.

34. Douwes JM, Humpl T, Bonnet D, et al. Acute vasodilator response in pediatric pulmonary arterial hypertension current clinical Practice from the TOPP registry. J Am Coll Cardiol 2016;67(11):1312–23.

35. Ulrich S, Fischler M, Speich R, et al. Wrist Actigraphy predicts outcome in patients with pulmonary hypertension. Respiration 2013;86(1). https://doi.org/10.1159/000342351.

36. Yetman AT, Taylor AL, Doran A, et al. Utility of cardiopulmonary stress testing in assessing disease severity in children with pulmonary arterial hypertension. Am J Cardiol 2005;95(5):697–9.

37. Wensel R, Francis DP, Meyer FJ, et al. Incremental prognostic value of cardiopulmonary exercise testing and resting haemodynamics in pulmonary arterial hypertension. Int J Cardiol 2013;167(4):1193–8.

38. Ivy D, Rosenzweig EB, Elliott C, et al. Risk assessment in pediatric patients with pulmonary arterial hypertension (PAH): Application of the REVEAL 2.0 risk calculator. Chest 2019;156(4):A169–71.

39. Zijlstra WMH, Douwes JM, Rosenzweig EB, et al. Survival differences in pediatric pulmonary arterial hypertension: Clues to a better understanding of outcome and optimal treatment strategies. J Am Coll Cardiol 2014;63(20):2159–69.

40. Abman SH, Hansmann G, Archer SL, et al. Pediatric pulmonary hypertension. Circulation 2015;132(21):2037–99.

41. Malhotra R, Hess D, Lewis GD, et al. Vasoreactivity to inhaled nitric oxide with oxygen predicts long-term survival in pulmonary arterial hypertension. Pulm Circ 2011;1(2):250–8.

42. Douwes JM, Van Loon RLE, Hoendermis ES, et al. Acute pulmonary vasodilator response in paediatric and adult pulmonary arterial hypertension: Occurrence and prognostic value when comparing three response criteria. Eur Heart J 2011;32(24):3137–46.

43. Davidson D, Barefield ES, Kattwinkel J, et al. Inhaled Nitric Oxide for the Early Treatment of Persistent Pulmonary Hypertension of the Term Newborn: A Randomized, Double-Masked, Placebo-Controlled, Dose-Response, Multicenter Study. Pediatrics. 101(3 Pt 1):32534.

44. Trachte AL, Lobato EB, Urdaneta F, et al. Oral sildenafil reduces pulmonary hypertension after cardiac surgery. Ann Thorac Surg 2005;79(1):194–7.

45. Galiè N, Barberà JA, Frost AE, et al. Initial Use of ambrisentan plus tadalafil in pulmonary arterial hypertension. N Engl J Med 2015;373(9):834–44.

46. Cohen JL, Nees SN, Valencia GA, et al. Sildenafil Use in children with pulmonary hypertension. J Pediatr 2019;205:29–34.e1.

47. Barst RJ, Ivy DD, Gaitan G, et al. A randomized, double-blind, placebo-controlled, dose-ranging study of oral sildenafil citrate in treatment-naive children with pulmonary arterial hypertension. Circulation 2012;125(2):324–34.

48. Barst RJ, Beghetti M, Pulido T, et al. STARTS-2: long-term survival with oral sildenafil monotherapy in treatment-naive pediatric pulmonary arterial hypertension. Circulation 2014;129(19):1914–23.

49. FDA drug safety communication: FDA clarifies Warning about pediatric Use of Revatio (sildenafil) for pulmonary arterial hypertension. Available at: https://www.fda.gov/drugs/drug-safety-and-availability/fda-drug-safety-communication-fda-clarifies-warning-about-pediatric-use-revatio-sildenafil-pulmonary. Accessed August 30, 2012.

50. Takatsuki S, Calderbank M, Ivy DD. Initial experience with tadalafil in pediatric pulmonary arterial hypertension. Pediatr Cardiol 2012;33(5):683–8.

51. Rosenzweig EB, Ivy DD, Widlitz A, et al. Effects of long-term Bosentan in children with pulmonary arterial hypertension. J Am Coll Cardiol 2005;46(4):697–704.

52. Hislop AA, Moledina S, Foster H, et al. Long-term efficacy of bosentan in treatment of pulmonary arterial hypertension in children. Eur Respir J 2011;38(1):70–7.

53. Takatsuki S, Rosenzweig EB, Zuckerman W, et al. Clinical safety, pharmacokinetics, and efficacy of ambrisentan therapy in children with pulmonary arterial hypertension. Pediatr Pulmonol 2013;48(1):27–34.

54. Schweintzger S, Koestenberger M, Schlagenhauf A, et al. Safety and efficacy of the endothelin receptor antagonist macitentan in pediatric pulmonary hypertension. Cardiovasc Diagn Ther 2020;10(5). https://doi.org/10.21037/cdt.2020.04.01.

55. Lammers AE, Hislop AA, Flynn Y, et al. Epoprostenol treatment in children with severe pulmonary hypertension. Heart 2007;93(6):739–43.

56. McLaughlin VV, Shillington A, Rich S. Survival in primary pulmonary hypertension: the impact of epoprostenol therapy. Circulation 2002;106(12):1477–82.

57. Ferdman DJ, Rosenzweig EB, Zuckerman WA, et al. Subcutaneous treprostinil for pulmonary hypertension in chronic lung disease of infancy. Pediatrics 2014;134(1). https://doi.org/10.1542/peds.2013-2330.

58. McLaughlin VV, Gaine SP, Barst RJ. Efficacy and safety of treprostinil: an epoprostenol analog for Primary pulmonary hypertension. J Cardiovasc Pharmacol 2003;41(2):293–9.

59. Feldman J, Habib N, Radosevich J, et al. Oral treprostinil in the treatment of pulmonary arterial hypertension. Expert Opin Pharmacother 2017;18(15): 1661–7.

60. Kanaan U, Varghese NP, Coleman RD, et al. Oral treprostinil use in children: a multicenter, observational experience. Pulm Circ 2019;9(3). https://doi.org/10.1177/2045894019862138.

61. Coghlan JG, Channick R, Chin K, et al. Targeting the prostacyclin pathway with selexipag in patients with pulmonary arterial hypertension Receiving double combination therapy: Insights from the randomized controlled GRIPHON study. Am J Cardiovasc Drugs 2018;18(1):37–47.

62. Sitbon O, Morrell NW. Pathways in pulmonary arterial hypertension: the future is here. Eur Respir Rev 2012;21(126):321–7.

63. Krishnan U, Takatsuki S, Ivy DD, et al. Effectiveness and safety of inhaled treprostinil for the treatment of pulmonary arterial hypertension in children. Am J Cardiol 2012;110(11):1704–9.

64. Olsson KM, Delcroix M, Ghofrani HA, et al. Anticoagulation and survival in pulmonary arterial hypertension: results from the comparative, prospective registry of newly initiated therapies for pulmonary hypertension (COMPERA). Circulation 2014;129(1): 57–65.

65. Preston IR, Roberts KE, Miller DP, et al. Effect of warfarin treatment on survival of patients with pulmonary arterial hypertension (PAH) in the registry to evaluate early and Long-Term PAH Disease Management (REVEAL). Circulation 2015;132(25): 2403–11.

66. Ghofrani HA, Morrell NW, Hoeper MM, et al. Imatinib in pulmonary arterial hypertension patients with inadequate response to established therapy. Am J Respir Crit Care Med 2010;182(9):1171–7.

67. Seyfarth HJ, Hammerschmidt S, Halank M, et al. Everolimus in patients with severe pulmonary hypertension: a safety and efficacy pilot trial. Pulm Circ 2013;3(3):632–8.

68. Callahan R, Esch JJ, Wang G, et al. Systemic Sirolimus to prevent in-Stent stenosis in pediatric pulmonary vein stenosis. Pediatr Cardiol 2020;41(2). https://doi.org/10.1007/s00246-019-02253-6.

69. Fukumoto Y, Matoba T, Ito A, et al. Acute vasodilator effects of a Rho-kinase inhibitor, fasudil, in patients with severe pulmonary hypertension. Heart 2005; 91(3):391–2.

70. Mcnamara PJ, Murthy P, Kantores C, et al. Acute vasodilator effects of Rho-kinase inhibitors in neonatal rats with pulmonary hypertension unresponsive to nitric oxide. Am J Physiol Lung Cell Mol Physiol 2008;294:205–13.

71. Said SI, Hamidi SA. Pharmacogenomics in pulmonary arterial hypertension: toward a mechanistic, target-based approach to therapy. Pulm Circ 2011; 1(3):383–8.

72. Chiu JS, Zuckerman WA, Turner ME, et al. Balloon atrial septostomy in pulmonary arterial hypertension: effect on survival and associated outcomes. J Hear Lung Transpl 2015;34(3):376–80.

73. Baruteau AE, Belli E, Boudjemline Y, et al. Palliative Potts shunt for the treatment of children with drug-refractory pulmonary arterial hypertension: updated data from the first 24 patients. Eur J Cardio-thoracic Surg 2015;47(3):e105–10.

74. Grady RM, Eghtesady P. Potts shunt and pediatric pulmonary hypertension: what We have learned. Ann Thorac Surg 2016;101(4):1539–43.

75. Esch JJ, Shah PB, Cockrill BA, et al. Transcatheter Potts shunt creation in patients with severe pulmonary arterial hypertension: initial clinical experience. J Hear Lung Transpl 2013;32(4):381–7.

76. Rosenzweig EB, Ankola A, Krishnan U, et al. A novel unidirectional-valved shunt approach for end-stage pulmonary arterial hypertension: Early experience in adolescents and adults. J Thorac Cardiovasc Surg 2021;161(4):1438–46.e2. https://doi.org/10.1016/j.jtcvs.2019.10.149.

77. Boudjemline Y, Sizarov A, Malekzadeh-Milani S, et al. Safety and feasibility of the transcatheter approach to Create a reverse Potts shunt in children with idiopathic pulmonary arterial hypertension. Can J Cardiol 2017;33(9):1188–96.

78. Lordan JL, Corris PA. Pulmonary arterial hypertension and lung transplantation. Expert Rev Respir Med 2011;5(3):441–54.

79. Galie N, Manes A, Palazzini M, et al. Management of pulmonary arterial hypertension associated with congenital systemic-to-pulmonary shunts and Eisenmenger's syndrome. Drugs 2008;68(8):1049–66.

Advanced Circulatory Support and Lung Transplantation in Pulmonary Hypertension

Marie M. Budev, DO, MPH, FCCP[a],*, James J. Yun, MD, PhD[b]

KEYWORDS

- Lung transplant • Heart–lung transplant • Pulmonary arterial hypertension • Right ventricular failure
- Mechanical circulatory support • Extracorporeal membrane oxygenation

KEY POINTS

- Lung transplantation is a therapeutic option for patients suffering from advanced pulmonary hypertension refractory to medical therapy or who are in WHO FC III or IV.
- Early referral for lung transplantation for patients with advanced disease is crucial to mitigate waitlist mortality and disease severity at the time of transplantation.
- Double lung transplant is the procedure of choice for patients with pulmonary arterial hypertension (PAH), with a resolution of secondary right ventricular failure in these patients.
- The use of extracorporeal life support for support of the deteriorating PAH patient is warranted if a clear treatment objective is present, including recovery or transplantation.
- The use of extracorporeal membrane support postoperatively may prevent graft failure. At experienced centers, the 1-year survival rates after lung transplantation for PAH exceed 90%.

INTRODUCTION

Pulmonary arterial hypertension (PAH) is a rare progressive disease that leads to pulmonary vascular remodeling and subsequent increase in pulmonary vascular resistance.[1] If left untreated, right ventricular failure can ensue due to the elevation in afterload and the inability of the right ventricle to adapt leading ultimately to death.[2] The advent of 5 classes of effective PAH targeted therapies, either used in combination or as monotherapy, have led to a more promising future for PAH care. Epoprostenol, initially introduced in the early 1990s, was the first drug to treat PAH, and improved 5-year survival in patients with familial and idiopathic PAH.[3,4] However, despite the advances in medical therapies, PAH is still associated with considerable morbidity and premature mortality. Patients with advanced PAH may fail combination or goal-directed therapies despite optimal medical treatments. Lung transplantation (LT) is an important therapeutic option for patients who fail medical therapy or remain in World Health Organization functional class (WHO FC) III and IV due to the high associated mortality rate.[5,6] Although, the timing of referral for LT can be challenging, early referral and assessment are strongly recommended to mitigate waitlist mortality and clinical severity at the time of transplantation.[6,7] Patients may deteriorate while on the waiting list, and mechanical support may be considered in appropriate patients as a bridge to transplant until a suitable donor is available.[8] Herein, we will focus on the role of transplantation in patients with PAH, predominantly idiopathic, or with congenital heart disease (CHD) with right ventricular failure, as these

^a Lung and Heart Lung Transplant Program, Respiratory Institute, Cleveland Clinic, 9500 Euclid Avenue, Desk A-90, Cleveland, OH 44195, USA; ^b Lung Transplant Program, Department of Thoracic and Cardiovascular Surgery, Cleveland Clinic, 9500 Euclid Avenue, Desk J4-1, Cleveland, OH 44195, USA
* Corresponding author.
E-mail address: BUDEVM@ccf.org

Cardiol Clin 40 (2022) 129–138
https://doi.org/10.1016/j.ccl.2021.09.001
0733-8651/22/© 2021 Elsevier Inc. All rights reserved.

cardiology.theclinics.com

are the primary patients considered for LT or heart–lung transplant (HLT). We will review the timing for referral and listing for transplantation, operative considerations including HLT versus LT for PAH, transplant-associated short-term and long-term outcomes, and options for bridging to transplantation including mechanical circulatory support.

REFERRAL AND LISTING FOR LUNG TRANSPLANTATION
Referral to a Transplant Center

The decision and timing for referral for LT can be challenging, since the disease rarely progresses uniformly. The advent of targeted therapies for PAH, although beneficial, has also reduced and delayed patient referral to lung transplant programs.[9,10] In patients with PAH, early referral to an experienced transplant center is important especially in those individuals who demonstrate an inadequate response to treatment with maximal combination therapy. In addition, early referral is recommended in disease variants of pulmonary hypertension including pulmonary veno-occlusive disease (PVOD) and pulmonary capillary haemangiomatosis (PCH) due to the limited or poor response to available medical therapy. The current recommendation is that patients with PVOD and PCH should be listed for transplantation at the time of diagnosis.[10] At our institution, similar to many other transplant centers around the country, early referral is encouraged based on the fact that delays in transplantation have been linked to higher waitlist mortality.[6] The evaluation for transplantation is complex, and whenever possible early referral is preferred and should begin before the need for transplant becomes urgent. Early referral allows the patient to understand the complexities of the transplant process, along with its requirements and outcomes. Early referral also offers the opportunity to modify and reduce risk factors (ie, obesity, malnutrition, frailty, or inadequate social support) and optimization of candidacy.[11] It is important to recognize that early referral does not necessarily translate to early listing, but instead allows for complete evaluation, allowing for the optimal timing for listing if deterioration in clinical condition occurs.[12] Since the 2014 International Society for Heart and Lung Transplantation Consensus (ISHLT) document on recipient selection, risk stratification in PAH has undergone a significant advancement, allowing for a better understanding of timing for referral and listing for lung transplant.[7,13] Galie and colleagues recommended in the most recent proceedings from the 2018 World Symposium on Pulmonary Hypertension (WHSPH), that a serial multiparametric risk

stratification approach be used to define PAH patients at low, intermediate, or high-risk status according to the expected 1-year mortality as PAH treatments are escalated. The goal of therapy based on the 2018 WHSPH is to achieve low-risk status either by the Registry to Evaluate Early and Long-term PAH Disease Management (REVEAL) risk score >7 or the ECS/ERS model.[14] Failure to achieve a low-risk status after the intensification of therapy after 3 to 6 months should lead to a transplant referral and listing.[8,10,12,13] Both predictive models do have limitations; therefore, clinical information and data including cardiopulmonary exercise testing, right ventricular assessment by cardiac MRI and serial echocardiograms may provide additional information on potential at-risk candidates for a clinical decline. In addition, clinical evidence of secondary organ dysfunction, including liver or kidney dysfunction or life-threatening hemoptysis, should prompt a rapid referral and listing.[15,16] Once patients are referred for LT and accepted for evaluation, a formal assessment for transplant candidacy by a multidisciplinary team is initiated. The patient evaluation is comprehensive to evaluate the suitability of a candidate including accounting for the contraindications to transplantation (Refer to **Box 1**).

Listing Pulmonary Arterial Hypertension Patients for Lung Transplant

After the transplant evaluation is completed, the decision will be made regarding when to list a patient for transplantation (Refer to **Table 1**). The patient should be mentally prepared to be transplanted at any time after being listed. Current recommendations are that PAH patients should be listed when they present at a high risk of death despite optimal combination therapy or an inadequate response to maximum medical therapy including intravenous or subcutaneous prostacyclin analogs.[12] Patients are deemed high risk according to the 2015 European Society of Cardiology (ESC)/European Respiratory Society (ERS) PH guidelines when the estimated 1-year mortality exceeds 10% or the REVEAL score is > 10 on appropriate PAH therapy, and may represent high-risk individuals whose expected mortality on medical therapy exceeds that of the expected mortality after transplantation, which is approximately 10% at 1-year posttransplantation.[10,17,18] The ISHLT recipient selection guidelines are presently under revision and will incorporate recommendations regarding timing for referral and listing of PAH patients.

Although on the waitlist, patients should be encouraged to remain active and participate in a

---

Box 1
Absolute contraindications to lung transplantation

- Severe obesity Class II or III (body mass index (BMI) $\geq$35 kg/m^2
- Recent history of malignancy, 2-yr disease-free interval with low risk for recurrence, 5-yr disease-free interval recommended for sarcoma, hematological malignancy melanoma, breast cancer, bladder, and kidney cancer
- Significant dysfunction of another major organ (heart, liver, brain, and kidney) unless a dual or multi-organ transplant is feasible
- Uncorrectable bleeding diathesis
- Acute sepsis or acute MI, medical instability, coronary disease not amenable to revascularization, end-organ ischemia, uncorrected atherosclerotic disease
- Chronic or poorly controlled infection with highly virulent or resistant microorganisms
- Active *Mycobacterium tuberculosis*
- Paucity of reliable or adequate support system
- Nonadherence history to medical therapy (current, prolonged, and repeated episodes)
- Psychiatric or psychological conditions associated with the inability to adhere to medical therapy or cooperate with the health care team
- Limited functional status with poor rehabilitation potential
- Ongoing substance abuse or dependence including tobacco, illicit substances

Data from Weill D, Benden C, Corris PA, et al. A consensus document for the selection of lung transplant candidates: 2014 an update from the Pulmonary Transplant Council of the International Society for Heart and Lung Transplantation. J Heart Lung Transplant 2015;34:1-15 and Bartolome S, Hoeper MM, Klepetko W. Advanced pulmonary arterial hypertension: mechanical support and lung transplantation. Eur Respir Rev 2017;26:170089.

---

formal pulmonary rehabilitation program in an effort to avoid deconditioning or a frail state.[19] Consideration of local waitlist times, which can depend on transplant center practices and geographic organ allocation factors, is important when listing any patient for LT for any disease state, not just PAH. In the United States, the policy for assigning organ allocation priority is based according to the lung allocation score (LAS), and a higher score corresponds to a greater priority for receiving an organ.[20] With the introduction of the LAS, waitlist mortality decreased for all disease states and transplant rates for almost all diseases increased. However, in a multivariable analysis comparing morality predicated by the LAS system to actual mortality in the REVEAL database, 2 additional variables were independently associated with increased mortality than the LAS, mean arterial pressure $\geq$ 14 mm Hg and 6-minute walk distance $\leq$300 m.[13] The LAS was further modified in 2015 to include these 2 factors along with the total bilirubin and cardiac index to reweight waitlist urgency and postsurvival benefit for patients with PAH, further improving the LAS to adequately reflect disease severity in PAH patients and allow for an equipoise between patients with different parenchymal lung diseases.[13,21] The current lung allocation system does allow for an exception score to be granted for PAH patients in whom LAS is thought not to adequately reflect disease severity or waitlist mortality. Certain specific criteria including patient deterioration on maximal therapy, right atrial pressure greater than 15 mm Hg or cardiac index less than 1.8 L/min/m^2 may qualify a candidate to receive a LAS to be at the national 90th percentile.[22]

OPERATIVE CONSIDERATIONS
Bilateral Sequential Lung Versus Heart–Lung Transplant

In 1981, the first HLT for PAH was performed at Stanford University, and the ensuing years were considered the primary procedure for PAH patients and CHD patients.[23] As per data from the ISHLT Registry, in 1989, the peak number of HLT was performed and then declined to less than 100 per year. The reason for this decline was partially due to the growing proportion of PAH patients receiving DLT, as well as a reduction in patients undergoing HLT for PAH. This change in proportion was due to several reasons including (1) scarcity of donor heart–lung blocs and (2) a growth in the number of heart recipients waiting for a suitable organ.[24] HLT is best reserved for patients with end-stage lung and heart failure, for example, in patients with Eisenmenger syndrome complicating complex CHD, failed CHD repair, uncorrectable CHD, and severe left ventricular failure.[25] Double lung transplant (DLT) is presently the procedure of choice for patients with PAH over HLT or single-lung transplants (SLTs). In 2001, a survey of 35 transplant and pulmonary hypertension centers reported that 83% of centers preferred DLT for PAH patients, with a minority reporting a preference of HLT for PAH.[26] In the 1990s, several studies described comparable short and long-term survival rates for DLT and

Table 1
Criteria for lung transplant referral and listing for PAH patients

Referral	• Early referral is preferred before clinical deterioration • ESC/ERS intermediate or high-risk REVEAL risk score > 7 on appropriate therapy • Significant RV dysfunction despite maximal PAH therapy • Signs of secondary liver or kidney dysfunction due to PAH • Worsening disease or recurrent hospitalizations for progressive PAH • Need for intravenous or subcutaneous prostacyclin • Know or suspected high-risk variants including PVOD, PCH, CTD-associated PAH (scleroderma), presence of giant pulmonary artery aneurysms, or presence of life-threatening hemoptysis
Listing	• ESC/ERS high risk or REVEAL risk score >10 on appropriate PAH therapy including intravenous or subcutaneous prostacyclin analogs • In PCH and PVOD patients, worsening hypoxemia • Progressive liver and kidney dysfunction, if end stage consider multiorgan transplantation if feasible • Life-threatening hemoptysis

Abbreviations: ERC, European Society of Cardiology; ERS, European Respiratory Society; REVEAL: Registry to Evaluate Early and Long Term Pulmonary Arterial Hypertension Disease Management; PCH, pulmonary capillary haemangiomatosis; PVOD: pulmonary veno-occlusive disease.

Data from Bartolome S, Hoeper MM, Klepetko W. Advanced pulmonary arterial hypertension: mechanical support and lung transplantation. Eur Respir Rev 2017;26:170089 and Hoeper MM, Benza RL, Corris P, et al. Intensive Care, right ventricular support and lung transplantation in patients with pulmonary hypertension. Eur Resp J 2019;53:1801906.

SLT for PAH. In addition, bypass time was noted to be reduced in the SLT performed for PAH; however, PAH was not reduced as effectively in SLT than DLT.[25,27] During the 1990s, the general thought was that if the left ventricular function was intact, an SLT was the procedure of choice for several reasons including primary shorter times under anesthesia and better allocation of organs.[25] Although SLT may be feasible, based on several studies and present clinical experience, most of the transplant centers presently favor DLT for PAH.[28–31] (Refer to **Table 2**) Immediately postoperatively in PAH recipients, the RV may need support to give it time to time to recover. Several studies have noted that RV remodeling and regression of both tricuspid valve regurgitation and right heart failure do occur after DLT, further supporting that HLT is not required for RV dysfunction associated with PAH except in the situations noted above.[18,35]

Another concern that has recently arisen in patients with PAH who undergoes DLT, is the exposure of occult left ventricular diastolic dysfunction (LVDD), which may be a result of the left ventricle being exposed to a higher cardiac output after transplant.[36] As a result, complications including pulmonary edema and acute hypoxemia can lead to the need for prolonged mechanical ventilation and thus, longer intensive care stays.[37] In an effort to avoid this issue, certain centers now advocate for HLTs in patients with severe PAH.[38] Arvriel and colleagues noted in a recent study of 116 PAH patients with LVDD who underwent LT, that patients with Grade 2 or higher diastolic dysfunction before transplant had a worse 1-year outcome than PAH patients with no LVDD. The presence of LVDD conferred a hazard ratio (HR) equal to 5.4 (95% confidence interval (CI): 1.3–22; $P = .02$).[37] The use of extracorporeal membrane oxygenation (ECMO) during the various phases of the transplant perioperative period and postoperative period has allowed for LV conditioning over time with an increase in ejection fraction, subsequent cardiac output, and improved LV dimensions early postoperatively.[39] Transplant centers may have variability in the selection of HLT versus DLT based on different thresholds for LVDD and RV dysfunction.[25,26]

LUNG TRANSPLANT OUTCOMES FOR PULMONARY ARTERIAL HYPERTENSION

In the era before the use of LT as an option for the treatment for severe PAH, the survival for PAH patients was poor, with a median survival of only 2.8 years.[40] However, with the development of epoprostenol therapy and the use of LT, the prognosis for this group of patients drastically improved. According to the 2019 ISHLT Registry data, between January 1995 and June 2018, 1863 transplants were performed worldwide for the indication of PAH (1768 DLT vs 95 SLT).[34] Registry data have demonstrated that patients transplanted for PAH have the highest mortality rates early after transplant. In transplants performed between 1990 and 2014, the mortality

Table 2
Pros and cons for single-lung transplant versus double lung transplant versus heart–lung transplant for pulmonary arterial hypertension

Transplant Type	Benefit	Risk	Median Survival
Single-Lung Transplant	Short anesthesia time Less bypass time Better donor organ allocation equity Less complicated dissection (one side only) Native lung may sustain patient with PGD of the transplanted organ	Native Lung may pose an infectious risk Pulmonary pressures may not be ameliorated as well as with DL Increased shunting and perfusion/ventilation mismatch early postop Hyperperfusion of the newly implanted lung increases the risk for PGD[32,33]	4.8 y (conditional to 1 y survival 6.5 y)* for all reasons for transplantation[34]
Double Lung Transplant	Better amelioration of pulmonary pressures vs SLT Improved Survival vs SLTx Better donor allocation equity than HLT Allows for intracardiac repair ASD, VSD, and Eisenmengers- PDA	Increased ischemic time Increased bypass time Longer operation than SLT	7.1 y[34]
Heart–Lung Transplant	Option for severe RV and LV function Option for complex CHD including uncorrectable CHD or single ventricle anatomy	Not offered at all transplant centers Allocation of dual organs may be difficult leading to long waitlist times Possible increased waitlist mortality due to longer waiting times Limited resource may not be an appropriate use of dual organ if a DLT or SLT could be performed instead Younger age cut off vs DLT	6.5 y[34]

Abbreviations: ASD, atrial septal defect; CHD, congenital heart disease; DLT, double lung transplant; HLT, heart lung transplant; LV, left ventricle; PDA, patent ductus arteriosus; RV, right ventricle; SLT, single lung transplant; VSD, ventricular septal defect.

Data from Schuba B, Michel S, Guenther S, et al. Lung transplantation in patients with severe pulmonary hypertension- Focus on right ventricular remodeling. Clinical Transplant 2019;33:e13586 and Sultan S, Tseng S, Agnese Stanziola A, et al. Pulmonary Hypertension. The role of lung transplantation. Heart Failure Clin 2018;14:327-31.

risk in the first 3 months was higher for PAH recipients (23%) than all other indications for LT including cystic fibrosis (CF) (9%) and chronic obstructive pulmonary disease (COPD) (9%).[24] However, in the last few years, specialized transplant centers with expertise in PAH have reported significant improvements in posttransplant survival rates at 3 months (100%) and 12 months (96%) due to improvements in the perioperative and postoperative care including the use of ECMO posttransplant.[39] For PAH patient who survive the early posttransplant period, long-term survival is frequently better than patients transplanted for other indications. ISHLT Registry data showed that for PAH transplant recipients who survived to 1 year, the conditional median survival was 10 years, which is superior to that of COPD patients) 7.0 yrs.[24]

In the early postoperative period, primary graft dysfunction (PGD) is one of the most common complications. PGD is defined as lung injury that occurs within the first 72 hours postoperatively. Although several recipient risk factors are known to contribute to the development of PGD, PAH has been repeatedly reported to increase the risk for developing PGD in several studies. Patients suffering from PH are at higher risk for developing PGD than other transplant indications.[41] Prophylactic extracorporeal life support in the first days after transplantation has recently been advocated to avoid severe PGD.[18] Severe PGD has been noted to be a contributing factor to reducing the 1-year survival of all lung transplant recipients and has been identified as a risk factor for the development of chronic rejection or chronic lung allograft disease (CLAD).[41,42] CLAD remains the leading cause of death for all lung transplant recipients and 41.5% of recipients within 5-years posttransplant would have developed CLAD.[43]

SUMMARY

Despite the advances in medical therapeutics that have evolved for the treatment of PAH, it still remains a chronic fatal disease with a high mortality rate in advanced cases. LT remains a viable therapeutic option for patients suffering from severe PAH and should be considered in appropriate candidates who do not respond to appropriate and optimized combination therapy or refractory disease. Transplant referral should be considered early to a transplant center with expertise in transplanting PAH patients and with an ECMO program for patients who may deteriorate while waiting for a suitable organ. BL transplant remains the procedure of choice for most patients with PAH. HL transplant should be reserved for a limited population of patients including patients with complex CHD or uncorrectable CHD or single ventricle anatomy and severe RV and LV dysfunction.

Advanced Circulatory Support and Lung Transplantation for Pulmonary Arterial Hypertension

In end-stage lung failure with pulmonary hypertension, advanced circulatory support is needed for pulmonary and/or right ventricular support when medical therapy is no longer effective.

Veno-Arterial ECMO

Extracorporeal membrane oxygenation—both veno-venous (VV) and veno-arterial (VA)—are used routinely at high-volume centers to bridge patients to lung transplant. Because VV ECMO corrects gas exchange but provides no right ventricular support, pulmonary hypertension patients with severe right ventricular dysfunction frequently require VA ECMO for the successful a bridge to transplant.[11] VA ECMO redirects blood flow away from the to the dysfunctional right ventricle, thereby reducing RV workload and overcoming low cardiac output by returning oxygenated blood directly to the systemic circulation. Chicotka and colleagues reviewed 50 patients with ILD and secondary PAH who were supported with VV or VA ECMO as bridge to transplant.[44] Initial use of VA ECMO resulted in a higher rate of successful bridging to transplant versus VV ECMO, and conversion from VV to VA ECMO increased survival while waiting for the transplant. In addition, the use of VA ECMO configurations with an arterial return to the upper body increased ambulation on ECMO, which in turn reduced mortality during ECMO support. However, complications associated with VA ECMO included limb ischemia, bleeding, stroke, renal failure, and vascular injury. A follow-up report from the same institution which reviewed results of VA ECMO as a bridge to transplant and recovery reaffirmed the importance of a multidisciplinary team for candidate selection, optimal medical therapy, and proper cannulation strategies to achieve best possible outcomes.[45] Our center and others have also used veno-arterial-venous (VAV) ECMO configurations when patients supported with VV ECMO require RV support beyond medical therapy; further study is needed to define the efficacy of this approach.

RVAD WITH OXYGENATOR

An alternative to VA ECMO support in cases of severe pulmonary hypertension and RV dysfunction is the use of a right ventricular assist device

(RVAD) with an oxygenator. Although no FDA approved, durable, completely implantable RVADs with oxygenation capability are currently available, a standard 2 cannula surgical RVAD or a single cannula Protek Duo cannula (Tandem Life, Pittsburgh, PA) can be linked in series to an oxygenator for use in the ICU setting. RVADs with oxygenators have been used successfully as a bridge to transplant[46] as well as intraoperative and postop lung transplant support in a case of absent inferior vena cava.[47] It should be noted, however, that in cases of severely elevated pulmonary vascular resistance (PVR), circulatory support with RVAD and oxygenator may be unsuccessful if the PVR is so high that RVAD support incurs lung injury from insurmountable RV afterload.[48] Gregoric and colleagues reported a case following emergent pulmonary embolectomy complicated by perioperative RV failure due to pulmonary hypertension in which RVAD therapy worsened PA hypertension and airway bleeding; conversion to VA ECMO therapy subsequently permitted successful bridge to heart–lung transplant.[49] In such cases, VA ECMO is favored because it offloads the right heart and permits the minimization of lung injury.

ATRIAL SEPTOSTOMY AND POTTS SHUNT

Nonmechanical circulatory options for the palliation of severe pulmonary hypertension include atrial septostomy and Pott's shunt. Atrial septostomy has been used to palliate severe pulmonary hypertension, and in select cases bridge patients to lung transplant. Rothman and colleagues reported a series of 12 technically successful atrial septostomies from 1990 to 1998 for either primary or secondary hypertension, with systemic oxygen saturation decrease ranging from 5% to 10%.[50] Half had clinical improvement with 5 of 6 eventually bridged to lung transplant; 6 others had no clinical improvement. The authors concluded that atrial septostomy was more effective in patients who were not in the terminal condition and could be most suited for patients not responding to escalating medical therapy.

Chiu and colleagues retrospectively reviewed 46 balloon atrial septostomies performed in 32 patients from 2002 to 2013 for right ventricular failure or syncope.[51] There were no procedural deaths, and lung transplant-free and repeat septostomy free survival were 87% at 30 days and 61% at 1 year. Seven of 32 patients were successfully bridged to lung transplant. The authors cited procedural experience at a high volume center as a reason for the reason for no procedural deaths and suggested that balloon trial septostomy could

be a therapeutic option in properly selected patients.

A recent meta-analysis of 16 balloon atrial septostomy studies including 212 patients total revealed that atrial septostomy was effective in reducing right atrial pressure and increasing cardiac index, while reducing systemic O_2 saturations an average of 8.5%.[52] Procedural and 30-day mortality were 4.8% and 14.6%, whereas long-term mortality (mean follow-up of 46.5 months) was 38%. Because septostomy improved hemodynamics and had low procedural mortality, but long-term mortality was less favorable, the authors suggested that septostomy might be best used as a bridge to definitive therapy, rather than a primary treatment for PAH. Notably, the authors also noted a ~24% spontaneous septostomy closure rate, significantly higher than previously reported in other studies.

The concept of a unidirectional (valved) Potts shunt was experimentally established by Bui and colleagues in France, who published the feasibility of a unidirectional valved shunt in pigs in 2011.[53,54] In recent years, interest in the Potts shunt in children for palliation of severe pulmonary hypertension and to delay the need for lung transplant has grown. Lancaster and colleagues recently reported mid-term outcomes of 23 Potts shunts performed in children since 2013 with suprasystemic pulmonary artery pressures despite maximal medical therapy.[53] Most often the Potts shunt was a surgical procedure (vs percutaneous ductus stenting) and performed via left thoracotomy. Of note, operative mortality was 20% in this challenging patient population, related most closely to the need for ECMO support and the presence of severe right ventricular dysfunction. As with atrial septostomy, the timing of intervention appeared important. When compared with 31 cases of lung transplant, there was no survival difference between Potts shunt and LT.

The first successful "modified" Potts shunt in an adult was reported in 2017 for palliation of severe idiopathic pulmonary hypertension; the patient was a 22-year-old woman who was not a candidate for the lung transplant due to medical noncompliance.[55] A 12 mm composite graft containing a valved bovine conduit was placed between the main pulmonary artery and descending aorta (with concomitant atrial septostomy closure) using cardiopulmonary bypass support. This resulted in a unidirectional shunt between the main pulmonary artery and aorta, which would relieve suprasystemic PA pressure while maintaining upper body oxygenation.

Further clinical experience is needed to determine the role of the Potts shunt in palliation of pulmonary hypertension, and as a bridge to lung transplant. The development of a pediatric international registry is an important first step toward this goal.[56]

CLINICS CARE POINTS

- PAH remains universally a fatal disease. Lung transplantation is a therapeutic option for appropriate candidates who have failed maximal combination medical therapies.

- Referral for lung transplantation should be made to a referral center with an expertise in transplanting PAH patients and with an ECMO program for bridging to transplant if a patient should deteriorate while waiting for suitable organs.

- Bilateral sequential lung transplants remain the procedure of choice for most patients with PAH.

- Heart lung transplants are only reserved for a patients with complex congenital heart disease or uncorrectable congenital heart disease, single ventricle anatomy of severe RV and LV dysfunction.

- Successful use of mechanical support to bridge patients with pulmonary hypertension or lung transplant requires multidisciplinary collaboration at experienced centers to properly select candidates and the type of circulatory support.

DISCLOSURE

The authors have nothing to disclose.

REFERENCES

1. Farber HW, Loscalzo J. Pulmonary arterial hypertension. N Engl J Med 2004;351:1655–65.
2. Price LC, Wort SJ, Finney SJ, et al. Pulmonary vascular and right ventricular dysfunction in adult critical care: current and emerging options for management of patients with severe pulmonary hypertension: a systematic literature review. Crit Care 2010;14:R169.
3. Sitbon O, Humbert M, Nunes H, et al. Long- term intravenous epoprostenol infusion in primary pulmonary hypertension: prognostic factors and survival. J Am Coll Cardiol 2002;40:780–8.
4. Barst RJ, Rubin LJ, Long WA, et al. A comparison of continuous epoprostenol (prostacyclin) with conventional therapy for primary pulmonary hypertension. N Engl J Med 1996;334:296–301.
5. Faber HW, Miller DP, Poms AD, et al. Five year outcomes of patients enrolled in REVEAL Registry. Chest 2015;148:1043–54.
6. Galie N, Corris PA, Frost A, et al. Updated treatment algorithm of pulmonary arterial hypertension. J Am Coll Cardio 2013;62:D60–72.
7. Weill D, Benden C, Corris PA, et al. A consensus document for the selection of lung transplant candidates: 2014 an update from the pulmonary transplant Council of the international society for heart and lung transplantation. J Heart Lung Transpl 2015;34:1–15.
8. Bartolome S, Hoeper MM, Klepetko W. Advanced pulmonary arterial hypertension: mechanical support and lung transplantation. Eur Respir Rev 2017;26:170089.
9. Keogh A, Benza RL, Corris P, et al. Interventional and surgical modalities of treatment in pulmonary arterial hypertension. J Am Coll Cardio 2009;54:S67.
10. Galie N, Humbert M, Vachiery JL, et al. 2015 ESC/ERS guidelines for the diagnosis and treatment of pulmonary hypertension. Eur Respir J 2015;46:903–75.
11. Ballie TJ, Granton JT. Lung transplantation for pulmonary hypertension and strategies to bridge to transplant. Semin Crit Care Med 2017;38:701–10.
12. Hoeper MM, Benza RL, Corris P, et al. Intensive care, right ventricular support and lung transplantation in patients with pulmonary hypertension. Eur Resp J 2019;53:1801906.
13. Benza RL, Miller DP, Frost A, et al. Analysis of the lung allocation score estimation of risk of death in patients with pulmonary arterial hypertension data from the REVEAL registry. Transplantation 2010;90:298–305.
14. Galie N, Channick RN, Frantz RP, et al. Risk stratification and medical therapy of pulmonary hypertension. Eur Resp J 2019;53:1801889.
15. Badagliacca R, Papa S, Poscia R, et al. The added value of cardiopulmonary exercise testing in the follow up pulmonary arterial hypertension. J Heart Lung Transpl 2019;38:306–14.
16. Van de Veerdonk MC, Kind T, Marcus JT, et al. Progressive right ventricular dysfunction in patients with pulmonary hypertension responding to therapy. J Am Coll Cardiol 2011;58:2511–9.
17. Galie N, Humbert M, Vachiery JL, et al. 2015 ESC/ERS guidelines for the diagnosis and treatment of pulmonary hypertension. Eur Respir J 2015;37:67–119.
18. Moser B, Jaksch P, Taghavi S, et al. Lung transplantation for idiopathic pulmonary arterial hypertension on intraoperative and postoperatively prolonged extracorporeal membrane oxygenation provides optimally controlled reperfusion and excellent outcome. Eur J Cardiothorac Surg 2018;53:178–85.

19. Wickerson L, Rozenburg D, Janaudis-Ferreira T, et al. Physical rehabilitation for lung transplant candidates and recipients: an evidence informed clinical approach. World J Transpl 2016;6:517–31.

20. Egan TM, Murry S, Bustami RT, et al. Development of the new lung allocation score in the United States. Am J Transpl 2006;6:1212–27.

21. Organ procurement and transplantation network LAS changes frequently asked questions. Available at: https://optn.transplant.hrsa.gov/media/1157/las_qa.pdf date last. Accessed April 23, 2021.

22. United Network of Organ Sharing. UNOS news heart/lung submitting lung allocation score requests for candidates diagnosed with pulmonary hypertension. Available at: https://unos.org/news/submitting-las-exception-requests-for-candidates-diagnosed-with-ph/%20Date%20last. Accessed April 23, 2021.

23. Reitz BA, Wallwork JL, Hunt SA, et al. Heart-lung transplantation: successful therapy for patients with pulmonary vascular disease. N Engl J Med 1982;306:557–64.

24. Yussen RD, Edwards LB, Kucheryavya Ay, et al. The registry of the international society for heart and lung transplantation: thirty-second official adult lung and heart lung transplantation report-2015;Focus theme:early graft failure. J Heart Lung Transpl 2015;34:1264–77.

25. Bando K, Armitage JM, Paradis IL, et al. Indications for and results of single, bilateral and heart lung transplantation for pulmonary hypertension. J Thorac Cardiovasc Surg 1994;108:1056–65.

26. Pielsticker EJ, Martinez FJ, Rubenfire M. Lung and heart lung transplant practice patterns in pulmonary hypertension centers. J Heart Lung Transpl 2001;12:1297–304.

27. Gammie JS, Keenan RJ, Pham SM, et al. Single versus double lung transplantation for pulmonary hypertension. J Thorac Cardiovasc Surg 1998;115:397–402.

28. Levin SM, Gibbons WJ, Bryan CL, et al. Single lung transplant for primary pulmonary hypertension. Chest 1990;98:1107–15.

29. Girard C, Mornex JF, Gamondes JP, et al. Single lung transplantation for primary pulmonary hypertension without cardiopulmonary bypass. Chest 1992;102:967–8.

30. Pasque MK, Trulock EP, Cooper JD, et al. Single lung transplantation for pulmonary hypertension. Single institution experience in 34 patients. Circulation 1995;92:2252–8.

31. Nasir BS, Mulvihill MS, Barac YD, et al. Single lung transplantation in patients with severe secondary pulmonary hypertension. J Heart Lung Transpl 2019;38:939–48.

32. Schuba B, Michel S, Guenther S, et al. Lung transplantation in patients with severe pulmonary hypertension- Focus on right ventricular remodeling. Clin Transpl 2019;33:e13586.

33. George MP, Hunter CC, Pilewski JM. Lung transplantation for pulmonary hypertension. Pulm Circ 2011;1:182–91.

34. Julliard WA, Meyer KC, De Oliveira NC, et al. The presence or severity of pulmonary hypertension does not affect outcomes for single lung transplantation. Thorax 2016;71:478–80.

35. Chambers D, Cherikh WS, Harhay MO, et al. The International Thoracic Organ Registry of the International Society for Heart and Lung Transplantation: thirty-sixth adult lung and heart lung transplantation report -2019;focus theme: donor and recipient size match. J Heart Lung Transpl 2019;38:1042–55.

36. Knight DS, Steeden JA, Moledina S, et al. Left ventricular diastolic dysfunction in pulmonary hypertension predicts functional capacity and clinical worsening : a tissue phase mapping study. J Cardiovasc Magn Reson 2015;17:116.

37. Avriel A, Klement AH, Johnson SR, et al. Impact of left ventricular diastolic dysfunction on lung transplantation outcomes in patients with pulmonary arterial. Am J Transpl 2017;17:2705–11.

38. Fadel E, Mercier O, Mussot S, et al. Long term outcomes of double lung and heart lung transplantation for pulmonary hypertension: a comparative retrospective study of 219 patients. Eur J Cardiothorac Surg 2010;38:277–84.

39. Tudorache I, Sommer W, Kuhn C, et al. Lung transplantation for severe pulmonary hypertension-awake extracorporeal membrane oxygenation for postoperative left ventricular remodeling. Transplantation 2015;99:451–8.

40. D'Alonzo GE, Barst RJ, Ayres SM, et al. Survival in patients with primary pulmonary hypertension. Results from a national prospective registry. Ann Intern Med 1991;115:343–9.

41. Van Raemdonck D, Hartwig MG, Hertz MI, et al. Report of the ISHLT working group on primary lung graft dysfunction Part IV: prevention and treatment: a 2016 consensus group statement of the international society for heart and lung transplantation. J Heart Lung Transpl 2017;36:1121–36.

42. Snell GI, Yusen RD, Weill D, et al. Report of the ISHLT working group on primary lung graft dysfunction, part I: definition and grading-A 2016 consensus group statement of the international society for heart and lung transplantation. J Heart Lung Transpl 2017;36:1097–103.

43. Yusen RD, Edwards LB, Dipchand A, et al. The registry of the international society for heart and lung transplantation: thirty third adult lung and heart lung transplant report -2016; focus theme: primary diagnostic indications for transplant. J Heart Lung Transpl 2016;35:1170–84.

44. Chicotka S, Pedroso FE, Agerstrand CL, et al. Increasing opportunity for lung transplant in

interstitial lung disease with pulmonary hypertension. Ann Thorac Surg 2018;106(6):1812–9.

45. Rosenzweig EB, Gannon WD, Madahar P, et al. Extracorporeal life support bridge for pulmonary hypertension: a high-volume single-center experience. J Heart Lung Transpl 2019;38(12):1275–85.

46. Oh DK, Shim TS, Jo KW, et al. Right ventricular assist device with an oxygenator using extracorporeal membrane oxygenation as a bridge to lung transplantation in a patient with severe respiratory failure and right heart decompensation. Acute Crit Care 2020;35(2):117–21.

47. Joubert K, Harano T, Pilewski J, et al. Oxy-RVAD support for lung transplant in the absence of inferior vena cava. J Card Surg 2020;35(12):3603–5.

48. Berman M, Tsui S, Vuylsteke A, et al. Life-threatening right ventricular failure in pulmonary hypertension: RVAD or ECMO? J Heart Lung Transpl 2008; 27(10):1188–9.

49. Gregoric ID, Chandra D, Myers TJ, et al. Extracorporeal membrane oxygenation as a bridge to emergency heart–lung transplantation in a patient with idiopathic pulmonary arterial hypertension. J Heart Lung Transpl 2008;27:466–8.

50. Rothman A, Sklansky MS, Lucas VW, et al. Atrial septostomy as a bridge to lung transplantation in patients with severe pulmonary hypertension. Am J Cardiol 1999;84(6):682–6.

51. Chiu J, Zuckerman W, Turner M, et al. Balloon atrial septostomy in pulmonary arterial hypertension: effect on survival and associated outcomes. J Heart Lung Transplant 2015;34(3):376–80.

52. Khan MS, Memon MM, Amin E, et al. Use of balloon atrial septostomy in patients with advanced pulmonary arterial hypertension: a systematic review and meta-analysis. Chest 2019;156(1):53–63.

53. Bui MT, Grollmus O, Ly M, et al. Surgical palliation of primary pulmonary arterial hypertension by a unidirectional valved Potts anastomosis in an animal model. J Thorac Cardiovasc Surg 2011;142(5): 1223–8.

54. Lancaster TS, Shahanavaz S, Balzer DT, et al. Midterm outcomes of the Potts shunt for pediatric pulmonary hypertension, with comparison to lung transplant. J Thorac Cardiovasc Surg 2021;161(3): 1139–48.

55. Salna M, van Boxtel B, Rosenzweig EB, et al. Modified Potts shunt in an adult with idiopathic pulmonary arterial hypertension. Ann Am Thorac Soc 2017; 14(4):607–9.

56. Grady RM. Beyond transplant: roles of atrial septostomy and Potts shunt in pediatric pulmonary hypertension. Pediatr Pulmonol 2021;56(3):656–60.

Moving?

Make sure your subscription moves with you!

To notify us of your new address, find your **Clinics Account Number** (located on your mailing label above your name), and contact customer service at:

Email: journalscustomerservice-usa@elsevier.com

800-654-2452 (subscribers in the U.S. & Canada)
314-447-8871 (subscribers outside of the U.S. & Canada)

Fax number: 314-447-8029

Elsevier Health Sciences Division
Subscription Customer Service
3251 Riverport Lane
Maryland Heights, MO 63043

ELSEVIER